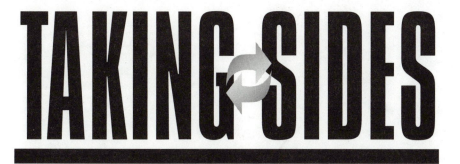

TAKING SIDES

Clashing Views on Controversial

Issues in Food and Nutrition

D0076203

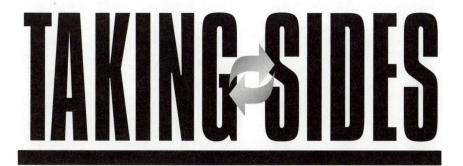

TAKING SIDES

Clashing Views on Controversial

Issues in Food and Nutrition

Selected, Edited, and with Introductions by

Marion Nestle
New York University

and

L. Beth Dixon
New York University

McGraw-Hill/Dushkin
A Division of The McGraw-Hill Companies

Photo Acknowledgment
Cover image: © 2004 by PhotoDisc, Inc.

Cover Art Acknowledgment
Charles Vitelli

Library of Congress Cataloging-in-Publication Data
Main entry under title:
Taking sides: clashing views on controversial issues in food and nutrition/selected, edited, and
with introductions by Marion Nestle and L. Beth Dixon.—1st ed.
Includes bibliographical references and index.
1. Nutrition—Health aspects. 2. Diet therapy. 3. Public health—United States.
4. Physical fitness—United States. 5. Vitamin therapy. 6. Genetically modified foods—
Popular works. 7. Food supply—Health aspects. 8. Health promotions—United States.
9. Herbs—Therapeutic use. 10. Dietary supplements. 11. Chronic disease—Nutritional aspects.
I. Nestle, Marion. II. Dixon, L. Beth. III. Title.
613.2
0-07-292211-7
ISSN 1547-1802

Printed on Recycled Paper

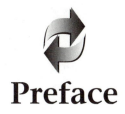

Preface

Taking Sides: Clashing Views on Controversial Issues in Food and Nutrition is designed with one principal purpose: to encourage critical thinking about current issues in these fields. The book consists of 34 previously published selections arranged in 17 sets of matched pairs, each taking a contrasting position on a particular issue. To simplify the nature of the controversy, each issue is expressed as a question; the selected readings address that question either affirmatively or negatively.

The selections cover scientific arguments related to basic dietary advice, intake of specific nutrients and supplements, associations of dietary factors to health, and societal concerns about hunger and irradiated or genetically modified foods. We chose selections that offer strong positions on the issues and are supported by strong arguments. We do not necessarily agree with the positions taken, but respect the authors' points of view.

We arranged the contents of the book into five parts that cover related issues. On the *part opener* pages we provide a brief overview of the issues. On the *On the Internet* pages we offer Internet sites that provide further information on those topics. We begin each issue with an *introduction* that provides a context for understanding the debate, needed background information, and guidance for reading the selections. We end each issue with a *postscript* that summarizes the debate, provides concluding observations, raises additional points, and suggests further readings on the subject. At the back of the book we identify the credentials and affiliations of the *contributors* to this volume—the scientists, physicians, professors, and journalists who debate the issues presented.

We hope that readers will use this book as a starting point for discovering and analyzing important issues in food and nutrition. We deliberately chose selections that address issues currently under active debate. We also hope that readers will use the contrasting opinions of authors as a starting point for analysis and evaluation, and as the basis for further discussion and understanding. Our goal is to broaden readers' knowledge and awareness of debates in food and nutrition, and to encourage critical thinking about these issues in the wider context of science and society as well as in the context of personal experience.

A word to the instructor An *Instructor's Manual With Test Questions* (both multiple-choice and essay) is available through the publisher for instructors using *Taking Sides* in the classroom. Also available is a general guidebook, *Using Taking Sides in the Classroom,* which discusses teaching techniques and methods for integrating the pro/con approach of *Taking Sides* into any classroom situation. An online version of *Using Taking Sides in the Classroom* and information for instructors who adopt *Taking Sides* can be found at http://www.dushkin.com/usingts/.

Taking Sides: Clashing Views on Controversial Issues in Food and Nutrition is only one title in the Taking Sides series. If you would like to see the table of contents for any of the other titles, please visit the Taking Sides Web site at http://www.dushkin.com/takingsides/.

Acknowledgments   We thank the students and faculty of the Department of Nutrition, Food Studies, and Public Health at New York University for their helpful suggestions at various stages of manuscript preparation. We especially thank Emily Adams and Ellen Fried for editorial assistance and helpful comments on the manuscript.

Marion Nestle
New York University

L. Beth Dixon
New York University

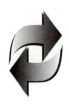

Contents In Brief

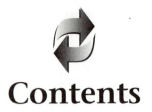

Contents

New York University nutrition professor Marion Nestle says that the U.S. Department of Agriculture (USDA) Food Guide Pyramid's hierarchical design and emphasis on plant-based diets represent a significant advance over previous federal food guides and that a few adjustments to the Pyramid's design would further strengthen its message and respond to most of the concerns of critics. Harvard School of Public Health nutrition professor Walter C. Willett and author P. J. Skerrett argue that the Pyramid at best offers "wishy-washy, scientifically unfounded advice" and at worst contributes to poor health. Overall, the Pyramid represents "a missed opportunity to improve the health of millions of people."

Nutrition professors Jeanne Freeland-Graves and Susan Nitzke speak for the American Dietetic Association (ADA) when they say that there is no such thing as a good or bad food: all foods can fit into healthful diets. Their approach to nutrition advice emphasizes the total diet, appropriate portion sizes, moderation and balance in food intake, obtaining nutrients from foods rather than supplements, and regular physical activity. Nutrition professor Suzanne Havala counters that some foods are better for health than others and that saying otherwise is just a way to rationalize the dietary status quo and protect the commercial interests of the food industry.

Nutrition professor Rebecca J. Bryant and her colleagues say that to prevent bone fractures, the recommended intake of dietary calcium should be 1,000 to 1,200 milligrams (1 to 1.2 grams) a day for adults. Biochemist B. E. Christopher Nordin says that calcium requirements are as much or more dependent on intake of other dietary factors than they are of calcium. Adults with low intakes of protein, phosphate, and sodium can maintain bone health on intakes as low as 400 milligrams of calcium per day.

PART 2   NUTRITION AND HEALTH   59

Issue 4.   Are Added Sugars Harmful to Health?   60

Researchers Barbara V. Howard and Judith Wylie-Rosett, representing the American Heart Association (AHA), state that high sugar consumption increases risk factors for heart disease and may adversely affect control of diabetes. Physician Anne L. Mardis, representing the U.S. Department of Agriculture's (USDA's) Center for Nutrition Policy and Promotion, says that the intake of sugar has no relation to the risk of heart disease or diabetes.

Issue 5.   Do Foods With a High Glycemic Index Increase Disease Risk?   74

Physician-scientist David S. Ludwig says that habitual consumption of foods with a high glycemic index alters metabolism in ways that increase the risk for obesity, type 2 diabetes, and heart disease. He maintains that the glycemic index should be used as a guide to food selection. Physician-scientist F. Xavier Pi-Sunyer says that research on the health effects of high-glycemic index foods is uncertain and inconclusive. He concludes that it would be a mistake to suggest avoiding foods just because they display a high glycemic index.

PART 3   DIET, PHYSICAL ACTIVITY, AND HEALTH   107

Issue 6.   Is Body Weight a Reliable Measurement of Overall Health?   108

Epidemiologist Alison E. Field and her team of investigators say that overweight adults are at increased risk of chronic disease, even if they are not obese. Health sociologist Annemarie Jutel says that the risks of overweight are exaggerated and that its cure—dieting—is a greater hazard.

Issue 7.   Can Low-Carbohydrate, Higher-Fat Diets Promote Health and Weight Loss?   128

Freelance science journalist Gary Taubes says that government advice to eat less fat produces the opposite of its intended effect; it makes Americans fatter. Instead, high-fat diets help people to lose weight and reduce chronic disease risk factors. Science journalist Bonnie Liebman, director of nutrition at the Center for Science in the Public Interest (CSPI), a consumer advocacy organization in Washington, D.C., counters that high-fat diets raise risks for heart disease and cancer and, when excessive in calories, induce weight gain.

Issue 8.   Must Exercise Be Daily and Intense to Prevent Chronic Disease?   150

To prevent weight gain and chronic disease, the Institute of Medicine of the National Academies recommends 60 minutes of daily physical activity of moderate intensity (such as walking at a rate of 4 to 5 miles per hour) in addition to activities normally performed as part of a sedentary lifestyle. Associate professor of the Harvard School of Public Health I-Min Lee and colleagues say that even light-to-moderate activity lowers heart disease rates among women and that as little as one hour of walking per week predicts lower risk.

Issue 9.   Do Education Campaigns Induce Communities to Change Their Diets and Improve Health?   174

West Virginia University researchers Bill Reger and Steven Booth-Butterfield and Center for Science in the Public Interest researcher Margo G. Wootan say that advertising and public relations campaigns can induce the public to make more healthful dietary choices. Researchers Stephen P. Fortmann and Ann N. Varady say that even long-term educational interventions in communities have little effect on overall trends in chronic disease risk.

PART 4   SUPPLEMENTS AND FUNCTIONAL FOODS   193

Physicians Robert H. Fletcher and Kathleen M. Fairfield say that even in populations where deficiencies are rare, "suboptimal" vitamin intakes are common, especially among the elderly; consequently, adults should take vitamin supplements to reduce their risk for chronic diseases. Cancer prevention researcher Demetrius Albanes argues that foods—not supplements—are associated with cancer prevention and that supplemental beta-carotene, for example, may have adverse effects on health. He argues that more evidence is needed before advising adults to take nutrient supplements.

Researcher Pierre L. Le Bars and his colleagues say that supplements of ginkgo biloba improve the cognitive and social functioning of people with Alzheimer's or other types of dementia. Researcher Paul R. Solomon and his colleagues say that ginkgo biloba has no beneficial effect on memory or cognitive function in healthy older adults.

Cyndi Thomson et al., representatives of the American Dietetic Association (ADA), say that fortified, enriched, or enhanced "functional" foods can improve health. The editors of *Consumer Reports on Health* say that the purpose of functional foods is not to improve health but rather to boost the profits of manufacturers.

PART 5 NUTRITION AND FOOD POLICY 253

Mark Nord et al., U.S. Department of Agriculture (USDA) economists, estimate that 11.5 million U.S. households do not have enough food to meet basic needs; of these, 3.5 million households sometimes go hungry for lack of resources to buy food. Robert E. Rector, policy analyst for the Heritage Foundation, a Washington, D.C.–based think tank, finds little evidence of hunger among the poor; on the contrary, he argues that their principal nutrition problems are overweight and obesity.

Johns Hopkins public health researcher Jean Humphrey and her Zimbabwe-based colleague Peter Iliff argue that the mortality risks of formula feeding are so high that infants of mothers infected with Human Immunodeficiency Virus (HIV), the virus that causes Acquired Immunodeficiency Syndrome (AIDS), have a better chance of survival if they are breastfed. Pediatrician Dorothy Mbori-Ngacha and her research colleagues argue that formula feeding is a safe alternative to breastfeeding and ensures longer survival of infants of HIV-infected mothers.

Agricultural researchers John P. Reganold and colleagues say that organic farming methods produce apples that are sweeter, less tart, more profitable, more energy efficient, and more environmentally and economically sustainable than those grown by conventional farming methods. Agricultural economist Dennis Avery counters that as a global food production system, organic farming would be an environmental disaster, an imminent danger to wildlife, and a hazard to public health.

Nutritionists Olivia Bennett Wood and Christine M. Bruhn, speaking for the American Dietetic Association (ADA), say that irradiation enhances the safety and quality of the food supply and helps protect consumers from foodborne illness. They maintain that officials should educate the public that irradiated foods are safe and offer a wider variety of such foods in the marketplace. Cancer researcher George L. Tritsch argues that the principal beneficiary of food irradiation is the food industry; the public derives no tangible benefit from this technology but bears all of its safety risks. He concludes that the long-term consequences of food irradiation will be far worse than any disease against which it may have been directed.

Scientist-official Robert B. Horsch, of the Monsanto Corporation, says that use of biotechnology will allow more food to be produced on less land with less depletion or damage to water resources and biodiversity. He insists that agricultural biotechnology is imperative for meeting growing demands for food. Scientist-official Margaret Mellon, of the Union of Concerned Scientists, says that science has yet to demonstrate that the benefits of food biotechnology outweigh the risks. She concludes that biotechnology is no panacea for world hunger and that it diverts attention from more effective methods for solving world food problems.

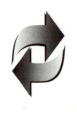

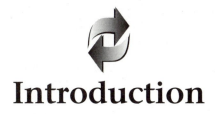

Introduction

Marion Nestle
L. Beth Dixon

Nearly every aspect of food and nutrition—from farm to fork and from science to policy—demands an exceptionally high level of critical thinking. This statement applies not only to the results of research studies but also to the *implications* of those studies for at least three areas: public health nutrition, government actions related to food and nutrition, and, of course, personal dietary practices. We developed *Taking Sides: Clashing Views on Controversial Issues in Food and Nutrition* to stimulate critical analysis of some of the most debated issues affecting these areas today.

The importance of food and nutrition is beyond question. Everyone eats, and diet profoundly affects health. People who do not have enough to eat lose weight and, in the most extreme situation, die of starvation. Those who eat too much gain weight and develop disease symptoms and conditions related to obesity. Such conditions, including coronary heart disease, cancer, diabetes, and stroke are leading causes of death and disability in most world populations today. Almost any one of the hundreds of chemical substances contained in foods—proteins, fats, carbohydrates, vitamins, minerals, trace elements, fiber, phytochemicals, additives, and contaminants—can affect health in one way or another.

If foods are complex, diets are even more so. They vary with geography, climate, economics, and culture. Even within one society, diets differ from day to day. Although societies throughout the world have found ways to construct healthful diets from available foods, the complexities of foods and dietary practices leave much room for uncertainty about the effects of any one dietary component on health. Uncertainty leaves room for controversy. Controversy demands critical thinking. In turn, critical thinking demands attention to the varying points of view—the stakeholder positions—expressed by the authors of the selections given here. Critical thinking also requires attention to the large number of factors that make research on diet, nutrition, and health particularly uncertain and inconclusive, and, therefore, controversial.

Stakeholder Issues

One further level of complexity is specific to the fields of food and nutrition. Because everyone eats, everyone holds a stake in the ways in which food is produced, consumed, and affects health. Stakeholders approach food and nutrition from their own self-interested perspectives. The debates in this book take place among five principal groups of stakeholders: food and nutrition professionals, officials of government agencies (and the groups that advise them), representatives of food companies and trade associations (known collectively as the food industry), consumer advocates, and journalists who write about food and nutrition issues. Nutrition and food professionals approach their fields from multiple standpoints, and they publish their research and opinions in journals that reflect those standpoints. For example, they view food and nutrition from the perspective of basic science (*Journal of Nutrition*), food science (*Food Technology*), clinical science (*American Journal of Clinical Nutrition*), medicine and epidemiology (*New England Journal of Medicine* or *Journal of the American Medical Association*), dietetics (*Journal of the American Dietetic Association*), education (*Journal of Nutrition Education and Behavior*), or public health (*American Journal of Public Health* and *Public Health Nutrition*), to name just a few. These multiple approaches suggest that professionals who work on problems related to mineral metabolism, for example, may view controversial issues in nutrition from a different perspective than professionals whose primary concern is nutrition education.

Government agencies are also heavily invested in food and nutrition. They issue dietary guidelines, monitor dietary intake and nutritional status, provide food assistance to the poor, support farm production, conduct food and nutrition research, regulate such food matters as labeling, advertising, irradiation, and biotechnology, and issue reports on all of these topics. Although nearly every federal agency has something to do with food or nutrition, the two most important are the United States Department of Agriculture (USDA) and the Department of Health and Human Services (HHS). The principal responsibility of the USDA is to promote sales and consumption of American agricultural products, but it also houses units that work on nutrition policy and advise the public about diet and health. Whereas one part of the USDA advises the public to avoid foods containing saturated fat, other parts promote increased consumption of meat (a principal dietary source of saturated fat) from American cattle producers. As discussed in Issue 1, these different functions can and do generate conflict. Similarly, the HHS includes several sub-agencies that deal with food and nutrition. The Food and Drug Administration (FDA), for example, regulates the safety and labeling of food products. The Centers for Disease Control and Prevention (CDC) conducts research and sponsors programs to prevent diet-related diseases. The National Institutes of Health (NIH) conducts and sponsors research on many aspects of nutrition and health. Other government or government-sponsored agencies investigate food and nutrition matters (for example, the General Accounting Office, which conducts research studies in response to congressional queries) or set standards for intake of essential nutrients (the Institute of Medicine of the National Academies). As we will see, these agencies act in their own self-interest and respond to political pressures, and they do not always agree with one another on controversial issues.

The food industry is a particularly influential stakeholder in matters pertaining to diet and health. Food is an enormous business that generates more than one trillion dollars in annual sales in the United States alone. Food must be produced, processed, distributed, and prepared before it is eaten, and each stage of food production, processing, and service is represented by its own segment of the food industry with its own special interests in influencing dietary advice and government regulations. Advice to avoid one or another category of food can have a large effect in decreasing sales or increasing production expenses, as can restrictive government regulations. Food companies are represented by trade associations such as the Food Marketing Institute (FMI), the National Restaurant Association (NRA), the National Food Processors Association (NFPA), the Council for Responsible Nutrition (representing makers of dietary supplements), and the Biotechnology Industry Organization (representing producers of genetically modified foods). These groups recruit lobbyists to help persuade government agencies and food and nutrition professionals to avoid issuing regulations or advice that might have an unfavorable effect on constituents' product sales.

Consumer advocacy organizations such as the Center for Science in the Public Interest in Washington D.C., and health-specific associations such as the American Heart Association, the American Cancer Society, and the American Diabetes Association attempt to promote the nutritional health of the public and, sometimes, counter the actions of food companies or the inactions of government. These organizations also hold a stake in matters related to food and nutrition, although they rarely enter the debate with financial resources as extensive as those of food companies.

Finally, the media hold a stake in food and nutrition issues. Stories about controversial issues attract readers and enhance the careers of journalists as well as of the researchers or groups that they write about. Research about the effects of food, nutrients, or agricultural practices on health often grabs front-page attention, and many leading journals issue press releases on studies likely to gain such attention. Reporters writing about food and nutrition issues of unusual interest win prizes and book contracts for their work. Because controversy makes news, media attention tends to focus on the differences rather than the similarities in points of view.

This book presents the opinions of people who work as nutrition researchers or as professionals who hold jobs in government agencies, food companies, food trade associations, and consumer advocacy groups, or who work as practicing journalists. When reading the opinions of anyone who discusses controversial matters in food and nutrition, it is often instructive to begin by identifying that person's stakeholder position. Stakeholder positions may well influence views about issues in food and nutrition because almost everyone holds fundamental beliefs and biases about diet and health, whether or not they recognize such biases. Beliefs about food issues may be based on matters such as religion (it is wrong to eat shellfish or pork), ethics (it is wrong to kill animals for food), philosophy (it is wrong to tamper with nature and irradiate or genetically modify foods), politics (the government is wrong to regulate dietary supplements), or economics (corporations have a right to profit from food sales). Such underlying beliefs are sometimes revealed by affiliations. For that reason, we identify the credentials and affiliations of the authors of these selections in the contributors section at the end of the book.

Research Issues

Nutrition research is complicated by genetic variations in individual nutritional requirements, the complexity of dietary intake, and interactions among dietary and other behavioral and lifestyle factors. It is also complicated by limitations in the ability to obtain accurate information about the dietary intake of individuals or populations. Proof of dietary causality—that sugar might have adverse affects on health (Issue 4) or that dietary supplements might improve health (Issues 10 and 11), for example—is difficult to demonstrate when health is affected by so many other genetic, environmental, and behavioral factors. The number and variety of factors that affect nutrients, foods, and diets make topics in food and nutrition especially difficult to study. As a result, much research in nutrition has tended to focus on the role of single nutrients in health. Such approaches isolate one nutrient from the context of foods or meals simply because its effects are easier to study that way. Such approaches are "reductionist" in that they appear to reduce—attribute—the effects of complicated dietary patterns to those associated with one nutrient. Examining single nutrients or food groups out of their "total diet" context, however, means that the studies require *interpretation*. Interpretation, in turn, requires critical thinking.

In practice, associations among dietary components and the risks of particular diseases are derived from many different types of studies. Some are conducted using laboratory animals. Others involve test-tube studies of cells or cell components. Those more directly related to human health involve epidemiological (population) approaches or clinical (medical) investigations. One fundamental problem in nutrition is that none of these methods are completely reliable—all have limitations. Animals are not people, and the results of animal studies may have little relevance to human health. Test-tube studies may not relate to living situations. Considered most compelling are epidemiological and clinical studies, but these also have limitations.

Epidemiologists identify associations between dietary factors and diseases across many different populations or within the same population. The results of such investigations often *associate* dietary factors to the risk of having a specific disease (but can never *prove* that the factor causes the disease). Issues 4, 5, and 7, for example, present epidemiological studies that associate the intake of certain dietary factors with the risk of breast cancer, diabetes, or heart disease. Such studies demonstrate that being overweight may increase the risk of certain forms of diabetes, but they do not prove that obesity causes diabetes. Other factors in addition to obesity may be equally or more important in influencing the development of that disease. Thus, such "observational" epidemiologic studies generate hypotheses that must be confirmed by further research.

One way to confirm observational hypotheses is through controlled clinical trials. In such trials, investigators study the associations of dietary factors with a disease over time. These studies are limited by high cost (and, therefore, the size of the population that can be studied) and all of the other factors (drinking, smoking, medications, exercise) that might affect the results of the study.

It is relatively easy to demonstrate that iron or any other single nutrient can prevent or treat the symptoms resulting from deficient intake of that nutrient, but it is far more difficult to show that beta-carotene protects against lung cancer (Issue 10), gingko supplements improve memory (Issue 11), or that the use of commercial infant formulas as a replacement for breast feeding prevents transmission of the virus that causes AIDS from infected mothers to their children (Issue 14). Such difficulties are especially evident in studies of the effects of dietary supplements on health. People who take such supplements are demonstrably healthier than those who do not, but the supplements may have less to do with their good health than with other differences between people who do and do not take supplements. As a group, supplement takers are generally wealthier and better educated, smoke fewer cigarettes, drink less alcohol, exercise more actively, and do more to take care of their health. A well-designed study must find ways to distinguish the effects of the supplement itself from the effects of these other aspects.

For such reasons, clinical studies must include a control group in order to distinguish the true effects of a dietary factor from those caused by something else. Control groups sometimes are given a placebo, a pill containing sugar or other components with no physiological effects. The dietary component must be shown to produce health benefits greater than those that can be obtained with placebos. Placebos are a powerful—though often unappreciated—force for healing in medicine, particularly because many illnesses resolve and get better by themselves. About 30 percent of people have the good fortune to be "placebo responders," meaning that just the act of taking a pill, even it if does not contain any medicine, makes their colds, aches and pains, feelings of tension or anxiety, and other such minor problems go away or become less severe. As a result, the most scientifically convincing evidence for an effect of a dietary factor on a disease comes from "randomized, double-blind, controlled trials" in which participants are assigned to the test or control groups (nutrient versus placebo or diet versus standard care) by a formal process of randomization, and neither the investigators nor the participants are told who is in which group during the many years that it takes for diseases to develop. The NO-side selection of Issue 10 describes several such studies of beta-carotene supplements and the risk of lung cancer. Overall, lengthy and complicated clinical studies do not easily recruit and retain participants, cost many millions of dollars, and rarely produce results that can be interpreted unambiguously.

Because of such limitations, associations between dietary factors and health risks are usually inferred from the *totality* of the available evidence. The associations are considered most compelling when data from all sources produce similar results, especially when the results of the studies are consistent, specific to the condition under investigation, dose-dependent (meaning that higher amounts of the nutrient produce stronger effects), and biologically plausible (meaning that the results make sense from a biological perspective). Inference from the totality of available evidence requires interpretation, attention to the points of view of the producers of that evidence, and, therefore, critical thinking.

Dietary Assessment Issues

Studies of diet and health depend on the ability of investigators to determine what people are actually eating. This is not as easy to do as it might seem. Try, for example, to list everything that you ate or drank yesterday and to estimate the precise amount of each item you consumed. Few people can do this with much accuracy. The most frequently used methods for evaluating dietary intake are to ask people to record what they ate or drank in the previous day (a 24-hour diet recall, done retrospectively), keep a record of what they eat for a day or more (diet record, prospective), or mark off on a list the foods they ate within the last day, week, month, or year (food frequency questionnaire, retrospective). These methods suffer from several systematic limitations. As already suggested, most people do not easily remember what they have eaten. They also may be uncomfortable reporting late-night snacks, alcohol, or the actual quantities of foods consumed. As a result, responses to dietary surveys tend to underestimate energy intake, the sizes of food portions, and the consumption of alcohol or other foods that people think are "bad" for them. In contrast, survey respondents tend to overestimate their intake of "good" foods. Thus, nutrition researchers typically debate whether one of the methods is better than another, whether collecting information on portion sizes is useful or necessary, or indeed whether any method can capture the complexities of diets that vary so much from person to person and from day to day.

A further problem is the translation of intake of foods into the amounts of energy (calories) and nutrients they contain. This translation requires use of computer software programs that associate data on food intake with similar foods listed in tables of food composition developed by the USDA. Studies of dietary factors and health risks depend on the reliability of the USDA food composition database. For example, to define standards of calcium intake that will protect the population against osteoporosis (Issue 3), it is necessary to determine how much calcium is consumed. This requires knowing how much calcium is available in dairy products as well as in vegetable sources of that nutrient. Carrots contain calcium, but is the calcium content of carrots grown in California the same as that of carrots grown in Arkansas or Massachusetts? Do carrots of a particular variety have the same calcium content as those of another variety? Are organically grown carrots more nutritious than conventionally grown carrots (Issue 15)? Resolving such questions requires careful attention to methods of sampling, preservation of samples throughout the testing process, and the reliability of laboratory tests for the calcium content of food. Food composition determinations are expensive and time-consuming, and the USDA has only a limited budget for such studies. Instead, it relies on composition information provided by food companies for the hundreds of thousands of packaged foods on the market and on collaborations with university researchers who analyze foods in laboratories or search the literature for values acquired during research studies. In many instances, companies are reluctant to provide information on the nutrient content of foods that they consider a proprietary "business interest." Such limitations do not necessarily mean that information about food composition and nutrient intake is incorrect, but it does mean that such information requires careful interpretation, skeptical attitudes, and much common sense.

Statistical Issues

Because so many factors other than the one under investigation can affect the results of nutrition studies, epidemiologists and clinical researchers use statistical tests to evaluate the data obtained. These tests are designed to probe the likelihood that the study results could have occurred by *chance* rather than as an actual effect of the dietary factor. Researchers use tests to decide whether the combined results of studies are likely to answer a specific question (are "statistically significant") or could have occurred by chance (are not statistically significant).

In such studies, a result is usually considered statistically significant if it has no more than a 5 percent probability of having occurred by chance—5 out of 100. This is expressed as a probability ($p = .05$). A result is even more likely to be statistically significant if the probability is no more than 1 percent (1 out of 100), expressed as $p = .01$. The use of 0.01 or 0.05 as cut points is arbitrary, but is generally agreed upon by scientists as a reasonable measure to use for testing study results. But like any other tests, these require interpretation. Although probabilities of .01 to .05 may reassure investigators that the results are what they claim to be, there is still a 1 percent to 5 percent chance that the results are misleading.

To evaluate how serious a diet-related health risk might be, epidemiologists use statistical tests to determine what they term a Relative Risk (RR) (or similar factors called Odds Ratios or Hazard Ratios). An RR of 1.0 means that a dietary factor has *no association* with risk. The results of epidemiologic studies involving dietary factors often yield Relative Risks that are quite low—in the range of 1.2 to 2.5—meaning that whatever factor is under investigation increases the risk of getting a disease by 20 percent to 150 percent ($1.2 - 1.0 = 0.2 \times 100 = 20$ percent; $2.5 - 1.0 = 1.5 \times 100 = 150$ percent). In the YES-side selection of Issue 6, for example, researchers determined that excess body weight increased the risk of certain diseases by Relative Risks of 1.5 to 2.5, or 50 percent to 150 percent. Although these percentages seem impressively large, they must be interpreted in the context of the number of cases involved. Consider this example: an increase in disease incidence from 1 to 2 cases per 1000 per year represents a 100 percent increase in risk. This increase may not mean much (except to that one individual), whereas an increase from 100 to 200 cases, also representing a 100 percent increase, carries much greater significance for the health of the population.

Context and Thematic Issues

This discussion should make it clear that nutrition studies must be interpreted in context with a dose of common sense. Food and nutrition are fields well suited to skepticism and critical analysis at every step of learning and interpretation, and they require an unusually high tolerance for ambiguity and uncertainty. The difficulties inherent in conducting and interpreting research studies, the historic emphasis of research (not to mention food advertising) on single nutrients instead of dietary patterns, and the interests of industry, government, and public stakeholders in the outcome of research, create ample opportunity for controversy. Debates about the meaning of nutrition research can best be resolved by viewing the issues in context, judging arguments on the basis of their plausibility and consistency with other sources of information, and using good common sense throughout this endeavor. The selections presented in this book represent just two points of view for an issue in situations where others may also be equally persuasive. If these readings suggest the benefits of other points of view, including your own, so much the better.

Organization of the Book

We present the issues debated in *Taking Sides: Clashing Views on Controversial Issues in Food and Nutrition* in five sections organized by category of debatable topics: Dietary Patterns and Guidelines, Nutrition and Health, Diet, Physical Activity, and Health, Supplements and Functional Foods, and Nutrition and Food Policy. These sections encompass debates about matters affecting the entire food chain, from production agriculture to advice about healthful diets. We deliberately selected topics to include debates about matters ranging from basic science to public policy, and we chose authors who are nutrition scientists, physicians, educators, practitioners, government officials, and policy analysts. Because so much public information about food and nutrition comes from the media, we also included one set of selections from practicing journalists. We chose these topics to illustrate the breadth of nutrition as a field of study, the ways in which food and nutrition debates affect public policy as well as personal and public health, and the extraordinary opportunities for ongoing discussion and further research that these fields not only permit but encourage.

A Note on Editing

To meet the series' requirements for length and content—and to improve readability—we edited nearly all of the selections in this book. We approached the editing task by changing the authors' words in only two ways. We occasionally added bracketed explanations of technical terms that we thought might be unfamiliar. Otherwise, our editing consisted solely of deletions. We deleted portions of the selections that we thought were not essential to a basic understanding of the argument, especially those that seemed technically complex. For example, we omitted many of the details of statistical and other methods as well as statistical tables, statistical data (such as confidence intervals, probability values, and correlation coefficients), data tables, complicated illustrations, and information about the authors' declarations of research sponsorship and statements of conflict of interest.

With considerable reluctance, we eliminated all reference citations in most articles. Space limitations governed this choice, particularly because such selections that involve scientific studies or reviews often cite more than 50 references. We indicate this omission with the phrase "references omitted." Our hesitancy about this choice derives from our strong belief that source material is a vitally important factor in determining the credibility of scientific arguments. The number of citations, the quality of the sources, and the ways in which the sources are used reveal much about the strength or weakness of an argument. Studies published in peer-reviewed journals, for example, carry more weight than newspaper accounts, simply because peer reviewers and editors have examined the authors' work and judged it worth publishing. Thus, the choice of reference materials should have a major influence on how we interpret an author's position in a debate. Whether done consciously or unconsciously, authors often tend to cite or exaggerate the significance of studies that bolster their arguments and to ignore, minimize, or misinterpret contrary studies. To determine whether such biases exist, it is necessary to read the cited references just as critically as one reads the selections themselves. Although we firmly believe that such an activity is highly instructive, that exercise goes well beyond the purposes of the Taking Sides series. We can only urge students to pick at least one edited selection, find the original unedited version (which often can be found online at university libraries), and look up and examine a few of the references. Students who accept this challenge will learn much about the ways in which nutrition opinions can be biased. This exercise also provides an opportunity to critically evaluate our editing. We tried to delete only those parts of the selections that seemed unnecessary to the debate. We encourage students to compare the edited against the unedited version and determine for themselves whether our editing succeeded in preserving an unbiased account of the authors' views.

The editors of certain selections would only permit reproduction of complete selections. In considering those selections, try to be aware of how the difference in presentation and the inclusion of statistical material, tables, and references might influence your view of the importance or credibility of the work. Might the absence of this material affect your perception of their arguments?

Finally, we believe that much of the excitement and enjoyment of studying food and nutrition derives from the complexity of the field and the many points of view that can be brought to bear on almost any aspect. Anyone interested in nutrition or food science—but also in history, sociology, anthropology, politics, biology, public health, medicine, law, or almost any other field of study—holds a legitimate stake in the issues debated in this book. Debates about food and nutrition are personal as well as political and for that reason are especially interesting, entertaining, and useful. We hope that readers will enjoy these debates and bring their own opinions and thoughts to the discussion.

Center for Nutrition Policy and Promotion (CNPP)

This Center for Nutrition Policy and Promotion (CNPP) Web site provides recent United States Department of Agriculture (USDA) publications on diet and health, including the USDA Pyramid graphic, brochure, and the history of its development; the Food Guide Pyramid for Children; the Dietary Guidelines for Americans; the Healthy Eating Index (a 10-component index of foods and nutrients designed to measure overall dietary quality); and data on the dietary intake of Americans. Click on the *Nutrition Insights* button to see especially, Insight 2, Escobar A., "Are All Food Pyramids Created Equal?" (April 1997).

http://www.usda.gov/cnpp/

Economic Research Service (ERS)

This Economic Research Service (ERS) research reports site offers the complete text of *America's Eating Habits: Changes & Consequences.* The site also offers a large range of USDA publications on food and nutrition policy.

http://www.ers.usda.gov/Publications/

The American Dietetic Association

The American Dietetic Association site is primarily designed for members, but it also offers information for the public about dozens of issues in nutrition, resources for studying those issues, legislation affecting food and nutrition, and nutrition careers.

http://www.eatright.org/Public/

The Centers for Disease Control and Prevention (CDC)

The Centers for Disease Control and Prevention (CDC) Web site is where to find the latest statistics on the national epidemic of overweight and obesity, organized by state, as well as information on definitions, health consequences, recommendations, and resources. Click on the "Obesity Trends" button to see how the prevalence of obesity in the United States has increased from 1985 to 2001.

http://www.cdc.gov/nccdphp/dnpa/obesity/index.htm

Institute of Medicine (IOM): Food and Nutrition Board

The Institute of Medicine (IOM): Food and Nutrition Board is responsible for developing the national standards for intake of essential nutrients, which is called the Dietary Reference Intakes. The full reports published to date (and additional information about their preparation) can be found at this site.

http://www.iom.edu/project.asp?id=4574

PART 1

Dietary Patterns and Guidelines

A *basic task of nutrition guidelines is to advise the public about diets that promote health and prevent disease. Throughout human history, people have constructed diets from foods that were available locally and through trade, and that were selected on the basis of culture as well as income, education, taste, and other factors that influence food choice. Diets are composed of a vast array of foods; foods contain dozens of individual nutrients essential for health. Therefore, nutrition recommendations can apply to dietary patterns (food guides), foods (dietary guidelines), or nutrients (dietary standards). This section addresses questions about each of these approaches to dietary advice. Can food guides describe a dietary pattern suitable for everyone in a population? Do factors other than science influence the content and wording of dietary guidelines? Do standards of intake of individual nutrients make sense outside of their dietary context? The selections in this part explain the basis of current debates about the value and meaning of recommendations for intake of diets, foods, and nutrients.*

- Does the USDA Pyramid Describe an Optimal Dietary Pattern?

- Can All Foods Fit Into a Healthful Diet?

- Are the New Dietary Reference Intakes for Calcium Appropriate?

1

ISSUE 1

Does the USDA Pyramid Describe an Optimal Dietary Pattern?

YES: Marion Nestle, from "In Defense of the USDA Food Guide Pyramid," *Nutrition Today* (September/October 1998)

NO: Walter C. Willett with P. J. Skerrett, from *Eat, Drink, and Be Healthy: The Harvard Medical School Guide to Healthy Eating* (Simon & Schuster, 2001)

ISSUE SUMMARY

YES: New York University nutrition professor Marion Nestle says that the U.S. Department of Agriculture (USDA) Food Guide Pyramid's hierarchical design and emphasis on plant-based diets represent a significant advance over previous federal food guides and that a few adjustments to the Pyramid's design would further strengthen its message and respond to most of the concerns of critics.

NO: Harvard School of Public Health nutrition professor Walter C. Willett and author P. J. Skerrett argue that the Pyramid at best offers "wishy-washy, scientifically unfounded advice" and at worst contributes to poor health. Overall, the Pyramid represents "a missed opportunity to improve the health of millions of people."

An optimal diet is one that provides enough calories and nutrients to support growth and reproduction, does so in the correct balance to promote health and prevent disease, and is available, affordable, and palatable so that people can and will consume it. Throughout human history, people have eaten foods available locally and through trade to meet their nutritional needs, yet dietary patterns and practices differ greatly among world populations. In the United States, a question of great interest to nutritionists, government health officials, and the public is, What kind of a diet best promotes health?

To answer that question, the U.S. Department of Agriculture (USDA) has issued dietary advice to the public since early in the twentieth century. At first, USDA nutritionists advised the public to be sure to eat foods every day from various groups: dairy, meat, fruits and vegetables, cereals, and sometimes fats and sweets. This advice was readily accepted and not at all controversial, largely because it met both of two distinct functions of the USDA: promoting consumption of American agricultural products and offering dietary advice. As long as the purpose of dietary advice was to encourage people to eat *more* of American agricultural products, the two functions did not come into conflict.

During the course of the twentieth century, however, disease patterns related to the dietary intake of Americans shifted. Early in the century, infectious diseases made worse by nutritional deficiencies were the leading causes of illness and death. By mid-century, *chronic* diseases such as coronary heart disease, cancer, diabetes, and high blood pressure began to predominate. To prevent chronic diseases, Americans would need to eat *less* of the dietary factors that increased risk for these conditions—fat, saturated fat, cholesterol, sugar, salt, and alcohol. This meant that people would need to eat less of the foods that contain these dietary substances. Advice to eat less of such foods, however, came into conflict with the interests of groups that produced or sold them. It also conflicted with the USDA's mission to promote greater consumption of American agricultural products. Thus, beginning in the mid-1970s, the history of USDA food guides for prevention of chronic diseases—as opposed to diseases caused by nutritional deficiencies—became one of nearly constant controversy.

As Marion Nestle explains, USDA nutritionists worked for many years to develop a Pyramid so well researched that it would be immune to controversy. Their research suggested that the Pyramid's hierarchical design would be understood by the public to mean that some foods should be eaten in greater amounts than others. The USDA nutritionists were surprised when the design proved controversial, and producers of foods in the narrower sectors of the Pyramid strongly objected to the placement of their products in the illustration. Nestle argues that given the political realities of dietary advising, the Pyramid represented a major forward step. Its strengths, she says, lie in its conceptual and research basis, its focus on consumption of plant foods, the strong scientific support for that focus, its representation of a dietary pattern more healthful than that currently consumed by the U.S. population, and its adaptability to a wide range of dietary preferences and cultural patterns.

In contrast, Walter C. Willett contends that the scientific foundation of the Pyramid is inadequate and does not reflect the current state of research on nutrition and health. He singles out several features for particular criticism. The Pyramid, he says, incorrectly implies that all fats are bad and all carbohydrates are good, all protein sources are equivalent, dairy products are essential, and potatoes are recommended. Instead, he says, a healthful diet demands attention to a *different* set of issues: body weight, type of fat and carbohydrate (with an emphasis on good fats and good carbohydrates), source of protein, avoidance of potatoes, alcohol in moderation (for adults), and multivitamins for nutritional insurance. He proposes an alternative pyramid that reflects these ideas.

This debate about the content and value of the USDA's Food Guide Pyramid raises fundamental questions about dietary advice. What are the most important dietary messages that a food guide should convey? Does either pyramid illustrate such messages adequately? What are the strengths of the two approaches? What are their limitations?

Marion Nestle

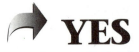 **YES**

In Defense of the USDA Food Guide Pyramid

Every 5 years since 1980, the US Department of Health and Human Services (HHS) and the US Department of Agriculture (USDA) have issued a joint statement of dietary guidance policy for health promotion and disease prevention—the *Dietary Guidelines for Americans.* The most recent edition appeared in 1995. It advises Americans to eat a variety of foods; to balance food intake with physical activity; to choose a diet with plenty of grain products, vegetables, and fruits but low in fat, saturated fat, and cholesterol and moderate in sugars, salt, and sodium; and to drink alcoholic beverages in moderation, if at all.

Although these Guidelines govern the content of all government nutrition programs and educational materials, they are not generally known or understood by the public. Thus, in 1992, USDA issued a *Food Guide Pyramid* to help people apply the Guidelines to their own diets. The Pyramid (see Fig. 1) depicts a hierarchical dietary pattern in which most daily food servings are from the grain, vegetable, and fruit groups, with fewer servings from the milk and meat groups, and even fewer from foods high in fat and sugar.

In its 6 years of existence, the Pyramid has become the most widely distributed and best recognized nutrition education device ever produced in this country. It appears in nutrition education materials, posters, and textbooks, in advertisements and package labels, in cookbooks, and on board games. It is recognized by an astonishing 67% or more of American adults. It is demonstrably iconographic as it has spawned numerous analogs illustrating specific dietary patterns. By any criterion of recognition or dissemination, the Pyramid has been highly influential.

This influence, however, has been achieved at the price of controversy. Even before its release, the Pyramid elicited intense criticism, and it has continued to stimulate lively debates. At first, producers of meat, dairy, and processed foods complained that the Pyramid's hierarchical design would diminish sales of their products. Other critics challenged its conceptual framework, scientific basis, and effectiveness as a teaching tool.

From Marion Nestle, "In Defense of the USDA Food Guide Pyramid," *Nutrition Today,* vol. 33, no. 5 (September/October 1998), pp. 189–195. Copyright © 1998 by *Nutrition Today.* Reprinted by permission of Lippincott Williams & Wilkins. References omitted.

Figure 1

Food Guide Pyramid: A Guide to Daily Food Choices

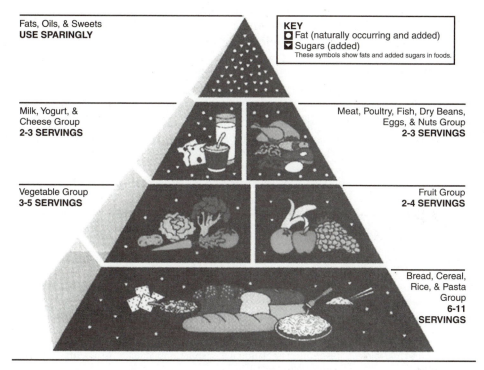

Source: U.S. Department of Agriculture/U.S. Department of Health and Human Services

More recent concerns about the Pyramid occur in the context of widespread public misunderstanding of the meaning of nutrition advice, of media research reports that appear to conflict with dietary advice, and of increasing confusion—even among experts—about the applicability of public health recommendations to the dietary practices of individuals. In this context, critics have challenged the value of even such basic advice as avoiding overweight or, as discussed previously, eating more fruits and vegetables. Alliances of nutrition societies, federal agencies, and food industry groups have only added to the confusion by arguing that no foods should be categorized as good or bad. Such advice implies that food group hierarchies, such as those in the Pyramid, may be inappropriate.

In 1996, USDA revised the Pyramid to reflect the 1995 Dietary Guidelines. As HHS and USDA develop the fifth Guidelines edition scheduled for 2000, it is worth reviewing the substantial advances in dietary guidance policy represented by the Pyramid's design and content, and considering ways to improve on its substantial strengths.

Historical Perspective

Table 1 summarizes key events in the Pyramid's history. This history begins in 1862 when Congress established the USDA with a mandate to advise the public about agricultural topics. In 1916, USDA began to issue food guides to help Americans prevent nutritional deficiencies. After World War II, as chronic diseases increasingly displaced deficiencies as the principal nutrition problems in the United States, new food guides were needed to address these conditions. USDA published its last food guide devoted solely to addressing nutrient deficiencies, known familiarly as the Basic Four, in 1958.

By that time, researchers already had associated diet with risks for coronary heart disease, and were providing dietary guidelines similar to those used today. Two decades later, as research increasingly supported the value of such advice, a Senate committee issued Dietary Goals with numerical targets for

Table 1

Key Events Relevant to the History of the USDA Food Guide Pyramid

1958	USDA issues *Daily Food Guide ("Basic Four")* to help the public prevent nutritional deficiencies.
1977	Senate Committee releases 1st and 2nd editions of *Dietary Goals for the United States* to prevent chronic diseases.
1979	USDA issues *Hassle-Free Guide to a Better Diet,* adding a 5th group to the *Basic Four* and emphasizing vegetables, fruits, grains.
1980	The Department of Health, Education, and Welfare (HEW) and USDA jointly issue *Dietary Guidelines for Americans.* The National Research Council (NRC) issues 9th edition of the *Recommended Dietary Allowances* (RDAs).
1981	USDA initiates a 3-year research program to design a food guidance system to meet RDAs and *Dietary Guidelines.*
1984	USDA presents research results as a *Food Wheel* for the American Red Cross.
1985	The Department of Health and Human Services (HHS) and USDA issue the 2nd edition of the *Dietary Guidelines.*
1988	USDA hires Porter-Novelli to develop and test graphic designs for the food guide; deems the Pyramid most effective. HHS issues *Surgeon General's Report on Nutrition and Health.*
1989	NRC publishes the 10th edition of the RDAs and the *Diet and Health* Report.
1990	USDA develops, submits for peer review, tests, and revises Pyramid brochure and graphic, completes clearance procedures. HHS and USDA issue 3rd edition of the *Dietary Guidelines.* Congress passes Nutrition Labeling and Education Act (NLEA).
1991	USDA withdraws Pyramid, hires Bell Associates to conduct further research.
1992	USDA issues *Food Guide Pyramid.*
1994	NLEA takes effect.
1995	HHS and USDA issue 4th edition of the *Dietary Guidelines.*
1996	USDA updates Pyramid to be consistent with the 1995 *Dietary Guidelines* and Daily Values on food labels.
1997	NRC issues the first set of Dietary Reference Intakes (DRIs) as replacements for RDAs. HHS and USDA request nominations for committee to develop 5th edition of the *Dietary Guidelines.*
1998	USDA and HHS announce appointment of 5th *Dietary Guidelines* Advisory Committee.

reducing fat, saturated fat, and cholesterol, and with suggestions for changes in food intake that would be needed to achieve the goals. USDA responded to this challenge by developing a food guide to prevent chronic as well as deficiency diseases in 1979; it rearranged the groups to emphasize those from plants, and suggested restrictions on a fifth group—fats/sweets/alcohol.

In 1980, federal agencies issued the first Dietary Guidelines; with minor word changes, the initial precepts have been retained throughout subsequent editions. Also in 1980, the National Research Council (NRC) issued the ninth revision of Recommended Dietary Allowances (RDAs) for intake of single nutrients that would prevent deficiencies in most healthy people.

Thus, by 1981, USDA nutritionists were well prepared to begin researching a food guide that would encompass Dietary Guidelines, RDAs, and dietary survey results, and would address prevention of nutrient excesses and imbalances as well as deficiencies. Three years later, USDA presented its research in the form of a Food Wheel designed for the American Red Cross. When it became clear that the Wheel was difficult for the public to understand, the agency recruited a marketing research firm, Porter-Novelli, to develop and test more comprehensible graphic designs.

Between 1981 and 1990, HHS and USDA issued the second and third editions of the Dietary Guidelines, the NRC released the 10th edition of the RDAs, HHS and NRC produced comprehensive reviews of the evidence linking diet to chronic disease risk, and Congress passed the Nutrition Labeling and Education Act—all of which influenced the Pyramid's design and content. From 1988 to 1990, USDA and Porter-Novelli developed, tested, peer-reviewed, and revised the Pyramid brochure, and completed all necessary federal reviews and clearances. In April 1991, the USDA Secretary abruptly canceled the Pyramid's publication on the grounds that it needed further testing with low-income adults and schoolchildren. Much evidence, however, suggested an alternative explanation—pressure from meat and milk producers concerned that the design was unfavorable to their products. The Pyramid's withdrawal led to unrelenting press reports of the apparent conflict between USDA's dual mandates to promote agricultural products and the health of the public. One year later, after completion of additional research, USDA finally issued the brochure.

In 1996, USDA revised the brochure to make it consistent with the 1995 Dietary Guidelines. Two recent events suggest that further revisions will most certainly be needed; the NRC is replacing RDAs with Dietary Reference Intakes, and HHS and USDA have appointed a committee to prepare the next Dietary Guidelines.

Critical Perspective

Upon release of the Pyramid in 1992, some nutrition and industry groups lauded it as an improvement over the Basic Four, but others criticized it. Table 2 classifies and summarizes the principal criticisms; these range from the trivial (*eg,* geometric, botanic) and flawed (some biochemical concerns), to the fundamental. Among the latter are questions about the assignment of certain foods to

Table 2

Principal Problem Categories and Criticisms of the 1992 USDA Food Guide Pyramid

Problem category	The Pyramid does not, but should:
Geometric	• Represent a pyramid (it is a triangle).
Botanic	• Classify fruits and vegetables appropriately (ie., tomatoes and peppers are fruits).
Ideologic	• Emphasize that all food groups are equivalent and that there are no good or bad foods.
Biochemical	• Recognize the biochemical equivalency of sugars and starches in the body.
	• Ensure adequate intake of essential fatty acids.
	• Distinguish the health impact of total fat relative to that of saturated, monosaturated, polyunsaturated, and trans-saturated fatty acids.
Gastronomic	• Emphasize whole, minimally processed—as opposed to refined—grains.
	• Separate beans (a vegetable) from meats.
	• Equate fresh beans (in vegetable group) with dried beans (meat group).
	• Distinguish high- from low-fat meat and dairy products.
	• Emphasize non-tropical oils opposed to tropical oils and animal fats.
	• Distinguish high- from low-fat cooking methods.
Pedagogic	• Guide educators to place commonly consumed foods in appropriate groups.
	• Explain serving sizes adequately or consistently.
	• Convey the complexities of information about nutrition and health.
Conceptual	• Distinguish serving recommendations that should be considered upper limits (meat and high-fat dairy foods) from those that should be considered lower limits (grain, fruit, and vegetable groups).
	• Meet the concerns and needs of vegetarians.
	• Reflect current *Dietary Guidelines,* emphasizing plant-based diets and including physical activity, salt, and appropriate use of alcohol.
	• Reflect replacement of Recommended Dietary Allowances (RDAs) by new Dietary References Intake (DRI) standards.

groups, definitions of serving sizes, and lack of distinctions among high- and low-fat foods, saturated and unsaturated fats, and servings meant to be upper limits (meat, milk, fat and sugar groups) from those meant to be lower limits (grains, fruits, vegetables). More recent concerns focus on the need to update the Pyramid to reflect a stronger emphasis on plant-based diets, and to include guidance about physical activity, salt, and alcohol.

It is difficult to imagine how any single graphic design might address the full range of such criticisms, or even those that are most valid. Other groups have attempted to correct some of the Pyramid's perceived inadequacies by creating their own versions to reflect, for example, Mediterranean, Asian, or vegetarian diets. Whether such alternatives may be complementary or competing, they solve some, but not all, of the problems of the USDA Pyramid and may well present others. It is always difficult to untangle science from values in developing clear and unambiguous dietary messages. Thus, the positive contributions of the USDA Pyramid are well worth review and emphasis.

Positive Contributions

The Pyramid derived from an 11-year process of conceptualization, research, and testing. Its dietary pattern is largely based on plant foods—grains, fruits, and vegetables—with fewer portions of foods from the meat and milk groups. That this pattern is far more healthful than diets typically consumed by Americans is well supported by recent research.

Conceptual Basis

USDA nutritionists intended the Pyramid to display a dietary pattern that would meet two goals at once: provide a balance and quantity of nutrients sufficient to meet RDAs, but also to meet targets for reduced intake of fat, saturated fat, cholesterol, salt, and sugar. Furthermore, USDA staff wanted the Pyramid to convey three key concepts: variety, moderation, and proportionality. They defined *variety* as the number of different kinds of foods within and among groups, *moderation* as the need to eat less of foods high in fat and sugar, and *proportionality* as the hierarchical—more servings should be consumed from some food groups than others. Thus, unlike previous USDA food guides, the Pyramid derived from an established conceptual framework.

Research Basis

The content and design of the Pyramid were established during three distinct phases of research. In the first phase (1981–1984), USDA nutritionists selected nutritional goals, defined food groups, calculated the number of daily servings, assigned serving sizes, and created the Food Wheel. Because this design did not readily convey moderation or proportionality, USDA soon abandoned it but continued to use the food groups and serving numbers in publications throughout the mid-1980s. In the second phase, which began in 1988, Porter-Novelli tested several designs for conveying key concepts to adults who had at least a high school education and average income. Focus-group research indicated that this audience preferred food groups to be displayed in bands within an equilateral triangle ("pyramid"), and that this design best conveyed the key concepts.

The third phase began in 1991 after USDA withdrew the Pyramid from publication. The agency contracted with a consulting firm, Bell Associates, to compare alternative designs among participants in food assistance programs. Bell used focus-group research to test the Pyramid against bowls, pie charts, and shopping carts among diverse groups of children and adults. This research found industry representatives to prefer pie chart and bowl designs that did not "stack" the food groups, but nutrition professionals to prefer pyramids that better conveyed the desired messages. At that point, the field narrowed to two design options, pyramids and bowls. Bell then collected opinions about pyramid and bowl shapes from more than 3000 children and low-income adults. Eventually, analysis of the results indicated that both designs effectively conveyed the need for variety in food intake, but the Pyramid better indicated moderation and proportionality.

Overall, USDA staff labored more than a decade to ensure that the Pyramid's principal features—food groups, serving numbers, and serving sizes—were substantiated by research, reviewed by experts, and understood by intended users. No food guide, USDA or other, has ever been researched to anywhere near this extent.

Scientific Support

Since 1992, the healthfulness of diets based largely on foods of plant origin has received increasing research support. Plant foods are the sole dietary sources of fiber, vitamin C, carotenoids, and phytochemicals, and are principal, although not exclusive, sources of folate, vitamins A and E, and other nutrients associated with prevention of chronic as well as deficiency diseases. Evidence for the substantial health benefits of exclusively or largely plant-based diets has been well reviewed. On the basis of such evidence, health authorities throughout the world consistently recommend Pyramid-like dietary patterns for overall health promotion, most notably for prevention of coronary heart disease and cancer.

Hierarchical Proportions

USDA's 1958 Basic Four guide displayed the milk, meat, fruit and vegetable, and bread and cereal groups as squares of roughly equivalent size. The 1979 Hassle-Free Guide was the first to introduce hierarchies in food groups. It displayed the groups stacked one above the other with vegetables/fruits at the top, followed in descending order by bread/cereals, milk/cheese, meat/poultry/fish/beans, and a fifth band at the bottom of fats/sweets/alcohol. In response to protests from producers of foods in the lower echelons, USDA soon ceased issuing this guide.

USDA staff intended the Pyramid as hierarchical to convey proportionality. More healthful diets are low in saturated fat and high in grains, fruits, and vegetables. The principal sources of saturated fat in American diets are fats and oils (41%), meat (26%), and milk-group foods (24%). The Pyramid illustrates hierarchies through the relative number of plant-group servings (11–20 in total) as compared to meat- and milk-group servings (4–6), and through the placement of meat, milk, and fats and oils in the narrower portions of the design.

Healthful Dietary Pattern

The dietary pattern displayed in the Pyramid represents an improvement over current food intakes in the United States. . . . USDA estimates that the US food supply provides about 9 daily grain servings per capita, 3 of vegetables, 1.5 of fruits, about 2 each of dairy and meat foods, but more fats, oils, and sugars than is recommended. Such data should not be interpreted as indicating a shortfall in food availability; per capita figures include infants and children as well as adults. They do suggest some imbalances in food production, however, that could be corrected by increasing the supply of fruits and vegetables and decreasing supplies of processed foods containing fat and sugar.

USDA 1996 survey data also indicate an imbalance between current and recommended dietary patterns. These data are constructed by disaggregating recipes for mixed dishes, and allocating weights of single food ingredients to appropriate Pyramid categories. Thus, the flour in cookies contributes to grain servings, apples in pies contribute to fruit servings, and potatoes in chips contribute to vegetable servings, as do tomatoes in ketchup. This method may yield more precise data on nutrient intake, but it shifts foods high in fat and sugar from the peak to the lower tiers of the Pyramid. Even so, these data reveal excessive intake of servings from the meat and fats/oils/sweets groups, but inadequate servings from the fruit and milk groups.

These data also reveal more specific dietary problems. Consumption of milk is especially low among teenagers who have replaced it with soft drinks. Vegetable servings may appear adequate, but only one-fourth serving comes from dark-green vegetables, and at least half the total derive from fast food garnishes—fresh and frozen potatoes, canned tomatoes, iceberg lettuce, and onions. Excluding fried potatoes reduces vegetable servings below three per day. A 1994 survey by the Beef Board identified even greater imbalances. Overall, diets could be improved by adding some servings of fruits and vegetables, and subtracting some servings of meat and other sources of saturated fat. Small dietary changes of this type are achievable and could greatly improve overall health.

Standard for Comparison

. . . [The] Pyramid proportions and servings constitute a convenient standard for evaluation of dietary intake patterns. Serving counts contribute to at least half the score of one index of healthy eating. Other researchers have used the Pyramid to assess the quality of foods advertised on children's television programs, and to evaluate its effect on advertising in culinary and health magazines. Such uses extend the influence of the Pyramid beyond dietary advice.

Adaptability

The Pyramid was designed to improve standard American eating patterns; if followed, it would do so. Its design is demonstrably easy to adapt to the particular food preferences and traditions of individuals, groups, and cultures. Pyramids for Mediterranean and vegetarian dietary patterns were developed from explicit conceptual systems; others diet Pyramids are more impressionistic. One vegetarian group, for example, suggests removal of the meat, milk, and fats/oils/sweets sectors, creating a Food Guide Trapezoid. Regardless of origin, all pyramids designed to advise the public about diet and health share a common emphasis on reducing saturated fat, and on consuming a greater proportion of food energy from plant sources.

Toward the Next Revision

At issue is whether the Pyramid represents an ideal dietary pattern and, if less than ideal, how it might be improved. Diets of widely varying composition—Asian versus Mediterranean patterns, for example—are associated with excellent health. Such patterns differ in characteristic foods, types and amounts of fat, and use of alcohol, but share a common reliance on grains, vegetables, and fruits as energy sources, with minimal use of foods high in saturated fat. The Pyramid readily encompasses both of these patterns, and others, with minimal modifications.

Although it is unlikely that any one graphic design can respond to the complexities of current information about diet and health, some adjustments to the Pyramid could further strengthen and clarify its messages. Revisions to the Pyramid might well incorporate design elements that:

- Clarify the food-group categorization of beans and nuts.
- Translate the fats, oils, and sweets category into foods that represent their principal dietary sources.
- Adjust the proportions of the food groups to place greater emphasis on grains, fruits, and vegetables, and to minimize servings that are major sources of saturated fat.
- Convert portion sizes and numbers to amounts that better reflect the typical daily intake of adults.

Such changes could make the Pyramid an even more useful vehicle for translation of research and policy into practical dietary advice to improve the health of Americans.

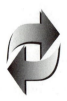

NO ↩

Walter C. Willett
with P. J. Skerrett

Eat, Drink, and Be Healthy

Introduction

We eat to live.

It's a simple, obvious truth. We need food for the basics of everyday life—to pump blood, move muscles, think thoughts.

But we can also eat to live well and live longer. By making the right choices, you will help yourself avoid some of the things we think of as the inevitable penalties of getting older. A healthy diet teamed up with regular exercise and no smoking can eliminate 50 percent of heart disease and 70 percent of some cancers. Making poor choices—eating too much of the wrong kinds of food and too little of the right kinds, or too much food altogether—increases your chances of developing cancer, heart disease, diabetes, digestive disorders, and aging-related loss of vision. An unhealthy diet during pregnancy can even cause some birth defects.

Separating what's good from what's bad can be a discouraging task. Each day you have to choose from an ever increasing number of foods and products, some good, most not so good. Maybe the time you have to prepare food, or even to eat, seems to shrink by the month. To make matters worse, you may feel overwhelmed by contradictory advice on what to eat. Your daily newspaper or TV newscast routinely serves up results from the latest nutrition studies. Magazines trumpet the hottest diets complete with heartfelt testimonials. One new diet or nutrition book hits the bookshelves every other day. Even supermarkets and fast-food restaurants offer advice, as do cereal boxes and a sea of Internet sites. This jumble of information quickly turns into nutritional white noise that many people tune out.

Turning to the USDA Pyramid Is a Mistake

For no-nonsense, rock-solid nutrition information, people often look to the Food Guide Pyramid developed by the U.S. Department of Agriculture (USDA). It is supposed to offer straight talk that rises above the jungle of misinformation and contradictory claims.

From Walter C. Willett with P. J. Skerrett, *Eat, Drink, and Be Healthy: The Harvard Medical School Guide to Healthy Eating* (Simon & Schuster, 2001), pp. 15–25. Copyright © 2001 by The President and Fellows of Harvard College. Reprinted by permission of Simon & Schuster Adult Publishing Group.

That's a shame, because the USDA Pyramid is wrong. It was built on shaky scientific ground back in 1992. Since then it has been steadily eroded by new research from all parts of the globe. Scores of large and small research projects have chipped away at the foundation (carbohydrates), the middle (meat and milk), and the apex (fats). The Dietary Guidelines for Americans, which are supposed to serve as the detailed blueprint for the USDA Pyramid, are a bit better. They are updated every five years and sometimes include ready-for-prime-time research. But the USDA Pyramid hasn't really changed in spite of important advances in what we know about nutrition and health.

At best, the USDA Pyramid offers wishy-washy, scientifically unfounded advice on an absolutely vital topic—what to eat. At worst, the misinformation contributes to overweight, poor health, and unnecessary early deaths. In either case it stands as a missed opportunity to improve the health of millions of people.

Rebuilding the Food Pyramid

. . . The Healthy Eating Pyramid (figure 1) is just as simple as the USDA Food Guide Pyramid. You don't have to weigh your food or tally up fat grams. There are no complicated food exchange tables to follow. You needn't eat odd combinations of foods or religiously avoid a particular type of food. Instead, our pyramid aims to nudge you toward eating mostly familiar foods that have been shown to improve health and reduce the risk of chronic disease. It involves simple changes you can make one at a time. Because it's an eating strategy aimed at improving your health instead of a diet aimed solely at helping you shed pounds, and because the changes suggested in this book can make your meals and snacks tastier, it is something you can stick with for years.

The Healthy Eating Pyramid isn't a single cute idea dolled up in a catchy graphic. It is the distillation of evidence from many different lines of research. This shouldn't be an important point, but it is. Few of the diets used by millions of Americans today are built on this kind of solid evidence. That was certainly clear from the "Great Nutrition Debate" sponsored by the USDA in February 2000. It brought together several authors of best-selling diet books for a lively, but mostly evidence-free, food fight. The wildly different recommendations presented in that three-hour session—eat lots of meat, don't eat any meat, eat lots of carbohydrates, don't eat any carbohydrates, cut your intake of fat to under 20 percent of calories, eat as much fat as you want, stay away from sugar, eat potatoes—neatly captured the chaos that we get in place of sound, sensible, and solid advice on healthy eating. This jumble of contradictions prompted USDA undersecretary Shirley Watkins to say afterward, "We will stand behind the Pyramid." But the USDA Pyramid isn't much better than most of these unsubstantiated diets!

The Holes in the USDA Pyramid

Some recommendations on diet and nutrition are misguided because they are based on inadequate or incomplete information. Not the USDA Pyramid. It is

Figure 1

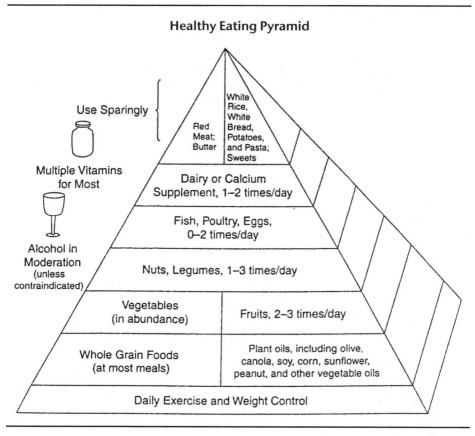

Healthy Eating Pyramid

wrong because it *ignores* the evidence that has been carefully assembled over the past forty years. Here are the USDA Pyramid's main and most health-damaging faults:

- *All fats are bad.* There's no question that two types of fat—saturated fat, the kind that's abundant in whole milk or red meat, and trans fats, which are found in many margarines and vegetable shortenings—contribute to the artery-clogging process that leads to heart disease, stroke, and other problems. But the USDA Pyramid's recommendation to use fats "sparingly" ignores the fact that two other kinds of fat—the monounsaturated and polyunsaturated fats found in olive oil and other vegetable oils, nuts, whole grains, other plant products, and fish—are *good* for your heart.

- *All "complex" carbohydrates are good.* Carbohydrates form the base of the USDA Pyramid. It suggests six to eleven servings of bread, cereal, rice, and pasta a day. But as with fats, this advice is too simplistic and overlooks essential research showing that the types of carbohydrates you eat matters a lot.

Most dietary guidelines recommend limiting simple carbohydrates (sugars) and eating plenty of complex carbohydrates (starches). White bread, potatoes, pasta, and white rice all fit this description and are the main sources of carbohydrates in the American diet. While the terms *simple* and *complex* have a specific chemical meaning, they don't mean much inside your body. In fact, your digestive system turns white bread, a baked potato, or white rice into glucose and pumps this sugar into the bloodstream almost as fast as it delivers the sugar in a cocktail of pure glucose. Swift, high spikes in blood sugar are followed by similar surges in insulin. As all this insulin forces glucose into muscle and fat cells, blood sugar levels plummet, triggering the unmistakable signals of hunger. To make matters worse, these high levels of blood sugar and insulin surges are now implicated as part of the perilous pathway to heart disease and diabetes. The harmful effects of these rapidly digested carbohydrates are especially serious for people who are overweight.

The carbohydrates that *should* form the keystones of a healthy diet come from whole grains, like brown rice or oats, from foods made with whole grains, like whole-wheat pasta or bread, or from beans. Your body takes longer to digest these carbohydrate packages, especially when they are coarsely ground or intact. That means they have a slow, low, and steady effect on blood sugar and insulin levels, which protects against heart disease and diabetes. They make you feel full longer and so keep you from getting hungry right away. They also give you important fiber plus plenty of vitamins and minerals.

The central message in the USDA Pyramid is that you should feel good about eating carbohydrates, especially if you are eating them in place of fats. But if you eat too much of the wrong kinds of carbohydrates and too little of the good kinds of fats, you can set yourself up for the same problems you may be trying to solve.

- *Protein is protein.* The protein group occupies one of the upper chambers of the USDA Pyramid. You need this type of nutrient every day and can get it from a variety of sources. The USDA Pyramid serves up as equals red meat, poultry, fish, eggs, beans, and nuts. All are excellent sources of protein. But red meat is a poor protein *package* because of all the saturated fat and cholesterol that come along. Red meat may also give you too much iron in a form you absorb whether you need it or not. Chicken and turkey give you less saturated fat. The same is true for fish, which delivers some important unsaturated fats as well. As protein sources, beans and nuts have some advantages over animal sources. They give you fiber, vitamins, minerals, and healthy unsaturated fats. Like fruits and vegetables, they also give you a host of phytochemicals, an ever expanding collection of plant products that help protect you from a variety of chronic diseases.

- *Dairy products are essential.* The USDA Pyramid includes two to three servings of dairy products a day. It's a message that the hip "Got Milk?" and even hipper "milk mustache" ads (all sponsored by the dairy industry) hammer home to every possible demographic group. As a prime source of calcium, dairy products have been enlisted to fight the so-called calcium emergency that is threatening Americans' bones. Only there isn't a calcium emergency. Americans get more calcium than the residents of almost every other country except Holland and the Scandinavian countries. And despite plenty of urgent public service announcements, there's little evidence that getting high amounts of calcium prevents broken bones in old age. Further complicating the issue are some studies suggesting that drinking or eating a lot of dairy products may increase a woman's chances of developing ovarian cancer or a man's chances of developing prostate cancer.

If you need extra calcium, there are cheaper, easier, and healthier ways to get it than dairy products. Whole-milk dairy products are loaded with the kind of saturated fat that is most powerful at raising cholesterol levels. One percent and skim milk are clearly better choices. Spinach, broccoli, tofu, and calcium-fortified orange juice and breakfast cereals are good sources of calcium and have other advantages—they are lower in unhealthy fat than most dairy products, and they give you many extra nutrients. Finally, dairy products are an expensive way to get calcium. Calcium supplements or calcium-based antacids cost pennies a day (and they are mostly calorie-free, to boot) compared with up to a dollar a day for two to three servings of dairy products.

- *Eat your potatoes.* According to the USDA, the average American eats 140 pounds of potatoes a year, making the spud the most popular vegetable in America. It is one of the few vegetables to be mentioned by name in the Dietary Guidelines—except it shouldn't be classified as a vegetable. Potatoes are mostly starch—easily digested starch at that—and so should be part of the carbohydrate group. While more than two hundred studies have shown that people who eat plenty of fruits and vegetables decrease their chances of having heart attacks or strokes, of developing a variety of cancers, or of suffering from constipation or other digestive problems, the same body of evidence shows that potatoes don't contribute to this benefit.

  Nutritionists and diet books alike often call potatoes a "perfect food." But while eating potatoes on a daily basis may be fine for lean people who exercise a lot or who do regular manual labor, for everyone else potatoes should be an occasional food consumed in modest amounts, not a daily vegetable. The venerable baked potato increases levels of blood sugar and insulin more quickly and to higher levels than an equal amount of calories from pure table sugar. French fries as they are usually sold do much the same thing, while also typically packing an unhealthy wallop of trans fats.

- *No guidance on weight, exercise, alcohol, and vitamins.* Like the Sphinx, the USDA Pyramid is silent on four things you need to know about—the importance of not gaining weight, the necessity of daily exercise, the potential health benefits of a daily alcoholic drink, and what you can gain by taking a daily multivitamin.

How the USDA Pyramid Got Its Shape

In Rudyard Kipling's classic children's story, the satiable Elephant's Child got its long trunk in a terrific tug-of-war, with Crocodile clamped on to its nose and Bi-Coloured-Python-Rock-Snake wrapped around its legs. That's pretty much how the USDA Pyramid got its structure—yanked this way and that by competing powerful interests, few of which had your health as a central goal.

The thing to keep in mind about the USDA Pyramid is that it comes from the Department of Agriculture, the agency responsible for promoting American agriculture, *not* from agencies established to monitor and protect our health, like the Department of Health and Human Services, or the National Institutes of Health, or the Institute of Medicine. And there's the root of the problem—what's good for some agricultural interests isn't necessarily good for the people who eat their products. (This schizophrenic split isn't unique to the USDA. The Nuclear Regulatory Commission, for example, is charged with the often contradictory tasks of promoting nuclear power and regulating its use.)

Serving two masters is tricky business, especially when one of them includes persuasive and well-connected representatives of the formidable meat, dairy, and sugar industries. The end result of their tug-of-war is a set of positive, feel-good, all-inclusive recommendations that completely distort what could be the single most important tool for improving your health and the health of the nation.

This Healthy Eating Pyramid Is Based on Science

You deserve more accurate, less biased, and more helpful information than that found in the USDA Pyramid. I have tried to collect exactly that in the Healthy Eating Pyramid. Without question, I have the advantage of starting with a lot more information than the USDA Pyramid builders had ten years ago. Equally important, I didn't have to negotiate with any special-interest groups when it came time to design this Pyramid.

The Healthy Eating Pyramid isn't set in stone. I don't have all the answers, nor can I predict what nutrition researchers will turn up in the decade ahead. But I can give you a solid sense of state-of-the-art healthy eating today and point out where things are heading. This isn't the only alternative to the USDA Food Guide Pyramid. The Asian, Latin, Mediterranean, and vegetarian pyramids promoted by Oldways Preservation and Exchange Trust are also good, evidence-based guides for healthy eating. But the Healthy Eating Pyramid takes advantage of even more extensive research and offers a broader guide that is not based on a specific culture.

About the only thing that the Healthy Eating Pyramid and the USDA Food Guide Pyramid share is their emphasis on vegetables and fruits. Other than that, they are different on almost every level.

. . . [T]he following list of the seven healthiest changes you can make in your diet offers an overview that describes how the Healthy Eating Pyramid differs from the USDA Pyramid. Topping the list is controlling your weight.

- *Watch your weight.* When it comes to long-term health, keeping your weight from creeping up on you is more important than the exact ratio of fats to carbohydrates or the types and amounts of antioxidants in your food. The lower and more stable your weight, the lower your chances of having or dying from a heart attack, stroke, or other type of cardiovascular disease; of developing high blood pressure, high cholesterol, or diabetes; of being diagnosed with post-menopausal breast cancer, cancer of the endometrium, colon, or kidney; or of being afflicted with some other chronic condition. Yes, it is possible to be too thin, as in the case of anorexia nervosa, but otherwise very few American adults fall into this category.
- *Eat fewer bad fats and more good fats.* One of the most striking differences is the placement of *healthy* fats in the foundation of the Healthy Eating Pyramid instead of relegating all fats to the "Use Sparingly" spot at the top. The message here is almost as simple as the USDA's and far better for you: Fats from nuts, seeds, grains, fish, and liquid oils (including olive, canola, soybean, corn, sunflower, peanut, and other vegetable oils) are good for you, especially when you eat them in place of saturated and trans fat.

  The all-fat-is-bad message has started a huge national experiment, with us as the guinea pigs. As people cut back on fat, they usually eat more carbohydrates. In America today, that means more highly refined or easily digested foods like sugar, white bread, white rice, and potatoes. This switch usually fails to yield the hoped-for weight loss or lower cholesterol levels. Instead it often leads to weight gain and potentially dangerous changes in blood fats—lower high-density lipoprotein (HDL), the so-called good or protective cholesterol, and higher triglycerides (a major type of blood fat).

  Substituting unsaturated fats for saturated fats, though, improves cholesterol levels across the board. It may also protect the heart against rhythm disturbances that can end in sudden death.

  The bottom line is this: It is perfectly fine to get more than 30 percent of your daily calories from fats *as long as most of those fats are unsaturated.* The Healthy Eating Pyramid highlights the importance of keeping saturated and trans fats to a minimum by putting red meat, whole-milk dairy products, butter, and hydrogenated vegetable oils in the "Use Sparingly" section at the top.
- *Eat fewer refined-grain carbohydrates and more whole-grain carbohydrates.* The Healthy Eating Pyramid has two carbohydrate building blocks— whole grains that are slowly digested as part of the foundation and highly refined, rapidly digested carbohydrates at the very top.

  For almost twenty years our research team has been one of several groups studying the health effects of foods made from refined and intact grains. The result of this work is compelling. Eating lots of carbohydrates that are quickly digested and absorbed increases levels of blood sugar and insulin, raises levels of triglycerides, and lowers levels of HDL cholesterol. Over the long run, these changes lead to cardiovascular disease and diabetes. In contrast, eating whole-grain foods is clearly better for long-term good health and offers protection against diabetes, heart disease, cancer, and gastrointestinal problems such as diverticulosis and constipation. Other research around the world points to the same conclusions.

- *Choose healthier sources of proteins.* In the Healthy Eating Pyramid, red meat occupies the pointy tip to highlight the fact that *something* about red meat—its particular combination of saturated fats or the potentially cancer-causing compounds that form when red meat is grilled or fried—is connected to a variety of chronic diseases. In this pyramid, the best sources of protein are beans and nuts, along with fish, poultry, and eggs. It separates vegetable and animal protein sources and makes the latter optional for people who want to follow a vegetarian diet.

- *Eat plenty of vegetables and fruits, but hold the potatoes.* Vegetables and fruits are essential ingredients in almost every cuisine. If you let them play starring roles in your diet, they will reward you with many benefits besides great taste, terrific textures, and welcome variety. A diet rich in fruits and vegetables will lower your blood pressure, decrease your chances of having a heart attack or stroke, help protect you against a variety of cancers, guard against constipation and other gastrointestinal problems, and limit your chances of developing aging-related problems like cataracts and macular degeneration, the most common causes of vision loss among people over age sixty-five. I've plucked potatoes out of the vegetable category and put them in the "Use Sparingly" category because of their dramatic effect on levels of blood sugar and insulin.

- *Use alcohol in moderation.* When the first reports appeared linking moderate alcohol consumption with lower rates of heart disease, many scientists thought that some other habit shared by drinkers, not the drinking, accounted for the benefit. Today the evidence strongly points to alcohol itself. Based on the best estimates available, one drink a day for women and one or two a day for men cuts the chances of having a heart attack or dying from heart disease by about a third and also decreases the risk of having a clot-caused (ischemic) stroke.

  Like many drugs, alcohol's effects depend on the dose. A little bit can be beneficial. A lot can eventually destroy the liver, lead to various cancers, boost blood pressure, trigger so-called bleeding (hemorrhagic) strokes, progressively weaken the heart muscle, scramble the brain, harm unborn children, and damage lives.

  The clear and ever present dangers of alcohol and alcohol addiction make the recommendation of moderate drinking a political hot potato. While I acknowledge the problems with alcohol, I think it is important to point out its possible benefits for middle-aged and older people.

  If you don't drink alcohol, you shouldn't feel compelled to start. You can get similar benefits by beginning to exercise (if you don't already) or boosting the intensity and duration of your physical activity, in addition to following the eating strategy we describe. But if you are an adult with no history of depression or alcoholism who is at high risk for heart disease, a daily alcoholic drink may help reduce that risk. This is especially true for people with type 2 diabetes or those with low HDL that just won't budge upward with diet and exercise. If you already drink alcohol, keep it moderate.

- *Take a multivitamin for insurance.* Several of the ingredients in a standard multivitamin—especially vitamins B_6 and B_{12}, folic acid, and vitamin D—are essential players in preventing heart disease, cancer, osteoporosis, and other chronic diseases. At about a nickel a day, a multivitamin is a cheap and effective genuine "life insurance" policy. It won't make up for the sins of an unhealthy diet, but it can fill in the nutritional holes that can plague even the most conscientious eaters. A daily multivitamin is especially important for people who have trouble absorbing vitamins from their food and for those who can't, or don't, get out in the sun every day. A daily multivitamin is also important for people who drink alcohol because it provides extra folic acid. Alcohol interferes with the metabolism of this key vitamin.

POSTSCRIPT

Does the USDA Pyramid Describe an Optimal Dietary Pattern?

By order of Congress, the U.S. government issues an official statement of nutrition policy, the *Dietary Guidelines for Americans,* every five years; it has done so since 1980. The guidelines state federal *policy*. The Pyramid is an *implementation guide* for food choices that fulfill that policy. In 2000 the dietary guidelines began with "Let the Pyramid guide your food choices," a sharp departure from "Eat a variety of foods," the statement given in the previous four editions. Including the USDA Pyramid as an integral part of the fifth edition of the guidelines reflects the familiarity of the Pyramid design to consumers, its attractiveness as a method for nutrition education, and its purpose: to encourage people to consume diets that follow the illustrated pattern.

In these selections, Nestle emphasizes the strengths of the USDA Pyramid, but Willett emphasizes its weaknesses. Both agree that the Pyramid is in need of revision, but they differ on the extent and content of those revisions. In Nestle's selection, she explains the history of the development of the Pyramid. She cites as a significant forward step that "the Pyramid was derived from an 11-year process of conceptualization, research, and testing" and suggests a few changes that would further clarify its messages. In contrast, Willett questions the fundamental basis of the research underlying the USDA Pyramid and, instead, suggests a different model—a Healthy Eating Pyramid—based on findings from research studies. He argues, "the only thing that the Healthy Eating Pyramid and the USDA Pyramid share is their emphasis on vegetables and fruits."

Willett raises issues related to the effectiveness of diets that adhere to the USDA Pyramid. His research group has produced studies demonstrating that people who consume Pyramid-like diets are not necessarily healthier; two such studies appeared in the *American Journal of Clinical Nutrition* in November 2000. On the basis of this research, Willett lists seven changes that Americans can make to improve their diets—and, therefore, their health. He argues that these changes are captured in the Healthy Eating Pyramid but not in the USDA Pyramid.

In sorting out the questions raised by these papers, it is important to note that much of the criticism of the USDA Pyramid is based on its graphic design, not on the text of the explanatory brochure that accompanies it. Neither the USDA Pyramid nor any other simple design can easily represent a complex food guidance system that deals with specific foods within groups; intakes of fat, added sugars, and other nutrients; energy levels; and serving sizes. Although not apparent in the design of the USDA Pyramid, the accompanying brochure recommends including dark green leafy vegetables and legumes in the diet several times a week and emphasizes consumption of good carbohydrates—whole grain breads and cereals—advice with which Willett agrees (see *Scientific American,* January 2003).

A commentary on Pyramids in the December 2001 issue of the *Berkeley Wellness Letter* suggests that dietary advice has become so sophisticated and complicated in recent years that a simple Pyramid diagram can only convey general principles and that "the nitty-gritty has to come from somewhere else." That writer prefers the way the USDA Pyramid handles fat, disagrees with Willett's concerns about potatoes and pasta, and concludes that "both pyramids are flawed. But one point is beyond dispute: a wide variety of fruits, vegetables and whole grains [is] the foundation of a healthy diet."

One additional point is beyond dispute: Americans do not follow the advice given by either Pyramid. National data show that only 1 to 3 percent of Americans consume the recommended number of Pyramid servings each day (*Journal of Nutrition*, February 2001). People especially neglect fruits, dark green and deep yellow vegetables, and whole grains, and they eat far more fat and added sugars than recommended.

Modifications to the USDA Pyramid might help clarify dietary messages. Since its publication in 1992, the Institute of Medicine has issued *Dietary Reference Intakes* for dozens of nutrients (National Academies Press, 1997–2003). The American Institute for Cancer Research (1997), the American Heart Association (*Circulation,* October 2000), and the American Diabetes Association (*Diabetes Care,* January 2002) have updated their own dietary guidelines, and national surveys have provided more recent information on what Americans are eating (http://www.cdc.gov/nchs/nhanes.htm). As a result, USDA nutritionists are reevaluating the Pyramid based on these new sources of nutrition information. Perhaps their revisions will bring the two food pyramids discussed here closer together.

ISSUE 2

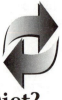

Can All Foods Fit Into a Healthful Diet?

YES: Jeanne Freeland-Graves and Susan Nitzke, from "Position of the American Dietetic Association: Total Diet Approach to Communicating Food and Nutrition Information," *Journal of the American Dietetic Association* (January 2002)

NO: Suzanne Havala, from *Good Foods, Bad Foods: What's Left to Eat?* (Chronimed Publishing, 1998)

ISSUE SUMMARY

YES: Nutrition professors Jeanne Freeland-Graves and Susan Nitzke speak for the American Dietetic Association (ADA) when they say that there is no such thing as a good or bad food: all foods can fit into healthful diets. Their approach to nutrition advice emphasizes the total diet, appropriate portion sizes, moderation and balance in food intake, obtaining nutrients from foods rather than supplements, and regular physical activity.

NO: Nutrition professor Suzanne Havala counters that some foods are better for health than others and that saying otherwise is just a way to rationalize the dietary status quo and protect the commercial interests of the food industry.

The U.S. food industry generates more than one trillion dollars in annual sales, about half for food prepared for consumption outside the home and sold in restaurants, fast food places, food carts, schools, and all other locations where meals are served. Food companies make more than 300,000 packaged food and beverage products available for purchase; supermarkets generally sell about 50,000 of them. How are people to make healthful choices from among this vast array of prepared, packaged, and fresh foods? With overweight and obesity now increasingly prominent as public health nutrition problems, how can people choose diets that will help them avoid gaining weight?

The Food Guide Pyramid, or the policy document that governs it, the *Dietary Guidelines for Americans,* reveals little prescriptive information that might guide choices of specific foods. The Pyramid illustrates the relative numbers of servings to be selected from the various food groups but does not specify or distinguish the nutritional quality of foods within those groups. Dietary guidelines also leave much room for interpretation, particularly because most of them refer to specific nutrient components—fat and sugar, for example—as sources of calories rather than to the foods that contain them. Furthermore, in a deliberate effort to avoid suggestions to restrict one or another food, the guidelines state advice in positive ("eat more") terms. They use words like *choose* and do not use words like *avoid* or *limit.*

The American Dietetic Association (ADA) supports this approach. The ADA represents more than 60,000 nutrition professionals who hold credentials as registered dietitians in the United States. As a matter of policy, the ADA has long maintained that singling out specific foods or food categories as "good" or "bad" is unlikely to help consumers choose more healthful diets. In alliance with government and food industry organizations, the ADA designed a campaign especially to counter the "good foods/bad foods myth." Instead, the ADA campaign promotes positive messages about diet and health that emphasize balance, variety, and moderation. The ADA views the labeling of foods as good or bad as overly simplistic and misleading—and more likely to promote than to prevent unhealthful dietary practices. The ADA campaign promotes the idea that all foods can fit into healthful diets, thereby empowering people to make choices within the context of their own dietary preferences. Although the ADA recognizes that some people might view the "total diet" approach as giving the food industry unlimited license to market fast foods and soft drinks, for example, the authors of its position paper believe that this problem can be overcome by educating consumers about appropriate portion sizes.

Suzanne Havala, although a member of the ADA, sharply disagrees with its dietary guidance policy on good and bad foods. Consumers, she says, want help with dietary choices: "straightforward advice with specific directions." If the ADA promotes a policy of "all foods can fit," it may be because it does so in alliance with trade associations for the meat, dairy, sugar, and processed food industries that stand to benefit from nonrestrictive dietary advice. As economists C. Edwin Young and Linda Scott Kantor explained in 1999 in *America's Eating Habits* (U.S. Department of Agriculture, Economic Research Service), the segments of the agriculture and food industries that produce "bad" foods would experience profound "adjustments" if people actually began to follow dietary advice to eat less of such products.

This debate touches on the theme of the interaction between science and politics in matters of nutrition advice and the difficulties of determining whom to trust in such matters. What does it mean to say that all foods can fit into healthful diets? What are the strengths and limitations of this approach? Freeland-Graves and Nitzke are members of an organization that accepts contributions from food companies. Do partnerships between nutrition professional groups and food companies compromise the integrity of policy statements? Havala is the author of several books on vegetarian nutrition. In what ways might vegetarian interests influence her views on this issue?

In the selections that follow, Freeland-Graves and Nitzke argue that terming foods as good or bad is inappropriate and counterproductive, but Havala views their approach as just a way to "resist, bargain, and rationalize" the need for dietary changes to improve health.

Jeanne Freeland-Graves and
Susan Nitzke

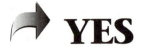 YES

Position of the American Dietetic Association: Total Diet Approach to Communicating Food and Nutrition Information

Abstract

It is the position of the American Dietetic Association that all foods can fit into a healthful eating style. The ADA strives to communicate healthful eating messages to the public that emphasize the total diet, or overall pattern of food eaten, rather than any one food or meal. If consumed in moderation with appropriate portion size and combined with regular physical activity, all foods can fit into a healthful diet. Public policies that support the total diet approach include Reference Dietary Intakes, Food Guide Pyramid, Dietary Guidelines for Americans, Nutrition Labeling and Healthy People 2010. The value of a food should be determined within the context of the total diet because classifying foods as "good" or "bad" may foster unhealthy eating behaviors. . . . Nutrition confusion can be reduced by emphasizing moderation, appropriate portion size, balance and adequacy of the total diet over time, the importance of obtaining nutrients from foods, and physical activity. . . .

Nutrition messages from dietetics professionals can be more effective if they focus on a positive image of healthy food choices over time, rather than individual foods to be avoided. This concept is not new, The American Dietetic Association strives to communicate that there are no good or bad foods, only good or bad diets or eating styles. No single food or type of food ensures good health, just as no single food or type of food is necessarily detrimental to health.

Research conducted for the Dietary Guidelines Alliance's "It's All about You" campaign suggests that the "good foods/bad foods" myth should not be perpetuated. The Alliance is a consortium of government and food industry organizations, including ADA, whose mission is to provide nutrition messages to help achieve healthy, active lifestyles. In order to boost effectiveness, it is recommended that food tips be kept positive, short, and simple and include examples of foods and activities that reflect the lifestyle, preferences, and culture of

From Jeanne Freeland-Graves and Susan Nitzke, "Position of the American Dietetic Association: Total Diet Approach to Communicating Food and Nutrition Information," *Journal of the American Dietetic Association,* vol. 102, no. 1 (January 2002). Copyright © 2002 by The American Dietetic Association. Reprinted by permission of Elsevier. References omitted.

the audience. The recent Food for Thought III survey reported that the news media are airing more positive messages about food and fewer negative messages. This positive approach empowers consumers to achieve the principles of a healthy diet as part of their overall lifestyle.

Positive messages help avoid the consumer confusion that results when messages from experts appear to be in disagreement, as well as the feelings of guilt that are associated with eating "less healthful foods." . . .

Federal Nutrition Guidance That Supports the Total Diet Approach

The Dietary Guidelines for Americans and the Food Guide Pyramid take a total diet approach to food guidance which form the basis of federal food, nutrition education, and information programs. From their inception in 1980, the Dietary Guidelines for Americans have recommended moderation for certain dietary components, such as fat and sugar, while continuing to emphasize nutrient adequacy. The Guidelines are reviewed every 5 years by a scientific advisory committee to ensure that they reflect the most current research that is available on diet and health. The science-based framework supporting the Food Guide Pyramid, originally developed in the early 1980s, incorporates dietary standards, including the Dietary Guidelines and data on food composition and food consumption practices of Americans. This research framework is updated continually by the USDA to ensure that Federal dietary guidance is based on the most accurate and current scientific data.

The developers of the Dietary Guidelines for Americans and the Food Guide Pyramid found that consumers and educators tend to prefer dietary guidance that allows consumers to eat in a way that suits their individual tastes and lifestyles. An illustration would be to balance a high-fat dessert such as rich ice cream with lower fat selections in other food groups to achieve an overall healthful diet. Exorbitant amounts of high-fat desserts would not be possible in a healthful diet, but limited quantities could be incorporated if low-fat selections of other foods were consumed in moderation. Another example is including French fries, a common fast-food item, within the context of the total diet.

Caution must be taken, however, to avoid a common misimpression; ie, that the "no bad foods" message gives people license to consume snack foods and desserts in unwarranted quantities. This does not invalidate the message that there are no inherently "bad" foods, but rather challenges educators to emphasize that the "all foods can fit" message includes an important concept of overall dietary balance. . . .

Successful Communication Campaigns and Programs

Teaching consumers to make wise food choices in the context of the total diet is not a simple process. A continuum of nutrition information, communication, promotion and intervention strategies must be integrated in order to design the most appropriate educational intervention. In addition, successful campaigns often include the coordinated efforts of a number of agencies and organizations with similar health-promotion goals. . . .

Social Marketing

"Social marketing" is a behaviorally focused process that adapts commercial marketing technologies to the analysis, planning, execution and evaluation of programs designed to influence the behavior of target audiences to improve their well-being. Social marketers work to create and maintain exchanges of target audience resources, such as money or time, for perceived benefits such as feeling better or having more independence. Just as educators may utilize a range of theoretical concepts to design effective interventions, marketing campaigns may also be more effective when important determinants of behavior are identified and utilized in a media campaign. Examples of such campaigns are "5-A-Day for Better Health" and "It's All About You."

The 5-A-Day for Better Health campaign was one of the first major health campaigns to follow the principles of social marketing theory. Using data from a variety of research interviews and surveys, designers of this campaign studied the preferences and habits of various audience segments and developed messages that would be perceived as relevant, comprehensible, and actionable by people in those subgroups. By adapting messages and distribution techniques to the needs of consumers in a variety of settings such as supermarkets, restaurants, and the Internet, this campaign has made progress toward the goal of increasing Americans' consumption of fruits and vegetables.

In the Dietary Guidelines Alliance's "It's All About You" campaign, educators were urged to customize information to the needs, likes and dislikes of the particular audience for maximum impact. The more focused and individualized the messages are, the more likely it is that consumers will act on them.

Social marketing is an important and powerful tool for communicating relatively simple messages such as "eat five servings of fruits and vegetables a day." However, unless the message is consistent with a total diet emphasis, the application of a strict marketing approach that focuses exclusively on specific behavioral outcomes may inadvertently lead to use of oversimplified messages such as good/bad food advice that may conflict with more comprehensive educational goals.

Psychosocial Consequences of "Good" and "Bad"

Categorizing foods as "good" or "bad" promotes dichotomous thinking. Dichotomous thinkers make judgments in terms of black/white, all/none or good/bad and do not incorporate abstract or complex options into their decision strategies.

The Magic Bullet Approach

Thinking in terms of dichotomous (black-and-white) categories is common in childhood. Almost all elementary-age school children believe that there are "good" and/or "bad" foods. Although the ability to think in more abstract and complex modes is better developed in adolescents and adults, consumers of all ages tend to rely on dichotomous thinking in certain situations.

An example of dichotomous thinking is the "quick fix" or "magic bullet" approach to weight control. As long as one stays on the diet (target behavior) the person feels a sense of perceived control (self-efficacy). However, when an individual encounters a high risk situation such as a tempting food (eg, ice cream), loss of control may occur, depending on the emotional state, interpersonal conflict and social pressure.

In this approach to food choice, ice cream would be regarded as a forbidden food and a dieter who yields to a desire for a few spoonfuls of ice cream would tend to say, "I ate the ice cream. I have blown my diet. I am going to finish the carton." This type of thinking has been associated with addictive or compulsive behaviors. Once a mistake is made (such as breaking abstinence for alcoholics or eating a large bowl of ice cream for bingers), the tendency is to abandon oneself to one's weaknesses and indulge in the forbidden behavior. This pessimistic approach becomes self-fulfilling, as the subject believes that there is not much that can be done once a loss of control occurs. . . .

When dichotomous thinking is taken to the extreme, it can become an underlying force for disordered eating behaviors such as chronic restriction (anorexia), bingeing, or purging. When these eating behaviors are severe, the concept of moderation tends to be ignored. Part of the therapy for these conditions is to expand the range of acceptable food items, with the ultimate goal of learning that foods cannot be classified as good or bad. . . .

All-Good or All-Bad Foods?

Milk, egg whites, tomatoes and soybeans are foods associated with healthful diets that can be used to illustrate the problems in perceiving a food/food component as all good or all bad. Milk is considered to be an excellent food, as it contributes calcium, high quality protein, and B vitamins to the diet. However, when young children rely too heavily on milk as a source of calories to the exclusion of other nutritious foods, iron deficiency anemia may result. For example, infants consuming nonfortified formula or whole cow's milk have a 30–40% risk of iron deficiency by 9–12 months of age compared to 20% in infants who are exclusively breastfed. Thus, even low-fat milk cannot be classified as either "good" or "bad," but rather its value is determined within the context of the total diet.

Egg white is a high quality protein, yet low in zinc and, when used in research studies as a primary source of protein in the diet, it can induce a zinc-deficiency. Tomatoes are a source of lycopene and other phytochemicals with antioxidant properties, but also an alkaloid that can be toxic to humans in high doses. Similarly, soybeans have n-3 fatty acids, flavonoids, and phytoestrogens with health-promoting properties, but they also contain trypsin and protease inhibitors that may interfere with digestion, as well as phytates that may interfere with absorption of zinc and iron. While these components are not a problem with cooked soybeans consumed in moderation, very large intakes of raw soybeans may be harmful.

Even when a well-accepted system such as nutrient density is the basis for good/bad categorization systems, the results can be arbitrary and misleading. Nutrient density gives a relatively simple indication of the amount of a nutrient or nutrients (vitamins, minerals, protein and/or fiber) provided by an individual food in relation to its concentration of energy (kilocalories). When this concept is stretched to a simpler system of classification wherein foods are determined to be good or bad, these distinctions tend to become ambiguous. For example, plain potatoes are good sources of vitamin C and potassium, and would usually be considered a "good" food because of their high nutrient density. However, French fries and potato chips are higher in fat and sodium, so these are more likely to be classified as "bad." When an individual adds salt, butter, margarine, sour cream, and/or bacon bits to a baked potato, the nutrient profile more closely resembles that of French fries. It would be nearly impossible to specify a point at which the potato would have been changed from good to bad. With over 40,000 food items in the average supermarket and an infinite array of recipe combinations, the futility of attempting to sort all food items into two categories becomes evident. Thus, the total diet approach, with its emphasis on long-term eating habits and a contextual approach to food judgments, provides more useful information to guide long-term eating patterns.

Controversies With the Total Diet Approach

One concern with the total diet approach is that it may be viewed by dietetics professionals as permitting the food industry an unlimited license to add fast foods and soft drinks to school meal, hospital, and other food service programs. In addition, there may be concern that the lack of limits for individuals may encourage overconsumption of foods that may have marginal nutritional value. In a study utilizing the Diet Quality Index (DQI) as a measure of healthful diet quality, heavy consumption of savory, high-fat snacks was associated with higher DQI scores (poor diet quality). Similarly, consumption of fats, sweets, and alcohol was inversely related to nutritional adequacy of diets in the Second National Health and Nutrition Examination Survey.

Consequently, dietetics professionals must emphasize the need to select appropriate portion sizes. Nutrition education is critical because few consumers intuitively know that 3 oz of beef is considered an appropriate portion size. Choosing sensible portion size is a basic tenet of the new 2000 Dietary Guidelines for Americans. If one thought that a restaurant portion of broiled beef rib steak (8 oz) was the most appropriate portion size the caloric content would be far higher (500 kcal) rather than the 188 kcal from the Food Guide Pyramid's recommended 3 oz portion. Therefore, it is imperative that the message of appropriate portion sizes be incorporated into the total diet approach.

Another controversy with the total diet approach is the emphasis on variety. Choosing a variety of foods was a cornerstone principle in the past editions of the Dietary Guidelines for Americans. It has been believed that a variety of foods is needed for optimal nutrition because there are more than 50 nutrients needed for growth, repair and maintenance of good health and there is no one food or even one food group that contains all these nutrients.

A problem with variety, however, may be that a diversity of foods tends to increase our desire to eat and may even lead to overeating. When McCrory and colleagues analyzed 1999 food consumption data, increases in energy intakes and body fatness were associated with ingestion of a high variety of sweets, snacks, condiments, entrees and carbohydrate foods, coupled with a small variety of vegetables. Another review of food consumption data by Krebs-Smith and colleagues observed that a variety of foods was associated with nutrient adequacy up to a certain point, beyond which there was no improvement. Coulston has suggested that escalating energy intakes from dietary variety may be one of the factors contributing to the spread of obesity in this country. In contrast, Drewnowski and colleagues found that a low level of dietary diversity was associated with low energy intakes and lower dietary quality scores. Thus, confusion exists as to whether dietitians should promote a variety of foods.

To address these concerns, the 2000 (5th) edition of the Dietary Guidelines for Americans states that there are many healthful eating patterns that allow maximum flexibility in food choices. In addition, the wording of the major headings has been modified from previous editions to replace the broader "Eat a variety of foods" recommendation with more specific advice to "Let the Pyramid guide your food choices." The current Dietary Guidelines for Americans also places greater emphasis on appropriate serving sizes and specifies the need for variety in one's choices of fruits, vegetables and grains. These changes are meant to obviate the mistaken impression that large quantities of high-fat and high-calorie foods become more acceptable when one eats many different kinds of these foods. . . .

Reducing Nutrition Confusion

Recognizing that many consumers are overwhelmed by the high volume and apparent inconsistencies of nutrition advice, the following principles are recommended as points to consider in designing nutrition education for the public:

- Promote moderation, appropriate portion size, balance and dietary adequacy as fundamental and interrelated principles that can be used as indicators of whether and how the typical food pattern of a person or group may be improved. Although the definition of "moderation" varies according to individual circumstances, it generally refers to eating a wide selection of foods within and among the major food groups, with a recognition that no one major food group is more or less important than any other food group. Moderation should also include appropriate portion size in order to minimize passive overeating. "Balance" and its corollary term, proportionality, refer to eating relatively more servings from the larger food groups at the bottom of the Food Guide Pyramid and fewer servings of foods from the smaller food groups at the top of the pyramid. Dietary adequacy can be achieved by including a variety of nutrient-dense foods, such as grains, fruits and vegetables, within the context of the total diet.

- Emphasize total diet over time or food patterns, rather than individual nutrients or individual foods, as key considerations in evaluating and planning one's food choices. Be aware of the social, cultural, economic and emotional meanings that may be attached to some foods and allow for flexibility whenever possible. Understanding these social and cultural aspects of food consumption is essential for planning educational programs to help correct nutritional problems of individuals and population groups.

- Stress the importance of obtaining nutrients from foods, rather than relying on supplements. Although supplements are recommended when food intake is inadequate to meet specific needs (eg, calcium, vitamin B12 and folic acid for some population groups), it is important to stress that a balanced diet remains the preferred overall source of nutrients. Numerous bioactive compounds in foods such as phytochemicals and ultra trace elements have been identified that have potential health benefits. Yet the precise role, dietary requirements, influence on other nutrients, and toxicity levels of these dietary components are still unclear. Furthermore, foods may contain additional nutritional substances that have not yet been discovered. Thus, appropriate food choices, rather than supplements, should be the foundation for achieving nutritional adequacy.

- Acknowledge the contribution of regular physical activity as an essential part of a healthy lifestyle. According to the US Centers for Disease Control and Prevention, more than 60% of American adults are not regularly active and 25% of the adult population are not active at all. Health experts now understand that physical activity complements a diet that is nutritionally adequate and consumed in moderation in reducing the risk of premature mortality, coronary heart disease, hypertension, colon cancer, and diabetes mellitus. Healthy People 2010 goals for the nation's health and the Dietary Guidelines for Americans recommend that Americans engage regularly, preferably daily, in moderate physical activity for at least 30 minutes per day.

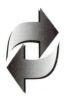

NO ⬅

Suzanne Havala

Good Foods, Bad Foods: What's Left to Eat

Talking Politics

The Politics of Your Plate

. . . It never really bothered anybody, say, back in the 1940s and 1950s, when the National Dairy Council produced its "Guide to Good Eating," which was used by elementary schools everywhere for decades to teach the fundamentals of nutrition. Based on the Basic Four Food Groups dietary model, it depicted dairy products—milk, cheese, ice cream—as one of the four cornerstones of a "balanced" diet. Never mind that the concept was the ultimate marketing tool for the dairy industry. The focus then was on preventing dietary deficiencies, and the nutritional merits of dairy products were emphasized exclusively. Recognition of and concerns about excesses in the American diet—too much fat, cholesterol, and protein—were many years away. Besides, milk was as American as apple pie. Who could find fault with that?

Fast forward to 1980, the year that the U.S. Departments of Agriculture (USDA) and Health and Human Services (HHS) jointly published the first Dietary Guidelines for Americans. Targeting every person over the age of two years, the Dietary Guidelines give advice about food choices that promote health and lessen the risk for disease. Revisions of the report were published in 1985, 1990, and 1995.

The Dietary Guidelines are the cornerstone of federal nutrition policy. As of 1990, legislation requires that the report be published every five years by the secretaries of USDA and HHS. The information is directed to the general public, must be based on the preponderance of scientific and medical knowledge current at the time of publication, and is to be promoted by USDA, HHS, and other federal agencies.

So the USDA is in the business of giving dietary advice to the American public. That's a sideline, however. The USDA's primary reason for being is to support American agriculture. The biggest players—and the most powerful, given their financial clout—are the meat and dairy industries. A conflict of interest? You bet. Does it influence what the Dietary Guidelines say? Absolutely. . . .

It has long been in industry's interest to support dietary guidelines that are relatively vague and "open to interpretation." The meat, dairy, and egg industries, in particular, would stand to lose if dietary guidelines were more specific and people began eating fewer of their products. It's that very ambiguity, however, that vexes the public and annoys consumer advocates. Without clear-cut guidelines that name names and give specific recommendations that get to the nitty-gritty of what people should eat, everyone is left standing at square one saying, "I've read the guidelines, and that's all well and good, but *what do* I *eat for dinner tonight?*". . .

The 1995 Dietary Guidelines Advisory Committee acknowledged that consumers have not been successful overall in translating the Dietary Guidelines into lifestyle changes and recommended that future revisions of the Dietary Guidelines take this problem into consideration. To investigate the issue further, the USDA and HHS sponsored consumer-based research in the spring of 1995. The findings: Consumers want straightforward advice with specific directions. Consumers do not have the time, energy or inclination to learn nutrition science before they can begin to eat a healthful diet. No surprise here.

In the meantime, an alliance of food industry and health organizations, in liaison with the federal government, was formed in 1996 to develop materials that will help consumers translate the Dietary Guidelines and put them into practice. Called the Dietary Guidelines Alliance, the group includes, along with the USDA and HHS, the American Dietetic Association, the Food Marketing Institute, the International Food Information Council, the National Dairy Council, the National Food Processors Association, the National Cattlemen's Beef Association, the Produce Marketing Association, the Sugar Association, the Wheat Foods Council, and the National Pork Producers Council.

Once again, that's the politics of your plate. . . .

No Good Foods, No Bad Foods

When nutritionists say there are "no good or bad foods, only good or bad diets," they often add the caveat that one cannot assign moral qualities to foods. Okay, so the salami isn't guilty of clogging your arteries. It was you who put it on your menu. As opponents of gun control will tell you, the hand that pulls the trigger is the guilty party, not the gun itself.

I look at the issue a little differently. Personally, when I say that a food is "good" or "bad," I am referring to the food's relative value in terms of health. A "good" food is one that promotes health. A "bad" food is one that is comparatively worse for you. A bad food is a food that, eaten in sufficient quantities, either contributes to nutritional excesses or displaces more valuable foods from the diet.

As Marian Burros, food writer for *The New York Times,* once opined, "Regarding good foods/bad foods: There are some foods that are better than others. If you don't want to use the term 'bad foods,' then there are foods and there are good foods. The good foods you can eat anytime and the foods you can eat occasionally."

Over the many years that I have been counseling people on diet and nutrition, one need has always risen above all others. That is, people want specific advice about what they should and should not eat, preferably with the emphasis on the good choices. They want to know what they can have for dinner tonight. They want concrete examples of good foods to order at restaurants, and they want lists of good snack ideas.

One of the ADA's "key messages" for National Nutrition Month 1996 was, "Any food in today's diverse marketplace fits in a healthful eating style." The theme for 1997 was "All foods can fit."

Sure. A chocolate chip cookie can be worked in each day if the rest of the diet is up to snuff. Dietary recommendations don't have to be strictly black or white, eat this and don't eat that. There is some gray area, some room for play and for individualizing the diet.

But most Americans are light years away from meeting current dietary recommendations. There are certainly some very specific tips that could be given that would be relevant to the majority. That means identifying some foods as being better choices than others. If the vague statements that are now the norm are not backed up strongly with specific recommendations that name names and define terms, then people will not be able to make the kinds of dietary changes that they need to make in order to see significant health benefits.

An article by Marian Burros in the November 15, 1995 issue of *The New York Times* explored the sticky issue of health professional associations accepting industry monies and in-kind services. She quoted Joan Gussow, Ph.D., a former head of the nutrition education program at Columbia University's Teachers College, who stated that the American Dietetic Association's dependence on industry money meant that "they never criticize the food industry." The ADA won't finger any particular food as being bad, unhealthful, or a poor choice. Even candy bars and soft drinks have a place, according to the ADA. "Actually, we could put our name on any McDonald's meal," said Dr. Doris Derelian, who was the current president of the American Dietetic Association.

In the same article, Dr. Gussow also stated, "If health professionals are led to agree that there are no 'good' or 'bad,' 'healthy' or 'unhealthy' foods, then we can't object to any food product that's put on the market, however wasteful or useless it may be."

She added, "The food critics of the '60s and '70s have been silenced, which is, of course, the point. The food industry prefers it that way."

"Variety, Balance, and Moderation Are the Keys"

Another of the ADA's key messages for National Nutrition Month 1996 was, "An eating style with food variety as well as balance and moderation maximizes life-long fitness." What does this mean?

The statement that there are no good or bad foods is often followed by the equally vague concept that variety, balance, and moderation are the keys to a healthful diet. What does this mean to a person for whom breakfast is a sausage-egg-and-cheese biscuit, lunch is a Big Mac and a Coke, and dinner consists of a "balanced" meal of a pork chop, mashed potatoes with gravy, iceberg lettuce salad with bleu cheese dressing, and a glass of milk? Does the salad balance the pork chop? Is moderation having a small Coke instead of a large? Does variety mean having chicken for dinner one night and beef the next?

The reality is that these terms mean little to anyone. We are a culture with such extremes in diet that a little tweaking here and there does not result in changes substantial enough to promote significant health benefits.

Politics enters into the frequent use of these terms as well. Take the term "moderation."

Bonnie Liebman, Director of Nutrition for the Center for Science in the Public Interest, has said, "I never use the term because it's too vague, and the food industry uses it as a smoke-screen to make people think whatever they're eating is okay."

Moderation. It seems so reasonable. So sane. It's a pacifier, especially when someone has the audacity to suggest that there might be something wrong with a steak at Morton's.

It bears repeating: If we were at the point of fine-tuning our diets, the term "moderation" might be relevant. But given the starting point for most people in our culture—such extremes in diet composition—the term loses its meaning.

Then there are "variety" and "balance." Increasingly, these words come into play when discussions about dietary recommendations get close to "naming names" and citing specific advice about food choices.

Why? Because the science is becoming difficult to ignore, and as research overwhelmingly points to the need for Americans to move to a more plant-based diet, this creates serious conflict. A move to a plant-based diet is a threat to the American way. Not only do we have an animal-based agricultural system, with many who stand to lose if meat and dairy products are relegated to the side of the plate or are pushed off all together, but we have a tradition of a certain way of eating.

Traditions are hard to shake. Ask anyone who has tried to overhaul his or her diet how difficult it is to change. Try eating out at a restaurant, inviting guests over for dinner, or being the guest in someone's else's home. Try finding a replacement for Aunt Dee's cream cheese brownies or simply letting go of the idea that a meal has to center around a piece of meat.

Changing lifelong habits and replacing old traditions with new ones is tough. It's uncomfortable. No wonder we all resist. We bargain. We rationalize. We grieve. We get angry. Ultimately, however, if we want to lose weight, to lower our cholesterol levels, and to be healthy, most of us will have to make the change.

So the terms "balance" and "moderation" are ways to resist, bargain, and rationalize.

"Sure, you can eat a cheeseburger. Just balance it with lower-fat foods the rest of the day."

"Extra-sharp cheddar cheese melted over your broccoli? Sure. All of that fat can be balanced with lower-fat choices elsewhere in the meal."

And so it goes. The idea is that by balancing high-fat foods with low-fat foods, it all evens out and everything is fine. The reality, of course, is that most people don't do a good enough job of the balancing act. They eat too much of too many high-fat foods. They don't eat enough plant matter—fruit, grains, vegetables, legumes. Most importantly, though, by not making more fundamental changes in the way they eat, they perpetuate a way of life that undermines their dietary goals and their health.

With the trend in dietary recommendations toward a more plant-based diet, the concept of "variety" is a trump card played by many in the food industry and in certain nutrition circles. "Eat a variety of foods" is often followed by warnings not to "omit entire food groups." The danger here, of course, is that people might get it into their heads that meat, eggs, cheese, and other dairy products should be limited. That wouldn't be good for business for many in the food industry, nor for their friends.

When all is said and done, "no good foods, no bad foods" and "variety, balance, and moderation" are words that sound like advice but don't actually have a useful meaning. They don't step on toes, they don't offend. They're friendly, feel-good words that don't disappoint. They don't elicit change. They perpetuate the status quo. . . .

Putting the Politics Into Perspective

The "politics" within groups of health professionals or government agencies are dynamic. Positions or statements made by organizations reflect what the current leadership thinks but may not be consistent with the opinions of some individuals or small groups within the organization. If those individuals and small groups persevere, they can eventually influence and change the voice of the organization as a whole.

. . . [E]xamples can be seen within groups of health professionals, such as the American Dietetic Association. The ADA leadership has a long history of protecting its relationships with industry groups, in part by not making any negative statements about particular foods. However, in recent years, a vegetarian nutrition dietetic practice group—a subgroup within the ADA—was organized by ADA members who want to explore nontraditional, plant-based diets. The practice group has worked to produce nutrition education materials that promote plant-based diets for the public and encourage people to consume fewer foods of animal origin. The group sponsors conference sessions at the ADA's annual meeting that focus on vegetarian diets, and the group produces a newsletter that is circulated among members.

The ADA is a large organization, and choices made by the leadership do not always speak for individual members or subgroups of the parent organization, some of which "politic" within the association for changes.

The point is, dietary recommendations are what they are, in part, because of politics. Because "politics" is the result of interactions among individuals and groups, the outcome is always changing. For now, though, you need to be aware of how the current political climate has influenced the dietary recommendations that you are hearing today. You need advice that has your best interests at heart—not the interests of industry groups or professional associations.

Let's peel back the layers of confusion produced by the politics of your plate and expose the truths behind recommendations about how you should eat. . . .

Summary: The Simple Truth . . .

Simple Keys to an Optimal Diet

The healthiest diet? That's the easy part. Remove the overlay of politics and cultural bias, and here you have it:

Eat a variety of foods   Make the bulk of the diet consist of whole-grain breads and cereal products, legumes such as beans and peas, vegetables, and fruits.

Get enough calories in your diet to meet your energy needs   Burn enough calories through regular physical activity to allow you to eat a reasonable volume of food, which, in turn, will help ensure that you will get all of the nutrients you need.

If you eat foods of animal origin, such as dairy products, eggs, and meat, make them no more than a side dish or minor ingredient in a dish   Animal products should be eaten as condiments rather than as a primary component in a meal. Most people would do best to weed these foods out of their diets, if not entirely, then considerably.

Limit the sweets and fatty, greasy, junk foods   Soft drinks and French fries are vegetarian, but they don't make for a nutritious diet. The more "empty calorie" foods you eat—foods that give you little nutrition for the calories—the more of the "good stuff" you displace or push off your plate. Most people can't afford to eat much junk without seriously compromising the nutritional quality of their diets.

Go easy on added fats in your diet, especially in the form of oils, margarine, butter, salad dressings, mayonnaise, fried foods, and fats that are added to foods in processing or preparation. Avoid them altogether if you can, particularly if weight control is an issue for you. A few nuts and seeds are fine if they are used as a garnish or very minor ingredient in a dish—a sprinkling here and there. This is especially true for children or people who are very physically active and need more calories. In these cases, added calories from plant sources of fat may be appropriate and desirable.

Choose foods as close to their natural state as possible   Processed foods are typically inferior to whole foods, since they have had fiber and nutrients removed or destroyed and often contain more sodium and other additives. Buy locally grown and organically grown produce when you have the choice.

If you feel uncertain about the nutritional adequacy of your diet or need individualized assistance, see a registered dietitian   I strongly advise you to find one that is familiar with plant-based or vegetarian diets. Call the American Dietetic Association's referral service (800-366-1655) to locate a vegetarian-friendly dietitian in your area. You can also call your health care provider, local vegetarian society, or community hospital for a referral.

POSTSCRIPT

Can All Foods Fit Into a Healthful Diet?

Underlying the arguments presented here is the observation that rates of overweight and obesity have increased dramatically in the United States, just within the past decade. As officials of the Centers for Disease Control and Prevention (CDC) explain in *Journal of the American Medical Association* (January 1, 2003), the increases in overweight—and in heart disease, diabetes, and other chronic conditions that accompany it—affect American adults of all ages, both sexes, all races, and all educational levels. To lose weight, people must consume fewer calories, become more active, or do both. What is the best way to advise people about how to accomplish these goals?

As Marion Nestle explains in *Food Politics: How the Food Industry Influences Nutrition and Health* (University of California Press, 2002), it is very much in the interest of food companies to form alliances with nutrition organizations, to sponsor nutrition research, and to fund nutrition conferences and journals. The book argues that such alliances compromise the ability of nutritionists to advise the public to eat less—particularly of highly marketed "junk" foods.

Havala offers an alternative set of dietary precepts that "remove the overlay of politics and cultural bias." The two approaches constitute an interesting comparison. Both sets of authors favor dietary adequacy (enough calories and nutrients) and physical activity. Although both recommend a variety of foods, their idea of the meaning of *variety* differs. Freeland-Graves and Nitzke argue that "no one major food group is more or less important than any other." In contrast, Havala says that the bulk of the diet should consist of whole-grain cereals, vegetables, and fruits, with foods of animal origin included in small amounts if at all. Furthermore, she suggests limits on sweet and fatty "junk" foods because they provide so many calories for so little nutritional value.

In sorting through these differing points of view, it is useful to note that practically everyone in the United States needs to eat less and be more active. The obesity epidemic and its health consequences have created an urgent need for methods to advise the public about diet, physical activity, and health. Epidemiologists Karin Michels and Alicja Wolk have shown that women who eat healthier foods are healthier and live longer than women who do not (*International Journal of Epidemiology*, August 2002). Furthermore, if people are to stop gaining weight, they must reduce their overall intake of calories, which means eating less and changing the way they make food choices. Havala is in no way suggesting that people completely avoid "junk" foods, but she does argue that people should eat less of them. When Freeland-Graves and Nitzke talk about moderation, balance, and choosing fewer servings of foods from the top of the Pyramid, they seem to be saying something quite similar.

ISSUE 3

Are the New Dietary Reference Intakes for Calcium Appropriate?

YES: Rebecca J. Bryant, Jo Cadogan, and Connie M. Weaver, from "The New Dietary Reference Intakes for Calcium: Implications for Osteoporosis," *Journal of the American College of Nutrition* (May 1999)

NO: B. E. Christopher Nordin, from "Calcium Requirement Is a Sliding Scale," *American Journal of Clinical Nutrition* (June 2000)

ISSUE SUMMARY

YES: Nutrition professor Rebecca J. Bryant and her colleagues say that to prevent bone fractures, the recommended intake of dietary calcium should be 1,000 to 1,200 milligrams (1 to 1.2 grams) a day for adults.

NO: Biochemist B. E. Christopher Nordin says that calcium requirements are as much or more dependent on intake of other dietary factors than they are of calcium. Adults with low intakes of protein, phosphate, and sodium can maintain bone health on intakes as low as 400 milligrams of calcium per day.

In designing food guides and dietary guidelines, nutritionists have two goals in mind. First, the advice should help people consume enough of each essential nutrient to prevent dietary deficiencies. At the same time, the advice must help people avoid eating too much of dietary factors that might lead to chronic disease if consumed in excess. In researching the basis of the Food Guide Pyramid, for example, U.S. Department of Agriculture (USDA) nutritionists calculated the numbers of servings from the various food groups needed to provide enough intake of vitamins and minerals to meet standards of nutritional adequacy but also to keep proportions of dietary fat and carbohydrate within recommended limits. Dietary advice must balance prevention of nutritional deficiencies against prevention of chronic diseases—heart disease and certain types of diabetes and cancer, for example—that might be caused by excess food intake.

The need for this kind of balance also applies to single nutrients. For any nutrient, inadequate intake leads to symptoms of deficiency, but too much can also be harmful. For each nutrient, a range of intake is optimal in preventing symptoms of deficiency and of excess. The ranges vary from one nutrient to another. Because people consume nutrients from food, because nutrient requirements vary from one person to another, and because nutrients interact with one another, establishing standards of appropriate nutrient intake for individuals and populations is an especially complicated business.

Since World War II, U.S. committees have established standards for intake of single nutrients—*Recommended Dietary Allowances* (RDAs)—at regular intervals. Through the tenth—and last—edition in 1989, the RDAs were based on the amounts of nutrients needed to prevent deficiency symptoms and were defined as "the levels of intake of essential nutrients . . . adequate to meet the known nutrient needs of practically all healthy persons." In 1997, as the role of nutrition in prevention of chronic diseases became more prominent, the Institute of Medicine (IOM) committee now in charge of the process began to issue new standards, *Dietary Reference Intakes* (DRIs). The DRIs are much more complex than the RDAs, and, in some ways, more controversial.

Calcium is a principal mineral in bone, and it is needed throughout life to prevent fractures due to osteoporosis, the loss of bone mineral density that occurs with aging. To maintain bone health, people (especially women) must consume enough calcium to replace the amounts that are excreted as a result of normal bone "turnover."

The level of calcium required to balance calcium losses is not simple to determine because it depends on activity levels and cigarette smoking habits, as well as on dietary intake. Some nutrients—magnesium, for example—promote calcium retention. Others, particularly protein, phosphorus, and sodium, promote calcium excretion. Thus, calcium standards have policy implications. Calcium is found in a wide variety of foods but in relatively small amounts in most. If the calcium standard is higher than amounts consumed by most people, dietary advice to consume more calcium tends to promote consumption of foods highest in calcium—dairy foods. The populations of many countries do not generally consume dairy foods, however, for reasons of culture or inability to digest their principal sugar, lactose. These populations obtain calcium from food plants or fish or other nondairy sources.

The research group headed by Rebecca J. Bryant says that 1,000 to 1,200 milligrams (mg)—1 to 1.2 grams—of calcium must be consumed daily by adults to maintain calcium balance, a level far higher than that commonly consumed by Americans, let alone international populations. The IOM committee bases this recommendation on studies demonstrating that amounts in this range are needed to reduce bone loss in the spine and to prevent bone fractures in the elderly.

B. E. Christopher Nordin disagrees. He says that people in many countries maintain calcium balance on much lower levels of intake and display no greater rates of osteoporosis. Instead, he says, calcium balance is so linked to intake of animal protein, phosphorus, and sodium, that only people with high intakes of those nutrients require so much calcium. People with low intakes of these nutrients require as little as 400 mg of calcium per day. The selections that follow provide the rationale for these positions.

Rebecca J. Bryant, Jo Cadogan,
and Connie M. Weaver

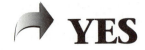 **YES**

The New Dietary Reference Intakes for Calcium: Implications for Osteoporosis

Dietary Reference Intakes

In August 1997, the Food and Nutrition Board of the Institute of Medicine, National Academy of Sciences, released the new Dietary Reference Intakes (DRIs) for calcium, magnesium, phosphorus, fluoride and vitamin D. The committee made recommendations aimed at helping individuals at different stages of life obtain enough of a nutrient to promote bone strength and to maintain normal nutritional status. The report for bone-related nutrients was the first in a series of reports presenting dietary reference values for the intake of nutrients by Americans and Canadians.

The DRIs supersede the Recommended Dietary Allowances (RDAs) that have been published since 1941 by the Food and Nutrition Board. The new recommendations were made by a group of more than 30 U.S. and Canadian scientists who examined the peer-reviewed literature on both the beneficial aspects of nutrients and the potential toxic effects of overconsumption. The DRIs were based upon current concepts about the role of nutrients and food components in long-term health, going beyond prevention of deficiencies. The relationship of calcium intake to bone health and osteoporosis prevention was the primary consideration for setting the new requirement. The four components of the new DRIs are Recommended Dietary Allowances (RDA), Estimated Average Requirements (EAR), Adequate Intakes (AI) and Tolerable Upper Intake Levels (UL).

The RDA is the average daily dietary intake level that is adequate to meet the nutrient requirement of approximately 97% to 98% of healthy individuals in a particular life stage, taking into consideration age and, if applicable, pregnancy and/or lactation. The sole purpose of the RDA for a nutrient is as a goal for daily dietary intake by individuals. It is not intended that it be used for nutritional assessment purposes, nor for planning diets for groups.

The EAR is defined as the nutrient intake value estimated to meet the requirement of fifty percent of the healthy individuals in a life-stage and gender group. For groups, it is used in conjunction with data on the group's distribution of intake, adjusted for day-to-day variation in intake. The EAR is the primary criterion for assessing adequacy of intake of groups. The EAR is also used

From Rebecca J. Bryant, Jo Cadogan, and Connie M. Weaver, "The New Dietary Reference Intakes for Calcium: Implications for Osteoporosis," *Journal of the American College of Nutrition,* vol. 18, no. 5 (May 1999), pp. 406S–411S. Copyright © 1999 by The American College of Nutrition. Reprinted by permission. References omitted.

to develop the RDAs, which are set at two standard deviations above the EAR when the standard deviation of the EAR is known.

An AI level was set for nutrients for which there was insufficient scientific data to establish an EAR and, therefore, an RDA. The AI is derived from observational or experimental estimates of nutrient intake, by a defined population or group, that apparently sustains a certain nutritional state. For calcium, the AI for each life-stage group is an experimentally derived approximate group mean value that appears to support maximal calcium retention, as determined by balance studies.

The UL is defined as the maximal level of daily nutrient intake that is likely to pose no risk of adverse health effects to almost all individuals in a specific life-stage and gender. As intake increases above the UL, the potential for adverse effects increases. The setting of an upper intake level was necessitated by the increasing use of dietary supplements among the population and the increased practice of food fortification with nutrients. The term "tolerable" was included in order to stress that the UL is not a recommended intake level; there are no established benefits for healthy individuals associated with consumption of nutrients above the RDA or AI.

The Calcium Requirement

Adequate calcium intake is thought to reduce the risk of a number of chronic diseases, but the relationship of calcium deficiency and osteoporosis is the most studied. The panel concluded that intakes which were optimal for bone health provided adequate protection for hypertension and colon cancer. Osteoporosis, a condition of reduced bone mass resulting in increased skeletal fragility, affects 25 to 30 million Americans. Approximately twenty-five percent of women of Anglo-Saxon origin over the age of fifty have osteoporosis. Within the female adult population there are more than 1.5 million bone fractures annually, resulting in healthcare costs in excess of $13 billion every year. The three sites most vulnerable to osteoporatic fracture are the spine, the wrist and the hip. Hip fractures are the most serious in terms of disability, loss of independence, mortality and medical costs.

Skeletal bone density is a marker for fracture risk at any age. The lower the skeletal bone density, the greater the risk for fracture. The goal for setting the calcium requirement was the intake which would promote development of maximal peak bone mass, or bone density, during growth and would minimize loss thereafter. This is the intake which maximizes calcium retention for highest bone strength within the genetic potential. To determine intakes which lead to maximal retention, a range of intakes needs to be studied. Longitudinal studies of bone density over a range of calcium intakes are unavailable. Therefore, for all ages for which data were available, balance studies were employed over a range of calcium intakes for the determination of maximal calcium retention. Calcium retention increases with intake until a plateau occurs beyond which there are little appreciable additional benefits.

In addition to maximal retention intake calculations, evidence used to set the calcium requirements came from randomized clinical trials, which measured changes in bone density and, to a lesser extent, cross-sectional and epidemiological studies. The calcium requirements are given in Table 1. . . . Calcium requirements across the life span are not uniform due to changes in skeletal growth and age-related changes in absorption and excretion. Calcium retention is high during growth and, ideally, is in balance with intake during adulthood, but becomes negative when calcium intakes are inadequate, since the skeleton serves as the primary mineral reservoir for the maintenance of serum calcium levels.

Table 1

Dietary Reference Intake Values for Calcium by Life-Stage Group for U.S. and Canada*

Life-Stage Group	(mg/day)
0 to 6 months	210
6 to 12 months	270
1 through 3 years	500
4 through 8 years	800
9 through 13 years	1300
14 through 18 years	1300
19 through 30 years	1000
31 through 50 years	1000
51 through 70 years	1200
> 70 years	1200
Pregnancy	
≤ 18 years	1300
19 through 50 years	1000
Lactation	
≤ 18 years	1300
19 through 50 years	1000

*Food and Nutrition Board, Institute of Medicine, National Academy Press, Washington, DC, 1997.

The Growing Years

Throughout childhood and adolescence, the calcium requirement is driven by high rates of bone mineral accretion. The peak rate of bone mass accrual occurs at age 13 in girls and 14.5 in boys. A recent cross-sectional study of 247 females aged between 11 and 32 years showed that approximately 90% of total body bone mineral content is achieved by age 17.9, 95% by 19.3 years and 99% by age 22.1 years. Furthermore, at sites of specific clinical interest, such as the femoral neck [part of a leg bone], bone gain may be complete by the end of longitudinal growth. Only approximately 4% of total body bone mineral content is achievable after age 20 years. Consequently, there is a limited window of opportunity for the attainment of maximal peak bone mass. Several randomized, controlled trials have shown that children and adolescents assigned to calcium intakes higher than control groups, whether provided by supplements, fortified foods or dairy products acquire higher bone density or mass than those assigned to the control group. Other characteristics including gender and race, as well as dietary factors other than calcium, could influence bone accretion.

The most important factor for determining the calcium required for children and adolescents is the attainment of peak bone mass within the genetic potential. At the end of consolidation, when the maximum amount of bone has been accumulated, certain sites may "peak" during adolescence or shortly thereafter. Maximizing peak bone density is thought important to protect against fracture later in life, but bone density may also predict fracture risk in children. Children aged 3 to 15 years who had suffered forearm fractures had substantially lower bone density than age-matched, non-fracture controls. The calcium intake which leads to maximal calcium retention in prepubertal children is 800 mg/day and 1300 mg/day for white adolescent girls as determined by balance studies over a range of calcium intakes.

Adulthood

In adults, total body bone mass remains relatively constant over the reproductive years, as decreases in the proximal femur [thighbone] and other sites after age 18 are offset by continued growth of the forearm, total spine and head. Bone loss proceeds at the rate of about 0.5% to 1% per year from the age of approximately 40 years in both genders, although in women this loss is increased in the first 3 to 5 years after menopause. Age-related decreases in calcium absorption and increases in urinary calcium contribute to this loss.

In premenopausal women supplementation with 1 g calcium significantly reduced vertebral bone loss and 2 g calcium supplementation provided no further benefit. In postmenopausal women, Dawson-Hughes reviewed the randomized clinical trials and concluded that calcium supplementation helped those on previously low intakes of calcium and was also beneficial when given more than five years post-menopausal. Recker *et al.* further found that increasing dietary calcium through supplementation or calcium-rich foods resulted in higher bone density and reduced incidence of fracture later in life. Calcium also augments the effect of hormone replacement therapy.

The calcium intake required by younger adults aged 19 to 50 years to achieve mean maximal retention or minimal loss was determined to be 1000 mg/day. In older adults aged 51 to 70, the calcium intake required to achieve maximal retention was 1200 mg/day, using the balance data of Spencer *et al.*

Pregnancy and Lactation

The criteria used to determine the calcium requirement for pregnant and lactating women was bone mineral content. No data suggests that parity [number of children] or lactation have permanent negative effects on bone density. Therefore, the panel set the AI for pregnant females less than 18 years to be the same as for nonpregnant adolescent females (1300 mg Ca/day). The AI for pregnant women aged 19 to 50 was also set at the same level (1000 mg Ca/day) as that for nonpregnant women and men in the same age category. At this time, calcium requirements are not higher due to pregnancy or lactation because calcium absorption efficiency and retention adjusts during the third trimester to accommodate skeletal needs of the fetus and during post-weaning periods. Net skeletal calcium loss during lactation is generally regained within six months *post partum* [after birth]. Furthermore, calcium supplementation does not appear to prevent lactation-induced bone loss. More research is needed to determine the effect of pregnancy and lactation on bone loss in adolescents and older mothers and the impact of inadequate calcium intake on bone mineral mass in the years following pregnancy and lactation. Requirements for some individuals may be higher during these altered states. Nevertheless, a larger public health concern is that calcium intakes of women are generally too low.

The Elderly

Adults aged 70 years or older have decreased physical activity which leads to reduced food intake. The tendency to spend most of their time indoors leads to lowered exposure to sunlight, which leads to reduced vitamin D status, a decline in calcium absorption efficiency and a decline in renal [kidney] calcium conservation. Hip fracture as well as nonvertebral fracture rates among elderly retirement home residents decreased when residents were supplemented with 1200 mg calcium and 800 IU [International Units] vitamin D daily. There was also a significant positive effect of calcium on the bone mineral density at the proximal femur in this study. In another randomized trial in men and women (mean age 71 years), Dawson-Hughes found that supplementation with 500 mg elemental calcium and 352 IU vitamin D significantly reduced nonvertebral fracture rates. Because there are very few data in men and women at high calcium intakes to allow an estimation of the intake above which no further gains in calcium retention occur, the AI was set at 1200 mg/day.

Achieving Adequate Calcium Intakes

Calcium intakes for most of the population from puberty and older are appreciably less than the requirement (Fig. 1). In the United States, the mean calcium intake of adolescents is likely inadequate to meet the demands of rapid skeletal growth, and they are destined to obtain a lower peak bone mass than their genetic potential. The mean calcium intake for boys in the U.S. aged 9 to 13 years is 980 mg/day and 889 mg/day for girls. The requirement of 1300 mg/day falls above the seventy-fifth percentile of calcium intake for boys and the ninetieth percentile of intake for girls. In older individuals, lower calcium intakes relative to the requirement typically lead to bone loss. The gap between actual calcium intake and AIs can be as high as hundreds of milligrams per day. Closing this gap is our responsibility and challenge as educators and health professionals.

Dairy foods provide 75% of the calcium in the American diet. Typically, it is at the crucial period of maximal skeletal accretion that adolescents, girls especially, decrease their intake of dairy products and replace milk with soft drinks as the primary beverage. Although calcium intake is an important determinant

Figure 1

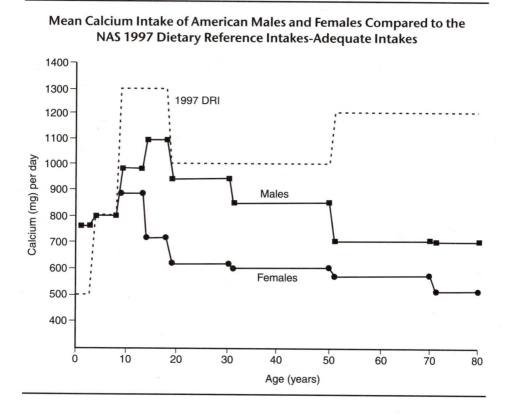

Mean Calcium Intake of American Males and Females Compared to the NAS 1997 Dietary Reference Intakes-Adequate Intakes

of peak bone mass, other lifestyle choices also affect bone including physical activity, anorexia and smoking, as well as intakes of other nutrients important for bone health, e.g., magnesium, phosphorus, protein and sodium. Without adequate dairy products, the diet may be inadequate in calcium, vitamin A, folate, riboflavin, vitamin B_6, magnesium and potassium. Certain vegetables and grains provide calcium, but the quantities required to replace the amount of calcium in even a single glass of milk practically limit the role of these foods. If intake of dairy products is limited or avoided, achieving adequate calcium intakes requires regular use of fortified foods and supplements.

Role of Genetics

Although environmental factors have a significant influence on the development of bone mass, sixty to eighty percent of peak bone mass is genetically determined. Some recent reports begin to illustrate the role of genetics in calcium and bone metabolism. O'Brien *et al.* hypothesized that bone turnover is less responsive to alterations in dietary calcium intake in both girls and adult women from families with histories of osteoporosis, compared to control families, in three generations of all families. They observed diminished responsiveness to calcium supplementation in girls from osteoporotic families due to an increased rate of resorption as well as formation compared to control girls from non-osteoporotic families. In these individuals, calcium requirements are likely higher to achieve desirable peak bone mass and to minimize skeletal loss.

The twin study of Johnston *et al.* evaluated the genetic effects on bone in female monozygotic [identical] and dizygotic [fraternal] twins. The intraclass correlation for monozygotic twins was found always to be significantly higher than the intraclass correlation for dizygotic twins, indicating a strong genetic contribution. Furthermore, this observation appeared to be true over a wide age range, suggesting calcium intake and lifestyle choices may have a greater influence on bone in individuals genetically predisposed to development of lower bone mineral density.

The interplay between genetic effects and diet on bone mass is unclear. . . . [G]enetic make-up in humans appears to influence ability to utilize nutrients. One wonders, with the advances being made in understanding the human genome, if nutrient requirements in the future will be differentiated by genetic typing at birth.

Racial Differences

An issue related to the role of genetics is possible racial differences in calcium requirements. The scientific data used to determine calcium requirements was collected primarily in Caucasians.

African Americans have generally been reported to have higher bone mass and lower incidence of fracture than whites. Although vertebral bone density did not differ between black and white girls before puberty, bone mineral content of the forearm was already higher in black than in white children by age one to six years. . . .

The incidence of osteoporosis, as reflected by the number of hip fractures, is rising in Asia and Japan. Usual calcium intakes do not decline with age in Asian countries as they do in America. Calcium intakes in China appear to be similar to intakes of elderly Americans, but lower in the younger adults than in their American counterparts. Vegetable calcium sources are more important in the Chinese diet than in the typical Western diet because of the lower intake of dairy products in the Chinese population. Vegetables and soy products provide 41% of the calcium intake of Chinese, in contrast to less than 10% for Americans. Calcium absorption from several commonly consumed Chinese vegetables was higher than from milk by almost 10%, although the amount of calcium in these vegetables on a per-serving basis would require ingesting, for example, upwards of two servings of Chinese cabbage or five servings of broccoli to equal the amount of calcium in a one-cup serving of milk. As Asians adopt more American-type diets, their incidence of osteoporosis would be expected to increase, as their consumption of high-quality calcium foods decreased.

More studies need to be done in black and Asian populations to determine how calcium metabolism and bone formation/resorption differ from those of whites on different dietary calcium intakes. This is essential in order to evaluate the appropriateness of the new AI for calcium for these populations.

Conclusion

Adequate calcium intake plays an important role in calcium retention, which dictates bone mass and, therefore, skeletal fragility. It is important to educate Americans that current calcium intakes fall far short of the recently established calcium requirements for most age groups. Many questions remain unanswered in our understanding of the requirements for calcium in individuals of different races and cultural environments. Comparative studies on calcium and bone metabolism with a sufficient sample size to have the necessary statistical power to detect differences are essential to expanding our knowledge and determining the adequacy of the AIs when considering blacks, Hispanics and Asians.

B. E. Christopher Nordin 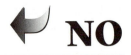 **NO**

Calcium Requirement Is a Sliding Scale[a,b]

Introduction

It must be a source of some surprise to rational scientists that the human requirement for calcium, an apparently inoffensive nutrient that contributes so much to our physical stability, arouses strong emotions in many breasts. Calcium requirements and allowances seem to attract more controversy and generate more heat than do the requirements and allowances for any other nutrient, the latest example of this being a recent controversy in the columns of the *New York Times* (1). The problem may be that calcium turnover is too slow and the effects of deprivation and replenishment too gradual to be easily demonstrated in humans; perhaps it is the very efficacy of the calcium homeostatic [balance] system that makes this system difficult to study. Whereas plasma concentrations of other nutrients (eg, sodium, potassium, phosphorus, and magnesium) can be lowered relatively easily and quickly by experimental deprivation (2), plasma (ionized) calcium is so well protected through access to the reserve stores in the skeleton that it cannot be used as a marker of calcium nutrition. Although there is overwhelming evidence that calcium deprivation causes osteoporosis in experimental animals (3), it would be both immoral and impractical to try to reproduce such experiments in humans. The calcium requirement therefore must be estimated by indirect means that, even if they satisfy many of the experts in the field, are open to criticism by others. Nonetheless, there is no smoke without fire and it may be that this controversy does reflect a deeper reality, although not perhaps the one that the critics of the calcium story envisage.

Experimental Background

The first step toward unraveling the effect of a nutritional deficiency is generally to study an experimental animal model. This has been done with calcium since 1885 when Pommer (4) first described and defined the histologic difference between osteomalacia (osteoid-covered bone) and osteoporosis (bone deficit with normal osteoid). Once that was established, it was shown in observational and experimental studies in dogs, cats, rats, rabbits, and other animals that calcium

From B. E. Christopher Nordin, "Calcium Requirement Is a Sliding Scale," *American Journal of Clinical Nutrition,* vol. 71 (June 2000), pp. 1381–1383. Copyright © 2000 by The American Society for Clinical Nutrition. Reprinted by permission. The American Society for Clinical Nutrition, Inc. does not endorse any commercial enterprise.

deficiency causes osteoporosis, at least in adult animals (3), and this is now the standard osteoporosis model alongside the oophorectomy model (5–8). The current consensus is that the same chain of events must occur in human adults if calcium intake falls short of requirement. At issue is what this requirement actually is and how much human osteoporosis can be attributed to calcium deficiency, ie, to a state of primary negative calcium balance, and how much to primary changes in bone with secondary negative calcium balance. Both types of osteoporosis must exist. In hyperthyroidism [a condition of excessive thyroid hormone], for example, there is agreement that the bone effects are primary and the negative calcium balance is the result rather than the cause of the bone disease. In the postmenopausal state, by contrast, there is reason to believe that the rise in urinary calcium (9) and the fall in calcium absorption (10, 11) are primary events and that the rise in bone resorption is essentially a response to this increased calcium requirement, exacerbated by the loss of some action of estrogen on bone (12). This interpretation of menopause is borne out by the effectiveness of calcium supplements in preventing postmenopausal bone loss (11) and in enhancing the bone effects of estrogen (13). The formulation of calcium requirements and allowances must be seen in this light.

Calcium Intake and Calcium Balance

For obvious reasons, we cannot reproduce in humans the calcium deficiency experiments performed in animals. To establish an incontrovertible experimental link between calcium deficiency and osteoporosis, we would have to ask volunteers to restrict their calcium intake for ≥ 1 y [a year or more] before we could hope to show a significant decrease in bone density. Deliberately withholding a nutrient for long periods would be unacceptable today, and when this was in fact done with Norwegian prisoners some 50 y ago (14), bone densitometry was not available to document the outcome. However, prolonged calcium balance studies can be regarded as a surrogate for bone densitometry; it is reasonable to assume that the mean calcium requirement is the mean calcium intake at which output and input are equal and that prolonged negative calcium balance must lead to osteoporosis. Thus, it is a critical fact that many of the Norwegian prisoners studied by Malm went into negative balance at calcium intakes less than ≈500 mg/d and remained in negative balance for ≥ 1 y. When the final calculations were made on the subjects at the end of the study, the mean calcium requirement of the fully adapted men was 420 mg/d (14). This relatively low value was achieved at the expense of an unspecified amount of bone loss.

Before Malm carried out this remarkable work, some hundreds of calcium balance studies had been published in the United States, yielding estimates of calcium requirements ranging from 400 to 800 mg/d, with a median value of ≈600 mg/d (15). It seems that when the FAO/WHO [Food and Agriculture Organization/World Health Organization of the United Nations] Expert Group met in Rome in 1960 and recommended an adult calcium allowance of 400–500 mg/d (16), few of these studies were available, apart from some short balance studies in Peruvian prisoners [which yielded an estimated requirement of 200 mg/d (17)] and Malm's Norwegian data referred to above. The Expert Group interpreted Malm's data to mean that humans could "adapt" to low calcium intakes by increasing their absorption, reducing their excretion of calcium, or both. The Expert Group was clearly also influenced by the prevalence of low calcium intakes without obvious injurious effect in many developing countries. The rather low recommendations of this group were followed by several countries (18), including the United Kingdom in 1969 (19). The United States adhered to the figure of 800 mg/d (20), whereas Australia recommended a less specific calcium intake of 400–800 mg/d (21). In the meantime, an analysis published in 1976 of 212 balance studies suggested a calcium requirement of 540 mg/d and an allowance of 800 mg/d (2). A balance study published in 1978 by Heaney et al (22) pointed to a requirement of 975 mg/d in premenopausal women. Since then, most national recommendations have crept up and are now 800 mg/d in Australia (23), 700 mg/d in the United Kingdom (24), 700 mg/d in the European Union (25), and 1000 mg/d in the United States and Canada (26).

In the meantime, 2 developments occurred that must influence scientific thinking on this subject. First, technically acceptable methods have emerged for the measurement of insensible calcium losses (eg, through the skin), which probably amount to ≥ 40 mg/d (27). Because of the kinetics of calcium absorption, this addition of 40 mg Ca to the body's obligatory losses through the bowel and kidneys needs to be offset by an increase in dietary calcium of some 200 mg, which increases the mean requirement from ≈ 550 to 750 mg/d (28) and must increase the recommended allowance from 800 to 1000 mg/d. The only authority to have taken this into account so far is the joint US and Canadian committee (26), which is one reason their recommendations are relatively high. Second, and even more importantly, it has become increasingly clear that obligatory urinary calcium, and therefore the calcium requirement, is strongly influenced by intakes of protein and sodium and possibly of other nutrients. These intakes need to be taken into account when calcium allowances are determined.

Published sources show that each gram of animal protein consumed increases urinary calcium by 1 mg (9, 11, 29–31) and that every gram of sodium ingested increases urinary calcium by ≈ 15 mg (9, 11, 32, 33). These may look like small effects at first glance but they signify that a 40-g reduction in animal protein intake reduces urinary calcium by ≈ 40 mg, which reduces the calcium requirement by ≈ 200 mg. Similarly, a reduction in dietary sodium of 2.3 g reduces urinary calcium by 40 mg, which reduces the calcium requirement accordingly. Differences of this order can occur in individuals from day to day, can be found between individuals within one culture, and without question are found between cultures. This has profound implications for the calculation of calcium requirements in different countries.

Implications

The implications of these data are particularly important at the transnational level. Although there is a shortage of data on the prevalence of osteoporosis in the developing world, there is evidence that hip fracture rates in many of these countries are much lower than in the West despite lower calcium intakes in developing countries (34, 35). Prentice et al (36) reported that despite the low daily calcium intake in The Gambia (360 mg), osteoporotic fractures are rare. Thus, there is a strong suggestion that the relatively low calcium intakes in many parts of the world are not accompanied by the increased prevalences of osteoporosis that might be expected.

This finding may be explained, at least in part, by the fact that animal protein intake varies across the world in parallel with calcium intake. The mean calcium intake in the developing world in 1990 was given as 344 mg/d, compared with 850 mg/d in the developed world (37); the corresponding total protein intakes were 59.9 and 103.0 g/d and animal protein intakes were 13.3 and 60.1 g/d. Thus, the paradox that calcium intakes are low where fracture rates are low and high where fracture rates are high probably signifies that high (animal) protein intakes increase the risk of osteoporosis because they increase urinary calcium (38, 39), as suggested by Hegsted (40) many years ago. This concept is supported by the results of a prospective study that showed that wrist fractures in American women were weakly but significantly related to animal protein intake (41). Dietary sodium is probably equally important but the shortage of international data on this nutrient makes it harder to define the worldwide implications of sodium intake. Note, however, that the effects of animal protein and sodium restriction on urinary calcium are likely to be additive because they exert their effects in different ways: sodium by competing with calcium for renal tubular reabsorption (32) and protein by virtue of its phosphate (and possibly sulfate) end products, which complex calcium in the renal tubules and take it out in the urine (9, 11). Thus, populations with low animal protein and sodium intakes are likely to have a very low calcium requirement.

From the available data, we can calculate what the calcium requirement might be at different animal protein or sodium intakes. These calculations show that a reduction in animal protein intake from a reference value of 60 to 20 g/d or a reduction in sodium intake from 150 to 50 mmol/d reduces the theoretical calcium requirement from ≈750 to 550 mg/d (29). The combination of both restrictions would reduce the calcium requirement to 400 mg/d (29). This suggests that the calcium requirements and allowances promulgated by developed nations in the past few years, although probably valid for their own countries and dietary cultures, cannot be extended to nations with different dietary cultures whose populations consume different amounts of animal protein or sodium. In addition, factors that influence calcium absorption may also need to be taken into account because this modality is such a central component of the calcium system. An example of such a factor is vitamin D, largely derived from sunlight, the supply of which depends mainly on latitude. Vitamin D may be another factor contributing to low fracture rates in developing countries at low latitudes (34). In fact, high calcium absorption (resulting from a high serum 1,25-dihydroxyvitamin D concentration) and low urinary calcium were reported in Gambian women (42–44) and these 2 factors in combination would greatly reduce the calcium requirement.

Although negative calcium balance must lead to osteoporosis, the amount of calcium required to prevent such negative balance varies not only from individual to individual but also from culture to culture. The conclusion is inescapable that there is no single, universal calcium requirement, only a requirement linked to the intake of other nutrients. Future recommendations—particularly those from international bodies—will need to take this into account despite the opinion of the US and Canadian committee that it is too early to do so (26).

Notes

[a]From the Division of Clinical Biochemistry, Institute of Medical and Veterinary Science, Adelaide, Australia.

[b]Address correspondence to BEC Nordin, Division of Clinical Biochemistry, Institute of Medical and Veterinary Science, PO Box 14 Rundle Mall, Adelaide, SA 5000, Australia. E-mail: christopher.nordin@imvs.sa.gov.au.

References

1. Murray M. Ads raise question about milk and bones. New York Times 1999 Sept 14:F1, F4.
2. Marshall DH, Nordin BEC, Speed R. Calcium, phosphorus and magnesium requirement. Proc Nutr Soc 1976;35:163–73.
3. Nordin BEC. Osteomalacia, osteoporosis and calcium deficiency. Clin Orthop 1960;17:235–58.
4. Pommer G. Rachitis und Osteomalacie. (Rickets and osteomalacia.) Leipzig, Germany: Vogel, 1885 (in German).
5. Hodgkinson A, Aaron JE, Horsman A, McLachlan MSF, Nordin BEC. Effect of oophorectomy and calcium deprivation on bone mass in the rat. Clin Sci Mol Med 1978;54:439–46.
6. Wronski TJ, Lowry PL, Walsh CC, Ignaszewski LA. Skeletal alterations in ovariectomized rats. Calcif Tissue Int 1985;37:324–8.
7. Shen V, Birchman R, Xu R, Lindsay R, Dempster DW. Short-term changes in histomorphometric and biochemical turnover markers and bone mineral density in estrogen- and/or dietary calcium-deficient rats. Bone 1995;16:149–56.
8. O'Loughlin PD, Morris HA. Oophorectomy in young rats impairs calcium balance by increasing intestinal calcium secretion. J Nutr 1994;124:726–31.
9. Nordin BEC, Polley KJ. Metabolic consequences of the menopause. A cross-sectional, longitudinal, and intervention study on 557 normal postmenopausal women. Calcif Tissue Int 1987;41:S1–60.
10. Heaney RP, Saville PD, Recker RR. Calcium absorption as a function of calcium intake. J Lab Clin Med 1975;85:881–90.
11. Nordin BEC. Calcium and osteoporosis. Nutrition 1997;13:664–86.
12. Nordin BEC, Need AG, Morris HA, Horowitz M. Biochemical variables in pre- and postmenopausal women: reconciling the calcium and estrogen hypotheses. Osteoporos Int 1999;9:351–7.
13. Nieves JW, Komar L, Cosman F, Lindsay R. Calcium potentiates the effect of estrogen and calcitonin on bone mass: review and analysis. Am J Clin Nutr 1998;67:18–24.
14. Malm OJ. Calcium requirement and adaptation in adult men. Scand J Clin Lab Invest 1958;10(suppl):1–289.
15. Nordin BEC. Nutritional considerations. In: Nordin BEC, ed. Calcium, phosphate and magnesium metabolism. Edinburgh: Churchill Livingstone, 1976:11–35.
16. FAO/WHO Expert Group. Calcium requirements. Rome: Food and Agriculture Organization, 1962.
17. Hegsted JM, Moscoso I, Collazos CHC. Study of minimum calcium requirements by adult men. J Nutr 1952;46:181–201.

18. Report of Committee 1/5 of the International Union of Nutritional Sciences. Recommended dietary intakes around the world. Nutr Abstr Rev 1983;53:939–1119.

19. Department of Health and Social Security. Recommended intakes of nutrients for the United Kingdom. London: Her Majesty's Stationery Office, 1969. (Report on Public Health and Medical Subjects no. 120.)

20. Committee on Dietary Allowances, Food and Nutrition Board, National Research Council. Recommended dietary allowances. 9th revised ed. Washington, DC: National Academy Press, 1980.

21. National Health and Medical Research Council. Dietary allowances for use in Australia. Canberra, Australia: Australian Government Publishing Service, 1970.

22. Heaney RP, Recker RR, Saville PD. Menopausal changes in calcium balance performance. J Lab Clin Med 1978;92:953–63.

23. National Health and Medical Research Council. Recommended dietary intakes for use in Australia. Canberra, Australia: Australian Government Publishing Service, 1991.

24. Department of Health. Dietary reference values for food energy and nutrients for the United Kingdom. Report of the Panel on Dietary Reference Values of the Committee on Medical Aspects of Food Policy. London: Her Majesty's Stationery Office, 1991.

25. Reports of the Scientific Committee for Food. Nutrient and energy intakes for the European Community. Luxembourg: Office for Official Publications of the European Communities, 1993. (31st series ISBN 92–826–6409–0.)

26. Food and Nutrition Board, Institute of Medicine. Dietary reference intakes for calcium, magnesium, vitamin D, and fluoride. Washington, DC: National Academy Press, 1997.

27. Jensen FT, Charles P, Mosekilde L, Hansen HH. Calcium metabolism evaluated by [47]calcium-kinetics: a physiological model with correction for faecal lag time and estimation of dermal calcium loss. Clin Physiol 1983;3:187–204.

28. Nordin BEC, Marshall DH. Dietary requirements for calcium. In: Nordin BEC, ed. Calcium in human biology. Berlin: Springer-Verlag, 1988:447–71.

29. Nordin BEC, Morris HA, Need AG, Horowitz M. Dietary calcium and osteoporosis. In: Pietinen P, Nishida C, Khaltaev N, eds. Proceedings of the 2nd WHO Symposium on Health Issues for the 21st Century: Nutrition and Quality of Life, Kobe, Japan 1993. Geneva: World Health Organization, 1996:181–98.

30. Kerstetter JE, Allen LH. Dietary protein increases urinary calcium. J Nutr 1989;120:134–6.

31. Heaney RP, Recker RR. Effects of nitrogen, phosphorus, and caffeine on calcium balance in women. J Lab Clin Med 1982; 99:46–55.

32. Nordin BEC, Need AG, Morris HA, Horowitz M. The nature and significance of the relation between urine sodium and urine calcium in women. J Nutr 1993;123:1615–22.

33. Goulding A, Lim PE. Effects of varying dietary intake on the fasting excretion of sodium, calcium and hydroxyproline in young women. N Z Med J 1983;96:853–4.

34. Nordin BEC. Calcium in health and disease. Food Nutr Agric 1997;20:13–24.

35. Kanis JA. Osteoporosis. Oxford, United Kingdom: Blackwell Science, 1994.

36. Prentice A, Shaw J, Laskey, MA, Cole TJ, Fraser DR. Bone and mineral content of British and rural Gambian women aged 18–80+ years. Bone Miner 1991;12:201–14.

37. Food and Agriculture Organization of the United Nations. Yearbook 1990. Vol 44. Rome: Food and Agriculture Organization, 1991.

38. Heaney RP. Protein intake and the calcium economy. J Am Diet Assoc 1993;93:1261–2.

39. Heaney RP. Bone mass, nutrition, and other lifestyle factors. Nutr Rev 1996;54:S3–10.

40. Hegsted DM. Calcium and osteoporosis. J Nutr 1986;116:2316−9.

41. Feskanich D, Willett WC, Stampfer MJ, Colditz GA. Protein consumption and bone fractures in women. Am J Epidemiol 1996; 143:472−9.

42. Prentice A, Jarjou LMA, Stirling DM, Buffenstein R, Fairweather-Tait S. Biochemical markers of calcium and bone metabolism during 18 months of lactation in Gambian women accustomed to a low calcium intake and in those consuming a calcium supplement. J Clin Endocrinol Metab 1998;83:1059−66.

43. Fairweather-Tait S, Prentice A, Heumann KG, et al. Effect of calcium supplements and stage of lactation on the calcium absorption efficiency of lactating women accustomed to low calcium intakes. Am J Clin Nutr 1995;62:1188−92.

44. Prentice A, Jarjou LMA, Cole TJ, Stirling DM, Dibba B, Fairweather-Tait S. Calcium requirements of lactating Gambian mothers: effects of a calcium supplement on breast-milk calcium concentration, maternal bone mineral content, and urinary calcium excretion. Am J Clin Nutr 1995;62:58−67.

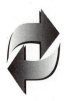

POSTSCRIPT

Are the New Dietary Reference Intakes for Calcium Appropriate?

Both authors agree that bone mass is established in childhood, that low intakes of calcium lead to bone demineralization and fractures, and that adults who do not consume excessive amounts of protein and sodium need far less calcium. According to Bryant et al., people must increase their intake of dairy products to meet the DRI for calcium; if they do not, they will need to consume fortified foods or supplements. Furthermore, postmenopausal women who are unwilling or unable to consume adequate calcium should be prescribed estrogen therapy, as this hormone promotes calcium retention. In January 2003, however, the Food and Drug Administration (FDA) began to require a warning label on estrogens used by postmenopausal women on the basis of studies suggesting that this therapy increased the risk of invasive breast cancer and cardiovascular disease in women who took such drugs (see http://www.fda.gov). Thus, the implication of the IOM committee report is that Americans of all ages should increase intake of foods from the dairy group of the Pyramid, calcium-fortified foods, and calcium supplements.

The dietary implications of Nordin's analysis are quite different. If, as he argues, diets high in protein and sodium are responsible for raising the requirement for calcium, then calcium balance could be improved by consuming less of foods high in animal protein (meat and dairy), replacing those foods with others lower in animal protein (fruits, vegetables, grains), and reducing intake of sodium by avoiding its primary sources: processed foods and salty snacks.

The implications of these approaches for food choice (and for the economic balance of the companies that produce dairy, meat, processed, and salted snack foods) explain some of the controversy associated with the DRI for calcium. Other commentators attribute the controversy to societal debates about the merits of vegetarian diets (see Robert Heaney's editorial in the *American Journal of Clinical Nutrition*, January 2001) or to unresolved scientific arguments about the effects of protein on bone mineralization (see debates by Linda Massey and her colleagues in the *Journal of Nutrition,* June 1998).

The calcium standard is especially controversial because it is set at a level higher than can easily be attained through usual food intake, but the scientific issues involved in studying any single nutrient—detached from its dietary context—will always be debatable. Such studies are inevitably "reductionist" in that they reduce our understanding of the health effects of dietary patterns to those produced by a single nutrient. Studies of single nutrients are easier to conduct than studies of dietary patterns, but they are open to varied interpretation.

On the Internet . . .

DUSHKIN ONLINE

The General Accounting Office (GAO)

In response to congressional requests, General Accounting Office (GAO) investigators produce reports on many issues related to agriculture, food, nutrition, and health. They also testify before Congress on these issues. This site provides the full text of GAO reports and testimony.

http://www.gao.gov

The American Diabetes Association

The American Diabetes Association promotes research, education, and advocacy to prevent, cure, and treat people with diabetes mellitus, type 1 ("juvenile-onset") and type 2 ("adult-onset"). This site provides information about these conditions for health professionals and the public. It also provides access to the association's journals, many of which publish articles on aspects of diet and diabetes prevention and control, such as the glycemic index.

http://www.diabetes.org/homepage.jsp

PART 2

Nutrition and Health

*E*veryone agrees that the overall diet has important effects on health, but arguments start as soon as the discussion focuses on associations between specific dietary factors and specific diseases. The selections in this part illustrate the complexities of research on diet and the reasons why research results are matters of interpretation as much as they are of science. These selections also reveal why advice about diet is so controversial. Much of the controversy is a result of the difficulties of conducting rigorously controlled research on human beings. For reasons of practicality as well as of ethics, scientists cannot turn people into laboratory rats—cage them, control their diets and activities, and observe them for many years. Instead, scientists must use other methods such as biochemical, animal, or epidemiological studies. The limitations of these methods leave much room for interpretation and, therefore, for differences of opinion. In this set of selections, methods play a critical role in establishing a basis for interpretation. Do research reviews provide more information than one carefully designed epidemiological study? Do the economic interests of scientific authors influence their opinions? Do disputes about methods mean that differences in opinions can never be reconciled? The selections in this part address these questions as they examine the effects of sugars and foods containing rapidly digested carbohydrate on risk factors for heart disease, diabetes, and obesity.

- Are Added Sugars Harmful to Health?

- Do Foods With a High Glycemic Index Increase Disease Risk?

ISSUE 4

Are Added Sugars Harmful to Health?

YES: Barbara V. Howard and Judith Wylie-Rosett, from "Sugar and Cardiovascular Disease," *Circulation* (July 23, 2002)

NO: Anne L. Mardis, from "Current Knowledge of the Health Effects of Sugar Intake," *Family Economics and Nutrition Review* (2001)

ISSUE SUMMARY

YES: Researchers Barbara V. Howard and Judith Wylie-Rosett, representing the American Heart Association (AHA), state that high sugar consumption increases risk factors for heart disease and may adversely affect control of diabetes.

NO: Physician Anne L. Mardis, representing the U.S. Department of Agriculture's (USDA's) Center for Nutrition Policy and Promotion, says that the intake of sugar has no relation to the risk of heart disease or diabetes.

Early in the twenty-first century, overweight and obesity emerged as predominant public health nutrition problems. By 2002 the *majority* of Americans were overweight or obese. Obesity raises the risk for multiple chronic diseases, most notably coronary heart disease, type 2 diabetes, and stroke. Overweight results from consuming more energy (calories) than is expended in daily activities. To maintain or to lose weight, people must consume fewer calories from food. Many experts believe that foods high in fats and sugars encourage weight gain—and increase the risk of chronic diseases—because people like the taste of such foods and are stimulated to eat more of them. Because the taste for sweetness is an innate genetic characteristic of humans, much attention has focused on sugars as a factor that raises chronic disease risk.

In 1980 the first edition of the *Dietary Guidelines for Americans* said, "*avoid* too much sugar." Twenty years later, the guideline read, "Choose beverages and foods to *moderate* your intake of sugars" (emphasis added in both). Foods high in sugars appear at the top of the Food Guide Pyramid, indicating that they should be consumed sparingly in healthful diets. The reasoning behind these recommendations is not in dispute: sugars (from cane, beets, or corn) provide calories but no vitamins or minerals. Furthermore, the quantity of sugars in the

U.S. food supply has increased over the years to a level of nearly half a pound per day per person, and the top six sources of added sugars in U.S. diets are, in order, carbonated soft drinks, fruit drinks, candy, cakes, ice cream, and sugar-coated cereals.

Very much in dispute, however, is whether or not high-sugar diets increase heart disease or its related risk factors, high blood cholesterol and triglycerides, high blood sugar, and obesity. The American Heart Association (AHA) was so concerned about the role of sugar in heart disease risk that it appointed a committee to examine the evidence. Barbara V. Howard and Judith Wylie-Rosett, writing for this committee, did not find studies directly linking sugars to heart disease, but they did find short-term studies that consistently revealed adverse effects of high-sugar diets. Such diets were clearly associated with lower levels of HDL (high-density lipoprotein cholesterol, the "good" kind), higher levels of blood triglycerides (a risk factor for heart disease), poor control of blood sugar (a symptom of diabetes), formation of certain sugar compounds that might lead to kidney disease, and promotion of weight gain. For these reasons, and because high-sugar foods add "empty calories that few Americans need," they suggest limiting intake of these foods as a means to improve health.

Anne L. Mardis draws different conclusions from a similar set of studies. She contends that human physiology cannot distinguish added sugars from those naturally occurring in fruits and vegetables or from any other form of carbohydrate, and that hereditary (genetic) factors leading to impaired metabolism account for increases in blood triglycerides. She notes that dietary factors other than sugars can account for excessive caloric intake, that water fluoridation and tooth brushing can prevent tooth decay, and that while people who consume high-sugar diets may decrease intake of some nutrients, they increase intake of others. The evidence, she says, does not support a role of sugar as an independent risk factor for any chronic disease.

In reading the following selections, note the ways in which the authors structure their arguments to support the different points of view. Their arguments agree on several key points but disagree on others. Are the points of disagreement matters of science or of interpretation? What might account for the disagreements? What are the implications of the two points of view for dietary advice to the public? What are the implications for the industries that produce sugar cane, sugar beets, corn sweeteners, or food products high in sugars?

**Barbara V. Howard and
Judith Wylie-Rosett**

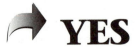

Sugar and Cardiovascular Disease

The purpose of this report is to review the effects of dietary sugar on health, with an emphasis on cardiovascular disease (CVD) and its risk factors. Although there are no dietary trials linking sugar consumption and CVD, there are several reasons why sugar consumption should be limited.

Definitions

There are many, sometimes confusing, terms used in the literature. *Simple carbohydrate* (sugar) refers to mono- and disaccharides; *complex carbohydrate* refers to polysaccharides such as starch. Common disaccharides are sucrose (glucose+fructose), found in sugar cane, sugar beets, honey, and corn syrup; lactose (glucose+galactose), found in milk products; and maltose (glucose+ glucose), from malt. The most common naturally occurring monosaccharide is fructose (found in fruits and vegetables). The term *dextrose* is used to refer to glucose. *Intrinsic* or *naturally occurring* sugar refers to the sugar that is an integral constituent of whole fruit, vegetable, and milk products; *extrinsic* or *added* sugar refers to sucrose or other refined sugars in soft drinks and incorporated into food, fruit drinks, and other beverages.

Sugar Consumption in the United States

Added sugar was not a significant component of the human diet until the advent of modern food-processing methods. Since then, the intake of sugar has risen steadily. The average US sugar utilization per capita on the basis of food disappearance data was 55 kg (120 lb) per year in 1970, and it reached 68 kg (150 lb) per year in 1995 (almost 0.5 lb per day). Sugar (simple carbohydrate) intake averages 25% of total energy intake. Data from the 1989 to 1991 Continuing Survey of Food Intake by Individuals indicate that soft drinks and sugars added at the table (eg, sugar/syrups and jams) are 2 of the top 4 carbohydrate sources for US adults.

From Barbara V. Howard and Judith Wylie-Rosett, "Sugar and Cardiovascular Disease," *Circulation,* vol. 106 (July 23, 2002), pp. 523–526. Copyright © 2002 by The American Heart Association, Inc. Reprinted by permission of Lippincott Williams & Wilkins. References omitted.

Sugar and Coronary Heart Disease

Yudkin and colleagues in the 1960s and 1970s found that a higher intake of sugar was associated with increased CVD in both within-country and cross-country comparisons. A few recent studies have examined the link between sugar consumption and coronary heart disease (CHD). The Iowa Women's Health Study showed no relation between the intake of sweets or desserts and risk of ischemic heart disease in 34 492 women monitored for 9 years. However, some major sources of sugar such as soft drinks were not considered. The Scottish Heart Health Study of 10 359 men and women found that neither extrinsic nor intrinsic sugars were significant independent correlates of prevalent CHD after adjustment for other major risk factors, but the data were not adjusted for other dietary variables. A recent report from the Nurses' Health Study showed that women who consumed diets with a high glycemic load* (increased blood glucose excursions associated with intake of sweets or highly processed starches and sweets) had an increased CHD risk, with those in the highest quintile [upper fifth] having a >2-fold risk during 10 years of follow-up. Simple carbohydrate alone was also predictive but did not reach statistical significance. This analysis controlled for total energy intake and other major dietary and nondietary risk factors.

Dietary Sugar and Plasma Lipoproteins

A number of studies link dietary sugar with adverse changes in lipoproteins [blood proteins associated with cholesterol]. Several studies have shown an inverse association between dietary sucrose and high-density lipoprotein (HDL) cholesterol [the "good" cholesterol]. Data from the Coronary Artery Risk Development In young Adults (CARDIA) study show a consistent inverse association between increased dietary sucrose intake and HDL cholesterol concentrations, in both cross-sectional [one point in time] and longitudinal [over a long time] analyses in blacks and whites, in both men and women, and after adjustment for other covariates.

A diet high in sucrose (ie, >20% of energy) is associated with an elevation of plasma triglyceride [fat] concentrations. This increase is due to both increased hepatic [liver] secretion and impaired clearance of very-low-density lipoprotein. Triglyceride response to dietary sugar may vary, however, according to the amount of sugar and the presence of other nutrients.

Dietary Sugar, Insulin Resistance, and Diabetes

Few epidemiological studies have directly examined the relationship between sugar intake and diabetes incidence. In general, prospective data show no association, and in fact, several dietary studies show an inverse association between

---

Glycemic load refers to a diet with many foods that have a high glycemic index. Glycemic index is a measure of the rise in glucose induced by ingestion of a carbohydrate. Foods that contain refined sugars make a major contribution to glycemic load; other contributors include refined starches, such as white bread and rice. It should be noted that glycemic index is determined by feeding individual foods.

total carbohydrate intake and diabetes incidence. This observation, however, is confounded because diets lower in carbohydrate are higher in fat (high fat intake predicts diabetes risk because of increased obesity). On the other hand, two recent prospective cohort studies have reported food frequency consumption data that showed that a history of consumption of foods with a high glycemic load predicts the development of type 2 diabetes in women and men.

No epidemiological study has examined the effects of dietary sugar on insulin resistance. Several clinical studies have shown that altering the proportion of carbohydrates in the diet for up to 4 months in humans does not influence insulin resistance, but the effects of varying sugar content per se were not examined.

It is widely believed that individuals with diabetes should avoid sugar to maintain glycemic control. However, there is considerable debate about whether high-sugar diets have adverse effects on glucose control in diabetic individuals. A number of studies that assessed the effects of single meals containing 12% to 25% of calories as sucrose found no adverse effects of sucrose on average glycemia [blood sugar levels]. Some long-term studies up to several months in duration showed that providing as much as 38% of calories as sucrose had no effect on average glucose control. Diabetic individuals, however, may experience fluctuations in blood glucose levels with a habitual diet that is high in concentrated sweets, especially if they make errors with regard to the amount of carbohydrates they consume.

Diet and Advanced Glycation End Products

Advanced glycation end products (AGEs) form when sugar is nonenzymatically linked to proteins, inducing cross-linking of the glycated proteins [super-protein complexes]. AGEs form at room temperature, but heating speeds up their formation; therefore, all cooked foods contain AGEs (formerly referred to as Maillard browning pigments). Dietary AGEs react with tissue proteins to form substances that reduce tissue elasticity and impede cellular function. AGEs have been identified as a pathogenic mechanism in diabetic nephropathy [kidney disease] and vascular complications. Approximately 10% of ingested AGEs enter the circulation, but only one third are excreted within 3 days of ingestion. Diabetes is associated with impairment in AGE excretion. In one study, urinary clearance of diet-derived AGE was 5% in diabetic individuals compared with 30% in the control group. Thus, caution is warranted with regard to the potential effects of a high sugar intake on AGE formation and increased risk of nephropathy. Additional research is needed to determine whether limiting intake of sugar in protein- and fat-containing foods reduces circulating AGE levels and risk of nephropathy.

Dietary Sugar and Overweight/Obesity

Because obesity has emerged as a major health problem in the United States and as a definite cause of cardiovascular morbidity and mortality, it is important to consider the potential impact of dietary sugar on weight gain. In human metabolic ward studies, the substitution of sucrose or other dietary carbohydrate for fat or protein in isocaloric diets shows no effect on weight or changes in energy expenditure. Some studies show that body mass index is correlated inversely with sugar consumption; however, this observation is confounded because dietary fat is correlated with obesity, and high-fat diets are lower in total and simple carbohydrate. Diets low in sugar have been associated with weight loss in some ad lib dietary studies [those in which subjects freely choose their own diets, *ad libitum*], perhaps as a result of lower total calorie consumption. Another relationship between sugar and obesity comes from studies of food preferences, which report that foods high in sugar are common choices of obese individuals. To lose weight, obese persons need to limit calorie intake; thus, limiting consumption of foods that are high in sugar (most of which have high energy density) can be a strategy for weight reduction.

Sugar and Other Health Problems

There have been a number of studies that link sugar consumption to hypertension [high blood pressure] in animals. In humans, there is one report that high dietary sugar intake enhances the risk of CHD in diabetic individuals who use diuretics [drugs that induce urination].

Sugar intake can increase carbohydrate fuel reserves and physical performance. However, this enhancement occurs only at exercise intensities and levels of physical activity associated with endurance performance of at least 30 minutes in duration. Blood glucose and liver and muscle glycogen provide the predominant fuels for muscle contraction. When these substances reach critically low amounts, fatigue may occur and consumption of sugar may rapidly return blood glucose levels to normal. For most low- to moderate-intensity activities like walking or housework, sugar consumption does not influence performance.

Another major area of interest has been the relationship between dietary sugar and behavior and cognitive function. The belief in a relationship between sugar and hyperactivity was based on two hypotheses. The first was a possible allergic response; the second was that hyperactive children might experience functional reactive hypoglycemia [low blood sugar]. Neither of these hypotheses has been proved, and a meta-analysis of 16 randomized trials in hyperactive children showed that decreasing the sugar content of the diet resulted in no improvement in degree of hyperactivity.

On the other hand, sugar is a well-established risk factor for dental caries. This observation is based on short-term cohort studies and comparisons of rates of dental caries across countries with wide variations in sugar consumption, although there is a lack of research findings regarding sugar consumption and periodontal disease.

High-Sugar Diets and Nutritional Adequacy

Diets high in sugar may adversely affect nutritional adequacy. Foods high in extrinsic sugar include soft drinks, candy, pastry, and cereals with high sugar

Table 1

Sugar Content of Typical Foods

Food Item	Amount	Sugar Content, g	Sugar Content, tsp
Table sugar, honey, or brown sugar	1 tsp	5	1
Jam/jelly	1 tbsp	10	2
Glazed doughnut	1 doughnut	10	2
Milkshake	10 oz	55	11
Fruit punch	12 oz	40	8
Cola	12 oz	40	8
Yogurt with fruit	1 cup	35	7
Candy bar	1	30	6
Apple pie	1 slice	15	3
Sweetened cereal	1 cup	15	3

Note: Sugar refers to both naturally occurring and added sugar.

Source: Sweetness and lite: Go easy on sugar and enjoy it. *Health Oasis, Mayo Clinic.* 1999. Available at: http://www.mayohealth.org/mayo/9606/htm/sugar.htm. Accessed June 8, 2000.

content (Table 1). Fat-free manufactured foods are often high in calories because of inclusion of high amounts of sugar. American Heart Association dietary guidelines stress consumption of fruits, vegetables, grains, and complex carbohydrates so that nutritional requirements for vitamins and minerals may be met by whole foods rather than by foods that are supplemented with vitamins. High-sugar foods displace whole foods (eg, soft drinks displace milk and juice consumption in children) and contribute to nutritional deficiencies, adding empty calories that few Americans need. Some studies that have assessed the nutritional adequacy of high-sugar diets do not necessarily show differences in vitamin and mineral intake because of the supplementation of these foods with vitamins and minerals instead of the preferred intake of these elements through the diet. Among children in the Bogalusa Heart Study, a linear decrease in the intake of many essential nutrients was associated with increasing total sugar intake.

The Role of Dietary Fructose, Sorbitol, and Mannitol

Sugars such as fructose (monosaccharide), sorbitol, and mannitol (sugar alcohols) are used to replace sucrose in food products and may lower the postprandial rise in glucose. In the 1970s, high-fructose syrup manufactured from [corn] starch began to be used as a replacement for sucrose in beverages and baked goods. Sorbitol and mannitol are used in a variety of "sugar-free" food products because they have fewer calories per gram than do either sucrose or fructose; in the liver they are readily converted to fructose. Fructose bypasses [certain] regulatory step[s] . . . [and] can increase very-low-density lipoprotein synthesis. In feeding studies, fructose has had inconsistent effects on plasma triglyceride levels, which may be related to factors such as the amount of fructose consumed; energy balance; and baseline triglyceride, insulin, and glucose levels. The postprandial [after eating] rise in triglyceride levels after fat intake may be augmented with the addition of fructose to a test meal. However, a study in individuals with type 2 diabetes showed a lack of significant variation in glucose, lipid, and insulin responses to three 28-day isocaloric [same calorie] feeding periods when 20% of calories were either fructose, sucrose, or starch. For most individuals, consuming fructose either free or in the form of sucrose has neither beneficial nor adverse effects.

Summary and Conclusion

As with most other dietary constituents, long-term trial data relating sugar consumption to the development of CVD events are unavailable. Longitudinal cohort studies relating sugar consumption to CVD are equivocal because of the many potential confounders that cannot be adequately controlled in the analyses. Shorter-term studies show consistent adverse effects of sugar consumption on HDL and triglyceride levels, which could accelerate atherosclerosis. High sugar consumption may worsen diabetes control, and the combination of sugar with protein and fats promotes formation of dietary AGEs, which may be especially detrimental to those with diabetes. Although increasing the amount of sugar in an isocaloric diet does not directly lead to changes in energy expenditure or weight gain in controlled feeding studies, high-sugar foods, which are sweet and calorie dense, may increase calorie consumption and lead to weight gain. Furthermore, replacement of whole foods with high-sugar foods compromises attainment of adequate dietary vitamin and mineral intake from whole food sources.

In the absence of definitive evidence, recommendations must rely on professional judgment. No data suggest that sugar intake per se is advantageous, and some data suggest it may be detrimental. The studies above, taken in total, indicate that high sugar intake should be avoided. Sugar has no nutritional value other than to provide calories. To improve the overall nutrient density of the diet and to help reduce the intake of excess calories, individuals should be sure foods high in added sugar are not displacing foods with essential nutrients or increasing calorie intake.

Anne L. Mardis

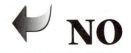

NO

Current Knowledge of the Health Effects of Sugar Intake

Twenty years ago, the common perception was that sugar intake was associated with several chronic diseases: Diabetes, coronary heart disease, obesity, and hyperactivity in children. Sugar was also thought to be the sole cause of dental caries. Recent advances in scientific knowledge, however, have shed some light on the role of sugar in chronic diseases and dental caries. The evidence indicates that sugar is not in itself associated with the aforementioned chronic diseases and is not the sole offender in the development of dental caries. This research brief discusses current scientific knowledge of the health effects of sugar.

Physiology

Despite having been labeled as "empty calories," sugars are truly important compounds from the perspective of the human organism. Humans have retained the ability to synthesize all forms of carbohydrates the body needs from simple sugars. This is not the case with the other dietary macronutrients, fats, and proteins. Following ingestion, all digestible complex dietary carbohydrates are broken down in the gut to simple sugars before they are absorbed into the body. Because simple sugars are all identical chemically, the absorption process cannot distinguish simple sugars resulting from the breakdown of complex dietary carbohydrates from corresponding simple sugars occurring naturally in the foods themselves or from corresponding simple sugars added to foods during processing. Within the body, most dietary sugars are converted to glucose, a major fuel used by all cells and the primary fuel required by brain tissue for normal function. Low levels of glucose in the blood will impair the brain and cause permanent mental impairment or worse—coma or death. The body can store a limited amount of glucose as glycogen, which it can draw upon for less than a day. After this, other sources such as proteins, from the breakdown of body tissues, must be used to synthesize glucose for the cells.

From Anne L. Mardis, "Current Knowledge of the Health Effects of Sugar Intake," *Family Economics and Nutrition Review,* vol. 13, no. 1 (2001), pp. 87–89. References and some notes omitted.

Diabetes

The relationship between dietary carbohydrates and insulin resistance (a risk factor for diabetes mellitus, ischemic heart disease, and hypertension) is not clear based on available research. In two studies based on a large, prospective study of U.S. women, sucrose and carbohydrate intake were not associated with an increased risk of diabetes. However, based on the same population, associations were found between a diet with high glycemic load[1] and high intake of refined grains and the risk of diabetes. The general consensus, based on epidemiological studies, is that sugar intake alone is not associated with the development of diabetes mellitus. Sugars fed at levels equivalent to those consumed by the U.S. population do not produce adverse glycemic effects in non-diabetics. The effects of sugar intake on glucose tolerance, insulin levels, and plasma lipids are confounded by other dietary components. The American Diabetes Association has also acknowledged, in its nutrition recommendations for people with diabetes, that there is no evidence that refined sugars such as sucrose behave any differently from other types of simple carbohydrates.

Heart Disease

The Sugars Task Force of the U.S. Food and Drug Administration presented a comprehensive review of epidemiological, clinical, and animal studies dealing with the relationship between sugar intake and heart disease or risk factors for heart disease. The report concluded that at current levels of consumption, sugar is not an adverse risk factor in heart disease. The same conclusion was made by the National Research Council in its report on chronic disease risk. There is no conclusive evidence that dietary sugar is an independent risk factor for coronary artery disease in the general population. However, hypertriglyceridemia[2] and central fat distribution,[3] consequences of abnormal glucose tolerance and diabetes mellitus, are independent risk factors for coronary heart disease. A 1996 randomized study of 32 hypertriglyceridemic patients provided evidence that an "extrinsic sugar-free" diet significantly lowers abnormally elevated plasma triglyceride levels. Evidence also suggests that insulin resistance and compensatory hyperinsulinemia[4] have major roles in the regulation of blood pressure in subjects predisposed to hypertension due to hereditary or environmental factors, possibly mediated by activity of the sympathetic nervous system. But there are multiple metabolic abnormalities associated with hyperinsulinemia in hypertensive patients that increase the risk of coronary heart disease.

Obesity

Despite popular belief that sugar causes obesity, a number of studies show an inverse relationship between reported sugar consumption and degree of overweight. An increase in the percentage of calories from sugar is, by definition, associated with a decreased consumption of calories from fat. Obesity is basically a consequence of higher energy intake than energy expenditure, where excess calories are stored as fat. The type of calories consumed is the subject of much study in obesity research. For instance, extra calories consumed as sugar cause an appropriate compensatory increase in carbohydrate oxidation (metabolism of carbohydrates for energy), whereas extra calories consumed as fat do not. Simply stated, obesity results from energy intake in excess of energy requirements. Many factors contribute to obesity, but evidence does not single out dietary sugar as a cause.

Hyperactivity

Many people still believe that sugar intake in children causes hyperactivity. A meta-analysis, however, of 16 different reports from 23 separate studies with 560 subjects showed virtually no effect of sugar intake on the hyperactivity in children. In a review of the literature, Krummel et al. reported that in 12 double-blind, placebo-controlled studies, no association was found between sugar intake and hyperactive behavior. Thus, despite numerous anecdotal perceptions to the contrary, systematic, controlled studies show that sugars do not cause hyperactivity.

Dental Caries

Dental caries is a chronic disease that has many causes. Sugar is involved in tooth decay, but it is one of many factors, including oral bacteria, saliva, tooth enamel, food substrate, and host susceptibility. All fermentable carbohydrates are potentially cariogenic. Other dietary factors such as the retention of food in the mouth affect cariogenic potential. Even starches, which may not taste sweet, are chains of glucose and are broken down to glucose in the mouth. Good oral hygiene, good genes, fluoridation of water, and restricting snacks between meals can prevent tooth decay, no matter how high the sugar consumption.

Nutrient Displacement

Research on the effects of sugar intake and nutrient displacement in the diet of children is inconclusive. In a review of the literature, Ruxton et al. found that higher intake of sugar did not negatively affect micronutrient intake. Gibney et al. found, in an analysis of the 1987–88 USDA Nationwide Food Consumption Survey, that high consumption of sugars was not associated with a poorer quality diet. In a study of 143 children ages 11 and 12 years, a 7-day weighed and recorded food inventory revealed that as the proportion of energy from sugars increased, there was no decline in dietary fiber or micronutrient intake, with the exception of niacin, which exceeded recommended levels. However, Linseisen et al. and Gibson did demonstrate intake of many micronutrients below recommended levels in persons in Germany and the United Kingdom who consumed high (energy-adjusted) amounts of sugar. In addition, high consumption of non-diet soft drinks, a significant source of added-sugar intake in children, is associated with lower consumption of milk and fruit juice and lower intake of riboflavin, vitamin A, calcium, phosphorus, and the ratio of calcium to phosphorus, which may be considered markers for milk consumption.

In an analysis of the Continuing Survey of Food Intakes by Individuals (1994–96), Bowman found that compared with Americans over 2 years of age with lower added sugar consumption as a percentage of total energy, individuals consuming greater than 18 percent of their total energy from added sugars did not meet the Recommended Daily Allowance (RDA) for many micronutrients. Farris et al. reported that as total sugar intake increased, a significant linear decrease occurred in mean intake of protein, fat, saturated fat, starch, cholesterol, sodium, vitamins B_6 and E, thiamin, niacin, iron, and zinc. Also, as total sugar intake increased, a significant linear increase occurred in mean intake of carbohydrate, fructose, lactose, sucrose, vitamin D, and calcium. But, the nutritional quality of the diet of children with higher sugar intake appeared to be adequate regarding vitamin and mineral intakes and were closer to meeting current recommendations for dietary fat. Nevertheless, a relationship between the consumption of sugars and nutrient displacement has not been observed consistently nor has there been consistency among the specific nutrients displaced when a relationship has been found. Thus, this issue remains unsettled and requires additional data from primary research.

Conclusion

Recent evidence shows that aside from dental caries, the intake of added sugars is not directly related to diabetes, heart disease, obesity, and hyperactivity, as was previously thought. This conclusion was also reached in a 1997 review of the literature on the health effects of sugar intake. Because high intake of sugars along with other factors can affect oral health and can displace important foods and nutrients in the diets of children when consumed as soft drinks, it seems prudent to limit excessive intake. But the focus on sugar as an independent risk factor for chronic disease and hyperactivity should be de-emphasized.

Notes

1. Glycemic load is a function of the effect of a carbohydrate meal on glucose levels in the blood.
2. Elevated blood levels of triglycerides: a form of fatty acid found in animal and vegetable fats.
3. A type of body fat distribution with a high ratio of waist or abdominal circumference to hip or gluteal circumference that is epidemiologically associated with heart disease and diabetes.
4. An increase in pancreatic secretion of insulin to compensate for cellular resistance to insulin.

POSTSCRIPT

Are Added Sugars Harmful to Health?

In this debate, representatives of two organizations that frequently issue dietary recommendations argue about the health effects of diets high in added sugars. The AHA, a professional organization devoted to prevention and control of coronary heart disease, maintains that sugars increase several risk factors for cardiovascular disease. Thus, the AHA suggests limits on intake of excess sugars. A representative of the USDA, a government agency responsible for promotion of the country's food supply as well as for nutrition policy, says sugars have no effect on chronic diseases except tooth decay (and even that problem can be overcome by good dental hygiene). Thus, there is no need to limit sugar intake to prevent chronic diseases.

It is difficult to separate science from politics in this debate. The idea that too much sugar is not good for health dates back many decades. Nevertheless, scientific questions about sugar and health have been difficult to resolve, mainly because studies cannot easily distinguish the effects of sugars (as a single dietary factor) from the effects of other dietary components consumed along with sugars—or of calories in general. Few studies have examined direct effects of sugars on heart disease, and studies of sugars and risk factors for heart disease and other chronic conditions often yield inconsistent or contradictory results. The authors of both selections agree that the science is uncertain. They also agree that sugar intake should be limited when it displaces more nutritious foods in the diet. Howard and Wylie-Rosett think that everyone would benefit from limiting sugar intake, but Mardis suggests limits only for children. Her review does not discuss the effects of sugars on HDL or triglyceride levels.

In this debate, the science itself is not nearly as much at issue as is the *interpretation* of the science, largely because of the economic and, therefore, political implications of the debate. Scientists at the Economic Research Service, another branch of the USDA, explain that following advice to reduce sugar intake would adversely affect the economic viability of growers of sugar cane, sugar beets, and corn, as well as the producers of food products high in sugars (see C. E. Young and L. S. Kantor in *America's Eating Habits: Changes & Consequences,* 1999). Sugar lobbying groups oppose advice to limit sugar intake and emphasize the research uncertainties. The Sugar Association, a trade organization of producers of table sugar (sucrose), for example, makes Mardis's paper available at http://www.sugar.org and refers to it as an authoritative source when challenging critics (see *Journal of the American Dietetic Association,* June 2002). The Sugar Association also promotes the idea that there are "no good or bad foods; all foods can fit into a healthy diet" and that portion size, sedentary lifestyle, and personal responsibility are more important than sugar intake in determining body weight. The Sugar Association carefully distinguishes sucrose (a double sugar of linked glucose and fructose) from corn sweeteners (glucose and fructose separated), even though enzymes in the body rapidly split sucrose into glucose and fructose.

To further confuse this debate, a committee cosponsored by the USDA is responsible for writing the *Dietary Guidelines for Americans*. Although this committee recommended in 2000 that the guideline say, "Choose beverages and foods to *limit* your intake of sugars," the USDA—reportedly under pressure from sugar lobbying groups—substituted the word *moderate*. More recently, sugar associations objected to a March 2003 report from the World Health Organization (WHO), *Diet, Nutrition and the Prevention of Chronic Diseases* (http://www.who.int/mediacentre/releases/2003/pr20/en/), which recommended that diets contain no more than 10 percent of caloric intake from added sugars. Sugar trade associations say that higher percentages are not unhealthy. The Web sites of the Sugar Association and of the WHO (http://www.who.org) provide information about this dispute. Susan Krebs-Smith, an official of the National Cancer Institute, discusses the quantitative aspects of sugar intake in a February 2001 supplement to the *Journal of Nutrition.* What level of sugar intake is moderate or should be limited? Her review concludes that Americans, and especially adolescents, consume added sugars far in excess of recommendations, and soft drinks, which are mainly made with corn sweeteners, are their major source. Few nutritionists would ever argue for a complete exclusion of sugars and soft drinks from the diet, but on the basis of calories alone, many people might view the placement of high-sugar foods at the top of the Pyramid to be a reasonable approach to dietary advice.

ISSUE 5

Do Foods With a High Glycemic Index Increase Disease Risk?

YES: David S. Ludwig, from "The Glycemic Index: Physiological Mechanisms Relating to Obesity, Diabetes, and Cardiovascular Disease," *Journal of the American Medical Association* (May 8, 2002)

NO: F. Xavier Pi-Sunyer, from "Glycemic Index and Disease," *American Journal of Clinical Nutrition* (July 2002)

ISSUE SUMMARY

YES: Physician-scientist David S. Ludwig says that habitual consumption of foods with a high glycemic index alters metabolism in ways that increase the risk for obesity, type 2 diabetes, and heart disease. He maintains that the glycemic index should be used as a guide to food selection.

NO: Physician-scientist F. Xavier Pi-Sunyer says that research on the health effects of high-glycemic index foods is uncertain and inconclusive. He concludes that it would be a mistake to suggest avoiding foods just because they display a high glycemic index.

One effect of the recent obesity epidemic has been to stimulate reexamination of long-standing advice about the composition of healthful diets. Despite the existence of dietary guidelines and food guides that recommend substitution of carbohydrate-rich foods for foods high in fat, Americans are gaining weight. Perhaps substituting carbohydrates for fat is not a good idea, especially if the carbohydrates are types that are digested and absorbed rapidly. Such carbohydrates are said to exhibit a high glycemic index, meaning that a certain amount of them causes blood sugar (glucose) levels to rise to nearly the same level as that caused by an equivalent amount of carbohydrate in a standard food, like a slice of white bread. The debate in the following selections is whether or not consuming foods containing carbohydrates with a high glycemic index alters metabolism in ways that promote weight gain and increase chronic disease risk.

In comparative tests, high-carbohydrate, bottom-of-the-Pyramid foods such as rice and potatoes display a high glycemic index. David S. Ludwig reviews evidence demonstrating that the carbohydrates in such foods raise blood glucose to levels as high as sugar itself. The pancreas responds by secreting insulin, which promotes uptake of glucose by muscle and fat cells. If there is too much glucose in the blood (hyperglycemia), then too much insulin is released (hyperinsulinemia), and blood glucose levels soon fall below normal (hypoglycemia). He maintains that hypoglycemia stimulates hunger, especially for carbohydrate foods of high glycemic index, thereby establishing a cycle that can lead to obesity. Furthermore, hyperinsulinemia increases fat deposition and also increases risks for cardiovascular disease as well as type 2 diabetes—the "adult" form in which the pancreas continues to secrete insulin but the cells resist the action of this hormone. Collectively, this complex of chronic disease risk factors is called *metabolic syndrome* or *syndrome X*. Ludwig attributes this syndrome to habitual consumption of foods of high glycemic index.

F. Xavier Pi-Sunyer, however, questions the clinical significance of the glycemic index. He argues that measurements of blood glucose after test meals vary widely, and they depend on time of day as well as on specific characteristics of the foods, such as ripeness, physical form, preparation method, and acidity. He finds little evidence for the idea that high insulin levels stimulate food intake and weight gain and finds puzzling the notion that eating high glycemic index foods might lead to syndrome X. He concludes that the strongest evidence for a role of the glycemic index in health derives from large epidemiological studies in which investigators collected information about dietary intake by means of a food frequency questionnaire (FFQ). He argues that FFQ methods are so flawed that no conclusions can be drawn about the relationship of the glycemic index to risks for heart disease and diabetes.

This debate has profound implications for dietary advice to the public. If rapidly absorbed carbohydrates do impair normal metabolic control of blood glucose and insulin levels to the point of increasing risks for obesity, heart disease, and diabetes, then recommendations to substitute carbohydrates for fat; to eat 6 to 11 daily servings of starchy foods (as recommended in the Food Guide Pyramid); and to substitute pasta, rice, bread, and potatoes for high-fat meat and dairy foods are not only wrong but dangerous to health. If, on the other hand, proponents of the glycemic index are overinterpreting its clinical effects, then dietary advice about obesity, heart disease, and diabetes should continue to focus on balancing caloric intake with expenditure, eating more fruits and vegetables, and eating foods lower in saturated fat.

The following selections should be read with questions in mind about points of agreement and disagreement but also with attention to some additional questions: Why do these authors, both physicians, disagree so strongly about the significance of the glycemic index for health? What is likely to happen to the glycemic index when carbohydrates are combined with fat or when foods are eaten in mixed meals? On what basis can one determine whether either set of arguments is sound or not?

In the following selections, Ludwig argues that high glycemic index foods are bad for health and should be avoided, but Pi-Sunyer insists that the evidence is too preliminary and contradictory to make such a suggestion.

David S. Ludwig 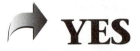 **YES**

The Glycemic Index: Physiological Mechanisms Relating to Obesity, Diabetes, and Cardiovascular Disease

All dietary carbohydrates, from starch to table sugar, share a basic biological property: they can be digested or converted into glucose. Digestion rate, and therefore blood glucose response, is commonly thought to be determined by saccharide chain length, giving rise to the terms *complex carbohydrate* and *simple sugar.* This view, which has its origins in the beginning of the century, receives at least tacit support from nutritional recommendations that advocate increased consumption of starchy foods and decreased consumption of sugar.

Throughout the past 25 years, however, the relevance of chain length in carbohydrate digestion rate has been questioned. Wahlqvist et al demonstrated similar changes in blood glucose, insulin, and fatty acid concentrations after glucose as a monosaccharide, disaccharide, oligosaccharide, or polysaccharide (starch) had been consumed. Bantle et al found no differences in blood glucose responses to meals with 25% sucrose compared with meals containing a similar amount of energy from either potato or wheat starch. Nevertheless, the physiological effects of carbohydrates may vary substantially, as demonstrated by marked differences in glycemic and insulinemic responses to ingestion of isoenergetic amounts of white bread vs. pasta (FIGURE 1). For this reason, Jenkins et al proposed the glycemic index as a system for classifying carbohydrate-containing foods according to glycemic response. This review examines the hormonal and metabolic events that occur following consumption of foods whose glycemic index differs and how these events might affect risk for or treatment of obesity, diabetes, and cardiovascular disease. . . .

Glycemic Index: A Physiological Basis for Classifying Carbohydrate

Glycemic index is defined as the incremental area under the glucose response curve after a standard amount of carbohydrate from a test food relative to that

Figure 1

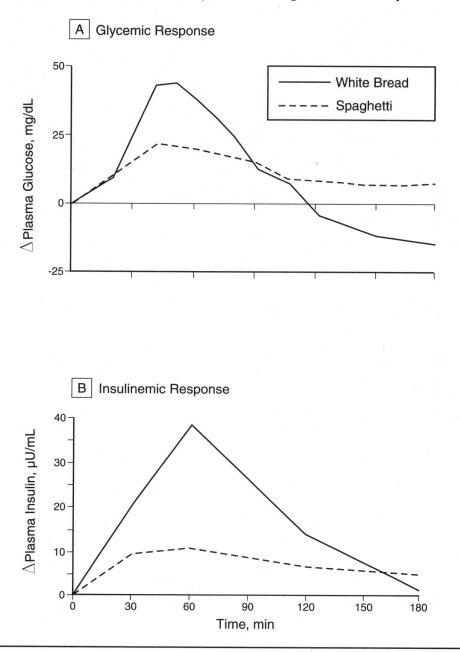

Glycemic and Insulinemic Responses After Ingestion of Carbohydrates

Responses were measured after ingestion of 50 g of carbohydrate as white bread or spaghetti made from identical ingredients. Qualitatively similar results were obtained after consumption of these foods as part of mixed meals, although nutrient interactions can modulate the magnitude of these responses to some degree. Adapted with permission from the *European Journal of Clinical Nutrition*.

of a control food (either white bread or glucose) is consumed. The glycemic index of a specific food or meal is determined primarily by the nature of the carbohydrate consumed and by other dietary factors that affect nutrient digestibility or insulin secretion. As shown in the TABLE, glycemic index values for common foods differ by more than 5-fold. In general, most refined starchy foods eaten in the United States have a high glycemic index, whereas nonstarchy vegetables, fruit, and legumes tend to have a low glycemic index. Coingestion of fat or protein lowers the glycemic index of individual foods somewhat but does not change their hierarchical relationship with regard to glycemic index. Despite initial concerns, the glycemic response to mixed meals can be predicted with reasonable accuracy from the glycemic index of constituent foods when standard methods are used. Regular consumption of high–glycemic index meals, compared with isoenergetic and nutrient-controlled low–glycemic index meals, results in higher average 24-hour blood glucose and insulin levels . . . in nondiabetic and diabetic individuals. The term *glycemic load,* defined as the weighted average glycemic index of individual foods multiplied by the percentage of dietary energy as carbohydrate, has been

Table 1

Glycemic Index and Glycemic Load Values of Representative Foods*

Food	Glycemic Index†	Glycemic Load‡
Instant rice	91	24.8 (110 g)
Baked potato	85	20.3 (110 g)
Corn flakes	84	21.0 (225 mL)
Carrot	71	3.8 (55 g)
White bread	70	21.0 (2 slices)
Rye bread	65	19.5 (2 slices)
Muesli	56	16.8 (110 mL)
Banana	53	13.3 (170 g)
Spaghetti	41	16.4 (55 g)
Apple	36	8.1 (170 g)
Lentil beans	29	5.7 (110 mL)
Milk	27	3.2 (225 mL)
Peanuts	14	0.7 (30 g)
Broccoli	. . .	. . .

*To determine the glycemic index of a specific food, subjects are given a test food and a control food on separate days, each food containing 50 g of available carbohydrate, and changes in blood glucose concentration are measured. Glycemic index is calculated with the trapezoidal rule as the incremental area under the blood glucose curve for 2 hours after the test food is eaten divided by the corresponding area after the control food is eaten, multiplied by 100%. Values for the most commonly consumed carbohydrate-containing foods have been determined and can be obtained from published lists. Ellipses indicate value not computed; the values for most nonstarchy vegetables are too low to measure.

†Glycemic index values are taken from Foster-Powell and Miller and expressed as a percentage of the value for glucose.

‡Glycemic load is calculated as the glycemic index multiplied by grams of carbohydrate per serving size, indicated in parentheses, divided by 100%.

proposed to characterize the impact of foods or dietary patterns with different macronutrient composition on glycemic response: thus, a carrot has a high glycemic index but a low glycemic load, in contrast to a potato, in which both are high (Table).

The glycemic index and glycemic load of the average diet in the United States appear to have risen in recent years because of increases in carbohydrate consumption and changes in food-processing technology. What effects might high–glycemic index diets have on health?

Acute Metabolic Events Following Consumption of a High-Glycemic Index Meal

The body has an obligatory requirement for glucose, approaching 200 g/d, determined largely by the metabolic demands of the brain. Should blood glucose concentration fall below 40 mg/dL (2.2 mmol/L), coma, seizure, or death may ensue. Conversely, blood glucose levels exceeding about 180 mg/dL (10.0 mmol/L) are associated with immediate and long-term consequences. For these reasons, blood glucose concentration is tightly regulated by homeostatic regulatory systems. Hyperglycemia [high blood sugar] stimulates insulin secretion, promoting uptake of glucose by muscle and adipose tissue. Hypoglycemia [low blood sugar] elicits secretion of . . . counterregulatory hormones that antagonize insulin action and restore normoglycemia.

The rapid absorption of glucose following consumption of a high-glycemic index meal challenges these homeostatic mechanisms. . . . Within the first 2 hours after a high–glycemic index meal (early postprandial period), integrated incremental blood glucose concentration can be at least twice that after a low–glycemic index meal containing identical nutrients and energy. This relative hyperglycemia, acting in concert with elevated concentrations of gut hormones . . . potently stimulates insulin release from pancreatic beta cells and inhibits glucagon release from alpha cells. The resultant high insulin-to-glucagon ratio would tend to exaggerate the normal anabolic responses to eating. . . . Between 2 and 4 hours after a high–glycemic index meal (middle postprandial period), nutrient absorption from the gastrointestinal tract declines, but the biological effects of the high insulin and low glucagon levels persist. Consequently, blood glucose concentration falls rapidly, often into the hypoglycemic range. . . . Approximately 4 to 6 hours after a high–glycemic index meal (late postprandial period), the low circulating concentrations of metabolic fuels trigger a counterregulatory hormone response that restores euglycemia [normal blood sugar] . . . and elevates free fatty acid concentration to levels well above those observed after a low–glycemic index meal. This combination . . . resembles a state of fasting normally reached only after many hours without food. After a low–glycemic index meal, by contrast, hypoglycemia and its hormonal sequelae do not occur during the postprandial period owing to continued absorption of nutrients from the gastrointestinal tract and rising hepatic glucose output. Thus, consumption of meals containing identical energy and nutrients can produce markedly different physiological responses throughout a 6-hour period.

Although genetic factors would be expected to influence individual response, postprandial hypoglycemia following consumption of high–glycemic index carbohydrate is so common as to be considered normal. For example, mean plasma glucose nadir was below the fasting level in the majority of 650 nondiabetic individuals who had an oral glucose tolerance test and was below 47 mg/dL (2.6 mmol/L) in 10% of the individuals. A similar phenomenon has been observed after consumption of mixed meals containing high–glycemic index foods. Moreover, postprandial hypoglycemia may be especially pronounced in obesity.

Obesity

The decreased circulating concentrations of metabolic fuels in the middle postprandial period after a high–glycemic index meal would be expected to result in increased hunger and food intake as the body attempts to restore energy homeostasis. For example, modest transient decreases in blood glucose concentration, either spontaneous or insulin-induced, were associated with hunger and initiation of feeding in rats and humans. Administration of 2-deoxyglucose, a compound that inhibits intracellular glucose use, increased hunger and food intake in nondiabetic subjects. Indeed, insulin-induced hypoglycemia appears to provoke prolonged hyperphagia [overeating], persisting well after restoration of normal blood glucose levels. Furthermore, hyperinsulinemia and hypoglycemia may preferentially stimulate consumption of high–glycemic index foods, leading to cycles of hypoglycemia and hyperphagia. Weight-loss efforts may exacerbate this phenomenon, as demonstrated by relatively severe postprandial hypoglycemia after overweight subjects on very low-calorie diets consumed high–glycemic index carbohydrate.

Experimental Evidence

There are no long-term clinical trials examining the effects of dietary glycemic index on body-weight regulation. However, numerous animal studies and short-term or small-scale studies in humans have addressed this issue. . . .

Among 16 single-day studies in humans, 15 found lower satiety, increased hunger, or higher voluntary food intake after consumption of high–compared with low–glycemic index meals. For example, obese children were given high–glycemic index instant oatmeal or low–glycemic index steel-cut oats with identical energy and macronutrient content at breakfast and lunch, and ad libitum energy consumption was monitored throughout the afternoon. Energy intake was 53% higher after the high–compared with the low–glycemic index meals.

Four groups studied the effects of dietary glycemic index in an outpatient setting. Slabber et al found significantly more weight loss in obese hyperinsulinemic women after 12 weeks of consuming an energy-restricted low–compared with high–glycemic index diet. . . . According to preliminary data,

Bouche et al found lower adiposity by DXA scan in 11 obese men after 5 weeks on an energy- and nutrient-controlled low–compared with high–glycemic index diet. . . . Spieth et al determined retrospectively that body mass index (BMI) decreased significantly more throughout an average of 4 months in children prescribed an ad libitum low–glycemic index diet compared with those prescribed an energy-restricted low-fat diet, after the effects of confounding factors were controlled. . . . In addition, Clapp found less maternal weight gain during pregnancy . . . and lower placental weight among nonobese women treated with controlled low–compared with high–glycemic index diets. Of particular note, infants born to women in the low–glycemic index group had lower adiposity. . . .

Diabetes Mellitus

. . . Calorie for calorie, high–glycemic index meals stimulate more insulin secretion than low–glycemic index meals. . . . This state of primary hyperinsulinemia may in turn cause insulin resistance. . . . These physiological changes, similar to those observed after muscle-specific inactivation of the insulin receptor gene, would . . . predispose to diabetes.

. . . Even a modest elevation in blood glucose concentration, . . . may produce insulin resistance in humans. Insulin resistance, in turn, generally leads to compensatory hyperinsulinemia. Thus, habitual consumption of high–glycemic index meals may initiate a cycle of hyperinsulinemia and insulin resistance. . . .

Experimental Evidence

. . . In humans, consumption of high–glycemic index meals compared with energy- and nutrient-controlled low–glycemic index meals adversely affects glucose tolerance at a subsequent meal. Net posthepatic glucose appearance was substantially higher 4.5 hours after ingestion of high–compared with low–glycemic index carbohydrate, suggesting resistance to insulin-stimulated uptake of glucose by the liver. However, studies of 3 to 4 weeks' duration of whole-body insulin resistance with diets differing in glycemic index yielded inconsistent results.

There are no long-term interventional studies examining the effects of dietary glycemic index in preventing diabetes mellitus, although 3 observational studies address this issue. The Nurses' Health Study and Health Professionals' Follow-up Study found that the risk of diabetes was higher among individuals in the highest quintile of glycemic index or glycemic load compared with those in the lowest quintile, after adjustment for BMI and other potentially confounding variables. By contrast, no meaningful associations were found between glycemic index or glycemic load and diabetes risk among women in the Iowa Women's Health Study.

Management of Type 1 and Type 2 Diabetes

A low–glycemic index diet may in theory improve management of diabetes by lowering early postprandial hyperglycemia and decreasing risk for postabsorptive hypoglycemia. Since 1988, 13 interventional studies have examined this possibility. . . . Twelve studies found improvement in at least 1 measure of glycemic control . . . with the low– vs high–glycemic index diet, 1 found no difference between diets, and none found improvement with the high– vs low–glycemic index diet. One of these studies reported a lower number of hypoglycemic events with the low–glycemic index diet. In addition, quality-of-life measures were higher among children who had type 1 diabetes and were counseled to follow a low–glycemic index diet compared with those who received standard dietary advice. . . . Recently, the American Diabetes Association, citing methodological issues with some of these studies, concluded that there is insufficient evidence of substantial long-term benefit to recommend use of glycemic index in the management of diabetes. Other professional associations do recognize a role for glycemic index in this regard.

Cardiovascular Disease

The higher postprandial blood glucose and insulin levels found in a high–glycemic index diet may affect risk for cardiovascular disease (CVD). . . .

Postprandial Hyperglycemia

Postprandial hyperglycemia has recently been recognized as an important risk factor for CVD not only among persons with diabetes, but also among the general population. . . .

Postprandial hyperglycemia appears to increase CVD risk by producing oxidative stress. . . . Administration of antioxidants can prevent or reverse these adverse effects. Thus, it is reasonable to hypothesize that habitual consumption of high–glycemic index meals increases the risk for CVD, at least in part by hyperglycemia-induced oxidative stress.

Hyperinsulinemia

A high–glycemic index diet may also affect the risk for CVD by increasing insulin levels. . . . Hyperinsulinemia is believed to mediate, in part, the increased risk for heart disease associated with the insulin resistance syndrome (also known as syndrome X or the metabolic syndrome). . . .

Experimental Evidence

Thirteen interventional studies have examined the effects of dietary GI on serum lipids under macronutrient-controlled conditions. . . . Of 6 observational studies, 5 demonstrated higher HDL cholesterol levels, lower triglyceride levels, or lower myocardial infarction rates among individuals in the lowest category of glycemic index or glycemic load compared with those in the highest category, after adjustment for potentially confounding factors. Two of these studies directly compared glycemic index and glycemic load with respect to serum lipid concentrations: one found that glycemic load had a greater effect; the other, that both had similar effects. The sixth observational study found no significant association between glycemic index and heart disease.

Controversies

The clinical relevance of glycemic index has been vigorously debated in recent years. Some experts argue that any beneficial effects of low–glycemic index diets on insulin resistance and related CVD risk factors are small in comparison with that of reduced-carbohydrate diets. Another concern is that the concept of glycemic index might be too complicated to be practical or that potentially simpler principles, such as energy density, effectively incorporate many of the advantageous aspects of low–glycemic index diets.

In response to these concerns, the following points should be considered. First, several dozen interventional studies have described statistically and clinically significant improvements in end points related to obesity, diabetes, or CVD among free-living subjects consuming self-selected low– vs. high–glycemic index diets. Second, observational studies link glycemic index to disease risk within prevailing dietary patterns. Third, several studies suggest that the beneficial effects of a low–glycemic index diet may be independent of, or additive to, that of other dietary manipulations involving carbohydrate content" or energy density. Fourth, low–glycemic index diets have no known adverse effects, in contrast with low-fat diets, for example, that may adversely affect serum HDL cholesterol and triglyceride concentrations. Fifth, whereas the concept of glycemic index may be complex from a food science perspective, its public health application can be simple: increase consumption of fruits, vegetables, and legumes, choose grain products processed according to traditional rather than modern methods (eg, pasta, stone-ground breads, old-fashioned oatmeal), and limit intake of potatoes and concentrated sugar. Indeed, these recommendations would tend to promote diets high in fiber, micronutrients, and antioxidants and low in energy density. . . .

Other questions remain unresolved: How do the long-term benefits of low–glycemic index and low–glycemic load diets compare with each other and with those of diets focused on other nutritional properties? To what extent do associated factors (eg, fiber, micronutrients, or antioxidants) contribute to the observed protective effects of low–glycemic index diets? How does glycemic index interact with genetic and lifestyle risk factors in the initiation and progression of disease? Mechanistically oriented studies, multicenter clinical trials, and prospective epidemiological analyses are needed to address these issues.

Conclusion

The rate of carbohydrate absorption after a meal, as quantified by glycemic index, has significant effects on postprandial hormonal and metabolic responses. . . . Thus, the habitual consumption of high–glycemic index foods may increase risk for obesity, type 2 diabetes, and heart disease, a hypothesis that derives considerable support from laboratory studies, clinical trials, and epidemiological analyses. Despite areas of continuing controversy, clinical use of glycemic index as a qualitative guide to food selection would seem to be prudent in view of the preponderance of evidence suggesting benefit and absence of adverse effects.

F. Xavier Pi-Sunyer

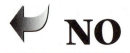

Glycemic Index and Disease[a-d]

Abstract

It has been suggested that foods with a high glycemic index are detrimental to health and that healthy people should be told to avoid these foods. This paper takes the position that not enough valid scientific data are available to launch a public health campaign to disseminate such a recommendation. This paper explores the glycemic index and its validity and discusses the effect of postprandial glucose and insulin responses on food intake, obesity, type 1 diabetes, and cardiovascular disease. Presented herein are the reasons why it is premature to recommend that the general population avoid foods with a high glycemic index. *Am J Clin Nutr* 2002;76:290S–8S.

Key Words

Glycemic index, glucose, insulin, obesity, diabetes, cardiovascular disease

Introduction

Although Otto et al (1, 2) first brought attention to the different glycemic effects of various foods, the glycemic index (GI) was initially conceived by Jenkins et al (3) as a tool for the dietary management of type 1 diabetes and, later, dyslipidemia [abnormal blood lipid levels] (4). Jenkins' initial studies compared 50-g portions of various carbohydrates (calculated from food tables) with 50 g glucose. Venous blood samples were taken fasting and at 30-min intervals for 2 h after the ingestion of carbohydrate. The area above (or below, as sometimes occurs) the fasting glucose concentration was calculated and was expressed as a percentage of the area obtained after the ingestion of 50 g glucose; the higher the area under the curve (AUC), the higher the GI of a food.

Subsequently, the standard against which foods are compared was changed to white bread (5, 6). This is unfortunate for 2 reasons: first, published GI values conflict; second, 50 g carbohydrate in white bread is more difficult to

From F. Xavier Pi-Sunyer, "Glycemic Index and Disease," *American Journal of Clinical Nutrition,* vol. 76, suppl. (July 2002), 290S–298S. Copyright © 2002 by The American Society for Clinical Nutrition. Reprinted by permission. The American Society for Clinical Nutrition, Inc. does not endorse any commercial enterprise.

determine accurately than is 50 g glucose. A comparative standard should be simple, accurate, and reproducible, and the one used to calculate GI is not.

It is important to remember in this debate that the GI was originally conceived as an inherent property of the food, and not as a metabolic response of an individual to the food. As such, any food would have a consistent and theoretically reproducible response from person to person, independent of other food with which it is ingested.

The question debated at the symposium *Is the Glycemic Index Important in Human Nutrition* was whether a diet that includes high-GI foods is detrimental to health. This report begins with the calculation of GI and then discusses the factors that influence the GI of a food and the "carbohydrate/insulin/disease" hypothesis. The discussion includes a critical review of some of the reports dealing with this concept, particularly as they relate to food intake, obesity, and diabetes.

Calculation of the Area Under the Curve for Glucose

Several technical limitations to the calculation of the GI must be considered when determining its worth as a nutritive marker for dietary recommendations. Glucose molecules are all the same and circulate in the bloodstream similarly. Is a glucose molecule that is considered to be below the fasting glucose concentration different from one above it? If not, why should the AUC for all of the available glucose not be used for the calculation? Several experts favor the use of the whole AUC as the real measure of glucose availability (7, 8). If the AUC is calculated in this manner, the differences in GIs between foods are greatly attenuated. For example, a person with a fasting glucose of 75 mg/dL ingests 2 foods, one with a GI of 100 and the other a GI of 72. If the GI is calculated by using the whole glucose AUC instead of the area above the fasting glucose, the values would be 100 and 92, respectively. The difference changes from an impressive 28 units to an unimpressive 8 units.

The postprandial disposal of glucose can take much longer than 2 h, especially in persons with diabetes (7). The choice to codify the glucose response using the 2-h standard made little sense because this standard was established only as a diagnostic tool for identifying type 2 diabetes and impaired glucose tolerance, not to mark the total period of postprandial glucose elevation. Patients with type 2 diabetes require much longer than 2 h for their blood glucose to return to normal concentrations, if at all. Gannon and Nuttall (7) showed that differences in GIs between foods greatly narrow as longer postprandial time frames are used to measure GI. Thus, the difference between 100 and 72 would be considerably less if the AUC were calculated for a more reasonable postprandial period of 4 h.

The GI has been defined as the testing of a person in the morning, after an overnight fast. However, AUCs differ if the test is given in the morning or as the second or third meal of the day (9–12). Had the standard been set to test for lunch rather than for breakfast, the differences in GIs between foods would be considerably less. A study by Brand-Miller (13) showed no difference between the glucose response to the second meal of the day whether it was a high-GI or a low-GI repast. This was also true of a study by Gannon et al (14). So, should we worry about GI primarily for breakfast?

Factors Affecting the Reproducibility of the GI

In tables compiled by Foster-Powell and Miller (15), the variability in the GI of glucose, the carbohydrate that can most accurately be measured, was 85–111 (ie, 25%). Even for foods that require no preparation (eg, cutting or cooking) before ingesting, such as whole milk and ice cream, the GI varied from 11 to 40 and from 36 to 68, respectively. In fact, the variability of GIs for many individual foods exceeds the calculated mixed-meal GI of the 5 population quintiles reported in the Nurses' Health Study, which ranged from 72 to 80 in one report (16) and from 64 to 77 in another (17). So, can we really tell people that the GI of a food is predictable?

Ripeness of Fruit

The ripeness of fruit affects the GI. As a fruit ripens, starch is changed to sugar. The starch generally has a higher GI than does the sugar, so as ripeness progresses, the GI decreases, such as was reported for bananas (18). So, are we going to tell the public that they can eat fruit at some points in their maturation and not in others?

Physical Form of Foods

Changing the particle size of some foods changes their GIs (19, 20). For example, the GI of a 1-inch cube of potato can increase by 25% just by mashing the cube (21). Consumption of whole apples, apple purée, and apple juice results in significantly different glucose and insulin excursions (22). So, are we going to tell the public that they can eat one physical form of a food but not another?

Variability Within Food Classes

The GI value of an individual food can vary widely depending on its type, the way it is processed, and the way it is prepared.

Type

Different types of a particular food can have different GIs. For example, different types of rice can have different GIs. The GI of rice is affected by the proportion of amylose to amylopectin in the grains. Amylose is a linear molecule with D-glucose units linked in an ($\alpha 1-4$) fashion. Amylopectin has both ($\alpha 1-4$) and (α-1–6) linkages (23), and is thereby a branched structure. The higher the proportion of amylopectin, the higher the GI, because amylopectin, which is made up of branched-starch molecules, is more easily hydrolyzed in the gut than is the single-strand amylose (24). Thus, 50-g equivalents of different rices produce

GIs ranging from 68 to 103 (15). So, are we going to specify for the public which kind of rice is eatable and which is not?

Pasta also produces different GIs depending on its type. The GIs of macaroni, star pastina, and spaghetti are 68, 54, and 45, respectively (25). Because different types of pasta can produce different glycemic responses, should we ban macaroni and allow spaghetti to be eaten? Even within a class of pasta, such as linguini, a different thickness will result in a different GI. Thin linguini has a GI of 87, and thick linguini has a GI of 68 (26). How would we advise the public about this major difference?

Processing

The method of processing of a single food can greatly change its GI. Starch exists in carbohydrate foods in the form of large granules. These granules must be disrupted so that the amylose or amylopectin starch macromolecules become available for hydrolysis. Grinding, rolling, pressing, or even thoroughly chewing a kernel or other starch food can disrupt the granules. Rolling or pressing foods, such as is done in the processing of many grains, disrupts the outer germ layer and granules and increases GI (27).

Chemically modifying a food also affects its GI. For instance, 1–2% acetylated potato starch decreases the GI (28), as does the addition of β-cyclodextrin to stabilize the carbohydrate (28).

The application of heat and moisture affects starch granules. Disorganization of the crystalline structure occurs as it encounters greater heat and moisture for a longer period of time. Gelatinization occurs first, with disruption of the crystalline structure, followed by a disruption of the granules. If the starch is then let stand, or stored for a time, so that cooling occurs, the starch becomes a gel, which will vary in structure depending on the amount of moisture, the amylose to amylopectin ratio and the time and temperature of storage (23). A crystallinity to the gel can occur that is called retrogradation of the starch. These starch complexes are insoluble and not amenable to hydrolysis in the small intestine. Repeated cycles of heating and cooling can further the retrogradation (29). Starch can also form insoluble complexes with proteins, such as occurs in the browning (Maillard) reaction, making it unavailable for digestion and absorption.

Preparation

The cooking method affects the GI beyond the effects of mashing or puréeing food, as mentioned above. For example, uncooked potato is resistant to hydrolysis, but when it is cooked the starch granules gelatinize and become readily digestible. When the potatoes are then cooled, the gelatinization reverses and some 12% of the potato starch is resistant to hydrolysis and cannot be absorbed (30).

The heat utilized, the amount of water, and the time of cooking, all have a significant effect on the GI (31, 32). Thus, the more a starch-containing food is heated, moisturized, ground, or pressed, the more it will be amenable to hydrolysis and digestion, except for the portion that forms insoluble complexes. This then, belies the concept that a food has a definitive GI, because the GI is dependent on the history of the processing, storing, ripening, cutting, and cooking of the food. So, shall we allow a grain to be eaten if processed or cooked in one manner but not if processed or cooked in another manner? Does a consumer need to know about retrogradation?

Effects of a Combination of Macronutrients on the GI

People do not generally eat single foods, they eat meals or snacks made up of ≥ 2 macronutrients. Several studies have investigated the effects of combinations of macronutrients on the GI and have shown 2 things: *1)* the higher the proportion of carbohydrate in a specific food, as opposed to protein and fat, the higher the GI; and *2)* a mixed meal of carbohydrate, protein, and fat will have a different and variable glucose response depending on the proportions of each nutrient. Thus, the glucose responses of a food eaten alone or in combination with other foods differ (33–35). Proponents of the GI have denied this (13, 36), but I have provided some examples below.

Protein, Fat, and Carbohydrate

Protein-rich foods are known to increase insulin secretion without augmenting glucose concentrations (37–39). Thus, whereas the glucose response does not change much or actually decreases, the insulin response increases. Therefore, as more protein is taken in conjunction with carbohydrate, the insulin response will increase, whereas postprandial glucose will not change much. Similarly, adding fat to a carbohydrate meal also enhances insulin secretion even though the plasma glucose response actually decreases (12, 40, 41). Also, all 3 macronutrients stimulate the release of several gut peptides, but to different degrees. Protein and fat are particularly efficacious in stimulating gut peptide release despite a small glucose effect (42). Thus, the insulin response to a carbohydrate food varies with the amount of fat, protein, or both, with which it is ingested.

There are many foods that do not contain carbohydrates only, but are mixed with other macronutrients. Thus, there may be foods that have a lower GI but would not be recommended for other reasons. For example, chocolate and cashews have low GIs but contain large amounts of fat. Other foods may have high GIs but be nutritionally more attractive because they are less energy dense and more nutritionally rich with micronutrients. An example is carrots.

Fiber

The extent to which the fiber in a particular food is responsible for its GI is a subject of much debate. Wolever (43) studied this relation in 25 foods and found that total dietary fiber was related to the GI ($r = 0.461$, $P < 0.05$), although weakly. Breaking it down, he found no significant relation between soluble fiber and GI, but found the strongest relation between insoluble fiber and GI ($r = 0.584$, $P < 0.001$); he attributed the effect to the uronic acids in insoluble fiber. However, he could only explain 50% of the variability by fiber differences. In contrast with the above findings, other studies in which fiber was added to a carbohydrate meal suggested that only soluble fiber has an effect on postprandial glucose concentrations and not the insoluble component (44). However, does the presence of naturally occurring fiber in foods affect the glucose response? It seems to have very little relation (3, 45). Comparisons between brown and white rice, brown and white spaghetti, and whole-wheat and white bread showed small differences in the GI, although the fiber contents were quite different. Jenkins et al (3), in testing several foods, found no relation at all between the GI and the fiber content of the food. Holt et al (46) found no relation between the postprandial insulin response to and the fiber content of a food. In persons with type 2 diabetes, no effect of fiber on glucose concentrations was found (44, 47). Long-term studies have not been done in nondiabetic subjects.

Sugar

In the past, diabetic patients were prohibited from eating dietary sucrose because it was thought to raise blood glucose concentrations inordinately. We now know that the GI of sucrose (using white bread as a standard) is relatively low at 65. The GI of glucose is 97, whereas those of fructose and lactose are 23 and 46, respectively (15). One would expect that adding sugar to a meal would lower the GI; however, Jenkins et al (3) found no relation between the sugar content in foods and the GI in 62 commonly eaten foods, nor did Brand-Miller (13). These findings remain unexplained, but they certainly complicate the entire GI issue.

Acidity

An increase in the acidity of a meal can greatly lower its GI. Increasing the amount of vinegar in a meal, for instance, will affect the glucose response. The addition of sourdough bread to a meal can result in different GIs, depending on its content of organic acids (48). These foods apparently affect the glucose response, at least partially, by slowing gastric emptying. So, should we alert consumers to check how much vinegar they put on their food and how much acid is in their bread?

Predictability of the Insulin Response

It has been widely assumed that the insulin response is proportional to the glucose response, and therefore that the glycemic response is an accurate predictor of the insulin response. This is not the case. For instance, as one increases the amount of a carbohydrate food ingested, the amount of insulin does not increase proportionately. Plasma insulin responses increase at a much faster rate than do plasma glucose responses (49). One cannot therefore predict that the insulin effect expected from a 50-g portion of a particular food would be doubled by ingesting a 100-g portion. Therefore, if the culprit we are trying to guard against is a high insulin response, it is a moving target that will depend considerably more on the portion size than on the GI of a food.

What is the best way to compare foods if one is looking for the insulin response? One could argue that it is better to compare normal serving sizes of a particular food or isoenergetic servings rather than to compare 50-g portions. Holt et al (46) compared the effect of isoenergetic amounts of foods on the insulin secretory response and found that the postprandial insulin responses were not closely related to the carbohydrate content or to the glycemic effects of the foods. Whereas the glycemic response was a significant predictor of the insulin response, it accounted for only 23% of the variability in the insulinemia. This implies that many factors other than an increase in glucose influence the secretory response of insulin. This is certainly not a surprise to anyone familiar with β-cell physiology.

Another way of looking at the insulin response is to compare the insulin response with the response to 1 g carbohydrate. The result of this comparison does not fit well with the GI hypothesis that high-GI foods, such as potatoes, are "bad." In fact, potatoes, baked beans, and lentils release insulin at rates of 284, 504, and 325 (pmol/L)$\cdot$g$^{-1}\cdot$ min^{-1}, respectively. Thus, of these foods, potatoes produce the least effect per gram carbohydrate (46).

Because the glycemic response can only predict 23% of the variability in the insulin response to an ingested food, other factors may be important. These factors include osmolality, gastric emptying, gut hormone release, and viscosity of gut contents (46); antecedent diet and degree of obesity (50); age (51); and even sex (12).

GI as the Cause of Disease

In recent years, the GI has been transformed by its popularizers from a potentially useful tool in planning diets for diabetic patients to a key player for the prevention of diabetes, dyslipidemia, cardiovascular disease, and even certain cancers in the general population. The debate concerns whether such a transformation is justified. That is, whether it is wise and reasonable to set as a public health policy for the entire population the avoidance of certain foods because of their high GI. To explore this question, one needs to examine the supporting data, their quantity and quality, their relation to causation, and the possible presence of confounders.

There are 2 theories about how high-GI foods increase food intake. The first is that it is a result of the elevation in glucose and the second, more commonly expressed recently, is that it is the result of a high insulin response. This high insulin response has been related to several phenomena: increased food intake leading to obesity (52), hyperinsulinemia leading to insulin resistance (53), β-cell exhaustion leading to type 2 diabetes (17, 54), dyslipidemia leading to coronary heart disease (CHD) (55), and unknown factors leading to certain kinds of cancers. What is the evidence for these suggested effects and how convincing is it?

Obesity

Single-Meal Studies

Several studies have examined whether a high postprandial glucose concentration is associated with satiety. In studies unrelated to the GI, results have generally shown that a high postprandial blood glucose concentration is associated with greater satiety (56–59). Also, several studies have tried to separate the effects of glucose and insulin on satiety (56–62) and most reported that glucose, rather than insulin, is the satiety signal.

Most of the data relating a high GI to increased food intake were collected in single-meal, experimental designs. The general pattern of investigation has been to give subjects a preload of a given carbohydrate food and observe the free food intake at a subsequent meal. Alternatively (and less satisfactorily), a preload was given but no measurement of meals followed; only a measure of hunger or satiety was ascertained by questionnaire. Many of these studies used liquid preloads and sugars rather than starches and some of the test meals that followed were liquid. At least 20 reports have measured hunger and satiety, but only 6 actually measured food intake.

Of the 20 studies that only measured subjective hunger or satiety rather than actual food intake, only 10 appear to be valid because they controlled for energy intake, energy density, and the palatability of the test meal (22, 24, 61, 63–69). In these studies, no consistent effect of a high-GI food compared with that of a low-GI food on hunger or satiety was shown. Four studies found a positive association between the low-GI food and greater satiety, reduced hunger, or both; 2 studies found a positive association between the high-GI food and greater hunger, reduced satiety, or both; and 4 studies found no difference. In 6 studies that actually measured intake at a subsequent meal, 3 found a significant effect of high-GI foods in increasing intake and 3 did not (64, 65, 68–71). Of the 3 that found significant effects, 2 compared only glucose and fructose, which is not a fair comparison of high- and low-GI foods because of other differential metabolic effects of these sugars that are unrelated to their GI effects.

Long-Term Studies

Long-term interventional studies are few, but worth reviewing, because the effect of a high- compared with a low-GI diet must surely be judged on the basis of its long-term effects on health and disease and not on the basis of a single-meal paradigm. The longest careful study was that by Kiens and Richter (72), who provided all food to lean volunteers who could eat as much as they wished for 30 d. After 30 d of consuming high- or low-GI diets in a crossover design, there was no difference in weight between the groups. This finding suggests that there was no significant difference in food intake between the groups. A shorter, 2–wk study, in which 6 healthy lean volunteers consumed high- or low-GI diets, also had no significant effect on body weight (9).

Insulin as a Hyperphagic Hormone

The experimental data that relate insulin to food intake suggest that insulin at physiologic concentrations reduces food intake (73). It is well known that insulin crosses the blood-brain barrier (74); that there are insulin receptors in the brain, and particularly in brain areas involved in energy homeostasis (75); that insulin suppresses food intake when injected directly into the brain (76); and that transgenic mice with a neuron-specific lack of insulin receptors become obese (77). Studies in rodents (78, 79) and primates (76) have shown that food intake and body weight decline when insulin is infused into the third ventricle.

Thus, there is no extant evidence that insulin at postprandial concentrations enhances food intake and body weight above normal. The belief that insulin increases body weight has grown out of the clinical experience of using large doses of insulin in type 2 diabetic patients. However, in these instances, insulin was given in amounts well above normal and systemically, not in the portal vein, which induces higher than usual circulating concentrations of the hormone. Also, investigators studying food intake regulation have given rodents large doses of insulin, enough to cause hypoglycemia, and have induced instances of overfeeding. However, nonphysiological amounts of the hormone were used. The theory that insulin, at physiologic concentrations, triggers weight gain has no evidence to support it (79). In fact, increased insulin secretion actually protects against subsequent weight gain in obese humans (80).

Postprandial Hyperglycemia and Hyperinsulinemia Leading to Insulin Resistance

The argument has been made that the hyperglycemia and hyperinsulinemia produced by a high-GI diet lead to insulin resistance, and that insulin resistance then leads to the development of diabetes, coronary artery disease, and other features of Syndrome X (81). This is a puzzling charge, given the available experimental data.

Two relatively long metabolic studies compared the association between high- and low-GI diets and increasing insulin resistance, one of which was the previously mentioned study by Kiens and Richter (72). In that study, healthy young men were fed isoenergetic high- or low- GI diets for 30 d. The mean GI for the low-GI diet was 24 units lower than that of the high-GI diet. The carbohydrate contents of the 2 diets was kept the same. Euglycemic hyperinsulinemic clamp procedures were performed before and at the end of the dietary study. Fasting glucose, fasting insulin, and fasting triacylglycerol concentrations were no different at the end of the study than at the beginning. The glucose disposal rate was similar with the 2 diets at an insulin infusion rate of 2.4 nmol/L, and it was significantly greater in the high-GI diet group at a higher insulin infusion rate of 370 pmol/L. Thus, there was no evidence of the development of greater insulin resistance with the high-GI diet than with the low-GI diet; in fact, the opposite effect occurred—lower insulin resistance was found with the high-GI diet.

The other study, conducted by Frost et al (53), is problematic. The study subjects were women who said they had no personal or family history of diabetes, hypertension, or other chronic disease. However, the report states that the subjects were divided into 2 groups, one with a parental history of CHD and one without. The subjects were not assigned randomly to high-GI, low-GI, or control diet groups. The control group comprised the women ($n = 33$) who refused to be randomly assigned, and the test group comprised the women ($n = 28$) who agreed to be assigned, half to the high-GI and half to the low-GI group for 3 wk. Some of these women had parental histories of cardiac disease and some did not. Those without a parental history of cardiac disease showed no difference in glucose uptake by fat cells taken from either subcutaneous or omental adipocytes. Those with parental histories of cardiac disease in the high-GI diet group had a significantly lower glucose uptake above baseline than did those in the low-GI diet group. A short intravenous insulin tolerance test of 15 min was done in some, but not all, of these women, with the slope of the plasma glucose decrease being measured between 3 and 15 min. Insulin sensitivity was significantly lower in both groups of women consuming the high-GI diet as compared with the low-GI diet. Because this study was poorly designed, did not randomly assign its subjects, and used an imprecise measurement of insulin sensitivity, particularly when not using arterialized blood samples, the significance of the study is unclear at best.

An older but better-designed study compared the effects of higher- and lower-carbohydrate diets. Thompson et al (82) showed that the higher-carbohydrate diet, fed for 10 d, resulted in greater insulin sensitivity than did the lower-carbohydrate diet. Thus, the diet with a greater glycemic load and a greater insulin demand resulted in greater insulin sensitivity. Two other interventional studies, conducted in healthy individuals and with durations of 3–5 and 21–28 d, also showed greater insulin sensitivity with a high-carbohydrate diet (83, 84); a third study showed no differences (85).

β-Cell Exhaustion Leading to Type 2 Diabetes

Although it is evident that β-cell exhaustion is one of the steps leading to the development of type 2 diabetes (86), it is considered in most cases to follow a period of insulin resistance (87, 88). Studies in Pima Indians have shown that the pathophysiology of type 2 diabetes begins with insulin resistance and, in those with the genetic predisposition, leads eventually to β-cell failure (89). Thus, to conclude that high-GI diets result in diabetes, it must first be definitively shown that these diets result in insulin resistance that in turn increases the insulin demand to such an extent that it eventually overwhelms and exhausts the pancreas. No such evidence exists, as noted previously. In fact, data from countries whose populations ingest high-carbohydrate diets and thus have an increased insulin demand, show a generally lower incidence of diabetes.

A High GI and Disease: Evidence From Epidemiologic Studies

Epidemiologic studies have been the primary impetus for the contention that high-GI diets lead to disease. The main epidemiologic studies purporting this contention are the Nurses' Health Study and the Health Professionals' Follow-Up Study (16, 17, 54). The Nurses' Health Study is a large, prospective cohort study of US women followed for several years, the duration depending on the study being reported. The cohort contained 121 700 female registered nurses aged 30–55 y at enrollment, residing in 11 states. Nutritional and outcome data were collected by means of mailed questionnaires. The Health Professionals' Follow-Up Study is another large, prospective longitudinal study of diet and lifestyle in relation to chronic diseases among 51 529 men aged 40–75 y at baseline in 1986 (54, 90). In the Nurses' Health Study, in 1980, a 61-item food-frequency questionnaire (FFQ) was used. In 1984, the questionnaire was expanded to 116 items. Similar questionnaires were again used in 1986 and 1990. The 1986 questionnaire was used as baseline and was completed by only 75 543 women. Women with ≥ 11 questionnaire items left blank, a total energy intake of < 2512 or > 14 654 kJ/d, or previously diagnosed disease (changing according to the report) were excluded. The final number of subjects valid for analysis was 65 173.

In the Health Professionals' Follow-Up Study, the FFQ given in 1986 included 131 items. Men were excluded if 70 of 131 total food items were left blank (even though "almost never" eaten was an option in the questionnaire). Thus, the persons who filled out the FFQs could ignore 61 of 131 items and still qualify. Persons reporting a calculated intake of < 800 or > 4200 kcal/d (54) were excluded. Also excluded were persons with a history of a disease that might have induced them to modify their diet. For the diabetes study, 42 759 men were found eligible and were followed for 6 y.

The FFQ required participants to estimate portion sizes and write down how often they ate a particular item of a particular size during the previous year. The authors stated that the reproducibility and validity of the FFQ were acceptable and provided information to support this contention in 5 validation reports (91–95). The validation plan has been the same for both men and women. A very small sample was chosen for the validation: 323 of 51 529 men (95) and 225 of 75 543 women (92). This was clearly not a representative sample, but a convenience sample in the Boston area. Of this sample, not all agreed to participate: only 127 men and 150 women did so. Two 1-wk diet records were kept ≈6–7 mo apart by the men and 4 were kept by the women in a given year. The first week's record was taken ≈3 mo after the first FFQ was administered and the second week's record ≈2–3 mo before the second FFQ was administered. Of the 1565 unique diet-record food codes, 348 were eliminated, "usually because they were not consumed frequently in this population" (95). Also, it is stated that "because of the small number of subjects ($n = 127$) relative to the number of food items, we collapsed the individual food items into 40 predefined food groups" (95). Some of the items collapsed into one category were all whole grains, all refined grains, all cold breakfast cereals, all fruit, and all fruit juices. It is difficult to believe that such a wholesale collapse of individual foods into large categories could produce a reliable measure of the GI of a diet. For example, Holt et al (46), who measured the GI of foods and placed them in categories, found a statistically significant difference between the foods within such food categories. Pearson correlation coefficients between the FFQs and the dietary records, corrected for week-to-week variation, ranged from 0.45 to 0.74. The actual range provided in the table was 0.21–0.83. The average dietary GI and the global dietary glycemic load were derived from the FFQs as follows

$$\text{Average dietary GI} = [(\text{carbohydrate content of each food item})$$
$$\times (\text{number of servings/d}) \times (\text{GI})]/$$
$$\text{total daily carbohydrate intake} \qquad (1)$$
$$\text{Global dietary glycemic load} = (\text{carbohydrate content of each food item})$$
$$\times (\text{number of servings/d}) \times (\text{GI}) \qquad (2)$$

Salmeron et al (17) stated that "the glycemic index, as a relative measure of glycemic response to a given amount of carbohydrate, does represent the quality of carbohydrate but does not take into account the quantity," whereas "In contrast, the total glycemic load represents the combination of quality as well as quantity of carbohydrate consumed, and may be interpreted as a measure of insulin demand." Let us look, then, at how these 2 values are calculated. The carbohydrate content of each food item was taken from food tables; however, we know that the carbohydrate content of a food varies. Clearly, the portion size is crucial to knowing the actual carbohydrate content. How is the portion size a person eats calculated? The person estimates it; the question gives "standard portions." The person also estimates the number of servings of the food item per year, and this amount is reduced by the investigators to the number of servings eaten per day. Finally, the GI is estimated for the particular food item from a table (for which a reference was not given). This estimate is then divided by the total amount of carbohydrate eaten per day, again derived from the FFQ, consolidating the carbohydrate contents of all foods eaten per year and reduced down to the amount eaten per day.

Thus, 4 very imprecise numbers are derived, 3 of which are then multiplied and divided by the fourth number. This process magnifies the imprecision even more. These values are then used to extrapolate to the effect of these nutrients on the development of disease. In addition, only one year's FFQ was used for the analysis in the diabetes studies—the one provided shortly after entry into the study. It is assumed that the diet then stays constant for the next 10 or more years, during which the appearance of disease is tracked. The persons being followed in these studies are all health professionals. Is it not possible that many would change their diet depending on the prevailing recommendations of the day? Can one be sure that these cohorts have maintained the same diets that they reported consuming 10 or more years before? In fact, one study suggests that over the period of the study, the nurses' diets improved significantly (96).

I believe that the final numbers derived for use in these widely quoted studies are extremely imprecise. In a laboratory-based report, the reliability of these measures would never be accepted, and the validation done would be considered inadequate. Tseng (97) identified the validation problem as follows: "validation of FFQ-based dietary patterns against dietary record based patterns with use of scales derived from factor analysis based on the same food items is comparable with validation of a scale against the same scale with individual items measured more accurately. In essence, the validation strategy presumes that the item level data are valid and uses these data rather than an independent indicator of each food pattern."

Despite the caveats in the methods used to derive the data from these prospective studies, let us look at the results of these studies concerning the development of diabetes. Categorized by quintiles of the GI of the diet eaten, the dietary glycemic load (ie, the measure of insulin demand) of the women was not significantly different across the quintiles (P < 0.09). The average dietary GI showed a significant trend ($P < 0.04$). In the men, neither the glycemic load ($P = 0.83$) nor the GI ($P = 0.12$) was significantly different across the quintiles. These are hardly convincing data.

It is also somewhat puzzling that there was no significant effect of the total amount of carbohydrate eaten on the development of diabetes in these 2 studies. One would think that if the glycemic load were the culprit, the insulin demand would have been greater the greater the carbohydrate intake and significantly correlated with the disease.

The results of several other long-term longitudinal studies do not agree with the above findings about the risk of the development of type 2 diabetes. These studies reported that populations ingesting a high-carbohydrate diet, which results in higher postprandial glucose concentrations and higher insulin demand, actually have a lower level of insulin resistance, diabetes mellitus, and cardiovascular disease. In the San Luis Valley Diabetes Study (98), for instance, a high-fat, low-carbohydrate diet, which by definition has a lower glycemic load, is associated with a higher incidence of diabetes than is a higher-carbohydrate diet that has a higher glycemic load. Also, in the Iowa Women's Health Study (99), no significant effect of high-carbohydrate diets on diabetes incidence was found.

Ecologic (100–103) and cross-sectional (98, 104) studies have also shown that a high-fat, low-carbohydrate diet increases the risk of diabetes. A case-control study by Himsworth and Marshall (105) and several prospective studies (106–108) also suggest that a high-fat, low-carbohydrate (ie, a low glycemic load) results in a higher incidence of diabetes.

What about the evidence for the development of CHD? In the Nurses' Health Study, glycemic load and GI were significantly related to risk of CHD (P for trend < 0.0001; 16). However, in reporting trends in CHD in relation to diet (96), the authors stated that the incidence of heart disease decreased during the study period, yet the glycemic load of the diet increased significantly ($P < 0.001$). How do these findings fit with their conclusions in the earlier report? Alternatively, the Puerto Rico Heart Health Program (109) showed that persons with a high carbohydrate intake (and thus a greater glycemic load) have a lower risk of CHD. Although the data on the association between the GI and the risk of CHD are intriguing and need to be followed up, the present data seem insufficient to warrant a public health recommendation.

Range of GIs in the Population

The GI quintiles for women in the Nurses' Health Study (17) and for the men in the Health Professionals' Follow-Up Study (54) are shown in Table 1. From the lowest to the highest quintile, the difference in GIs for women is only 13 units (from 64 to 77) and for men is 14 (from 65 to 79). The confidence limits for

Table 1

Median Glycemic Index Quintiles of Women in the Nurses' Health Study and of Men in the Health Professionals' Follow-Up Study

	Quintile				
	1	2	3	4	5
Women[1]	64	68	71	73	77
Men[2]	65	70	73	75	79

[1]From reference 17.
[2]From reference 54.

each quintile are wide. Because we know that the GIs for starches cluster in a relatively small range, it seems both impractical and unreasonable to try to move the GI down a few units for the US population. Furthermore, the quintiles reported in these 2 studies indicate that persons who consume a diet with the highest GI also consume the highest amount of carbohydrates, both in total grams and as a proportion of the total macronutrient content. Can we be sure that changing the GI will have the desired effect if the total carbohydrate intake, and thereby much of the glycemic load of the diet, stays the same?

Epidemiologic Studies and Causation

By its nature, an epidemiologic study can detect an association between 2 variables but cannot prove causation. To make public health decisions about what the optimal diet is for a population, some scientific evidence of cause and effect should be available. Although a certain amount of evidence can be accrued from investigations using animal models, epidemiologic studies, and clinical investigations, only controlled clinical trials can provide proof of causality (110).

Controlled clinical trials are expensive and difficult to conduct. As a result, epidemiologic studies take on more importance because of the lack of more definitive information. However, we must be assured that the methods used in epidemiologic studies are sound and that we can trust the results obtained as being relatively definitive. I do not have faith in the results of the studies mentioned previously that used FFQs. I am not convinced that the methods used in these studies were sound. The database used to derive the GIs is fraught with uncertainty and irreproducibility.

Because of the many uncertainties regarding the validity of the GI for determining what foods are "good" or "bad" for one's health, I believe it would be a mistake to initiate a public health campaign stating that certain widely consumed carbohydrates should be avoided. Much more definitive data are needed before any such dietary recommendations are made and controlled clinical trials are the best way to proceed.

There are many more worthwhile issues relating to diet and health that merit the focus of a public health effort. The prevention of type 2 diabetes is a critical public health priority given that the prevalence of diabetes in the US population has increased from 8.9% to 12.3% in 11 y (111), and continues to increase (112). The rate of obesity, a primary predictor of diabetes, is skyrocketing (113). As a matter of public health, the message is clear: decrease total energy intakes and increase physical activity (114). To decrease the incidence of cardiovascular disease, lifestyle changes and low saturated fat intakes are recommended (115). These are recommendations that we can all agree on, and much work is still needed to promote them to the US population.

Notes

[a]From the Obesity Research Center, St Luke's–Roosevelt Hospital Center, Columbia University College of Physicians and Surgeons, New York.

[b]Presented at a symposium held at Experimental Biology 2001, Orlando, FL, 1 April 2001.

[c]Supported by the National Institutes of Health (grant P 30 DK 26687).

[d]Address reprint requests to F Xavier Pi-Sunyer, Obesity Research Center, St. Luke's–Roosevelt Hospital Center, 1111 Amsterdam Avenue, New York, NY 10025. E-mail: fxp1@columbia.edu.

References

1. Otto H, Bleyer G, Pennartz M, Sabin G, Schauberger G, Spaethe K. Kohlenhydrataustausch nach biologischen aquivalenten. (Carbohydrate exchange according to biological equivalents.) Diatetik bei diabetes mellitus. Bern, Switzerland: Huber 1973:41–50 (in German).

2. Otto H, Niklas L. Differences d'action sur la glycemie d'ailments contenant des hydrates de carbone: consequences pour le traitment dietetique du diabete sucre. (The different actions on glycemia of foods containing carbohydrates: consequences for the nutritional treatment of diabetes mellitus.) Med Hyg 1980; 38:3424–9 (in French).

3. Jenkins DJ, Wolever TM, Taylor RH, et al. Glycemic index of foods: a physiological basis for carbohydrate exchange. Am J Clin Nutr 1981;34:362–6.

4. Jenkins DJ, Wolever TM, Kalmusky J, et al. Low glycemic index foods in the management of hyperlipidemia. Am J Clin Nutr 1985; 42:604–17.

5. Jenkins D. Starchy foods and glycemic index. Diabetes Care 1988; 11:149–59.

6. Brand-Miller J, Pang E, Broomhead L. The glycemic index of foods containing sugars: comparison of foods with naturally occurring v. added sugars. Br J Nutr 1995;73:613–23.

7. Gannon M, Nuttall FQ. Factors affecting interpretation of postprandial glucose and insulin areas. Diabetes Care 1987;10:759–63.

8. Crapo P, Insel J, Sperling M, Kolterman OG. Comparison of serum glucose, insulin, and glucagon responses to different types of complex carbohydrate in noninsulin-dependent diabetic patients. Am J Clin Nutr 1981;34:184–90.

9. Jenkins DJ, Wolever TM, Collier GR, et al. Metabolic effects of a low-glycemic-index diet. Am J Clin Nutr 1987;46:968–75.

10. Ercan N, Nuttall FQ, Gannon M. Effect of added fat on the plasma glucose and insulin response to ingested potato given in various combinations as two meals in normal individuals. Diabetes Care 1994;17:1453–9.

11. Ahmed M, Gannon M, Nuttall FQ. Postprandial glucose, insulin, glucagon and triglyceride responses to a standard diet in normal subjects. Diabetologia 1976;12:61–7.

12. Nuttall FQ, Gannon M, Wald J, Ahmed M. Plasma glucose and insulin profiles in normal subjects ingesting diets of varying carbohydrate, fat and protein content. J Am Coll Nutr 1985;4:437–50.

13. Miller JC. Importance of glycemic index in diabetes. Am J Clin Nutr 1994;59(suppl):747S–52S.

14. Gannon MC, Nuttall FQ, Westphal SA Fang S, Ercan-Fang N. Acute metabolic response to high-carbohydrate, high-starch meals compared with moderate-carbohydrate, low-starch meals in subjects with type 2 diabetes. Diabetes Care 1998;21:1619–26.

15. Foster-Powell K, Miller JB. International tables of glycemic index. Am J Clin Nutr 1995;62(suppl):871S–93S.

16. Liu S, Willett WC, Stampfer MJ, et al. A prospective study of dietary glycemic load, carbohydrate intake, and risk of coronary heart disease in US women. Am J Clin Nutr 2000;71:1455–61.

17. Salmeron J, Manson J, Stampfer M, Colditz G, Wing A, Willett W. Dietary fiber, glycemic load, and risk of non-insulin-dependent diabetes mellitus in women. JAMA 1997;277:472–7.

18. Englyst HN, Cummings JH. Digestion of the carbohydrates of the banana (*Musa paradisiaca sapientum*) in the human small intestine. Am J Clin Nutr 1986; 44:42–50.

19. O'Dea K, Nestel PJ, Antonoff L. Physical factors influencing postprandial glucose and insulin responses to starch. Am J Clin Nutr 1980;33:760–5.

20. Collier G, O'Dea K. Effect of physical form of carbohydrate on the postprandial glucose, insulin, and gastric inhibitory polypeptide responses in type 2 diabetes. Am J Clin Nutr 1982;36:10–4.

21. Wolever T, Katzman-Relle L, Jenkins A, Vuksan V, Josse RG, Jenkins D. Glycaemic index of 102 complex carbohydrate foods in patients with diabetes. Nutr Res 2001;14:651–69.

22. Haber G, Heaton K, Murphy D, Burroughs L. Depletion and disruption of dietary fibre. Effects of satiety, plasma-glucose and serum-insulin. Lancet 1977; 2:679–82.

23. Annison G, Topping DL. Nutritional role of resistant starch: chemical structure vs physiological function. Annu Rev Nutr 1994;14: 297–320.

24. van Amelsvoort JM, Weststrate JA. Amylose-amylopectin ratio in a meal affects postprandial variables in male volunteers. Am J Clin Nutr 1992;55:712–8.

25. Wolever T, Jenkins DJ, Kalmusky J, et al. Glycemic response to pasta: effect of surface area, degree of cooking, and protein enrichment. Diabetes Care 1986;9:401–4.

26. Granfeldt Y, Bjorck I, Hagander B. On the importance of processing conditions, product thickness and egg addition for the glycaemic and hormonal responses to pasta: a comparison with bread made from 'pasta ingredients.' Eur J Clin Nutr 1991;45:489–99.

27. Asp N-G. Definition and analysis of dietary fibre. Scand J Gastroenterol Suppl 1987;129:16–20.

28. Raben A, Andersen K, Karberg MA, Holst JJ, Astrup A. Acetylation of or beta-cyclodextrin addition to potato starch: beneficial effect on glucose metabolism and appetite sensations. Am J Clin Nutr 1997; 66:304–14.

29. Sievert D, Czuchajowska A, Pomeranz Y. Enzyme resistant starch. III. X-ray diffraction of autoclaved amylomaize. Cereal Chem 1991; 68:86–91.

30. Englyst HN, Cummings JH. Digestion of polysaccharides of potato in the small intestine of man. Am J Clin Nutr 1987;45:423–31.

31. Vaaler S, Hanssen KE, Aagenaes O. The effect of cooking upon the blood glucose response to ingested carrots and potatoes. Diabetes Care 1984;7:221–3.

32. Collings P, Williams C, MacDonald I. Effect of cooking on serum glucose and insulin responses to starch. Br Med J 1981;282:1032–3.

33. Coulston AM, Hollenbeck C, Reaven GM. Utility of studies measuring glucose and insulin responses to various carbohydrate-containing foods. Am J Clin Nutr 1984;39:163–7.

34. Calle-Pascual AL, Gomez V, Leon F, Bordiu E. Foods with a low glycemic index do not improve glycemic control of both type 1 and type 2 diabetic patients after one month of therapy. Diabetic Metab 1988;14:629–33.

35. Laine D, Thomas W, Levitt M, Bantle J. Comparison of predictive capabilities of diabetic exchange lists and glycemic index of foods. Diabetes Care 1987; 10:3387–94.

36. Wolever T. The glycemic index: flogging a dead horse? Diabetes Care 1997; 20:452–6.

37. Simpson RW, McDonald J, Wahlqvist ML, Altey L, Outch K. Macronutrients have different metabolic effects in nondiabetics and diabetics. Am J Clin Nutr 1985;42:449–53.

38. Nuttall FQ, Mooradian A, Gannon M, Bartosh N. Effect of protein ingestion on the glucose and insulin response to a standardized oral glucose load. Diabetes Care 1984;7:465–70.

39. Krezowski PA, Nuttall FQ, Gannon MC, Bartosh NH. The effect of protein ingestion on the metabolic response to oral glucose in normal individuals. Am J Clin Nutr 1986;44:847–56.

40. Collier G, McLean A, O'Dea K. Effect of co-ingestion of fat on the metabolic responses to slowly and rapidly absorbed carbohydrates. Diabetologia 1984; 26:50–4.

41. Gannon M, Ercan N, Westphal S, Nuttall FQ. Effect of added fat on plasma glucose and insulin response to ingested potato in individuals with NIDDM. Diabetes Care 1993;16:874–80.

42. Morgan L. Insulin secretion and the entero-insular axis. Nutrient regulation of insulin secretion. London: Portland Press Ltd, 1992.

43. Wolever TM. Relationship between dietary fiber content and composition in foods and the glycemic index. Am J Clin Nutr 1990; 51:72–5.

44. Nuttall FQ. Dietary fiber in the management of diabetes. Diabetes 1993; 42:503–8.

45. Kay RM, Stitt S. Food form, postprandial glycemia, and satiety. Am J Clin Nutr 1978;31:738–9.

46. Holt SH, Miller JC, Petocz P. An insulin index of foods: the insulin demand generated by 1000–kJ portions of common foods. Am J Clin Nutr 1997;66:1264–76.

47. Tattersall R, Mansell P. Fibre in the management of diabetes. 2. Benefits of fibre itself are uncertain. BMJ 1990;300:1336–7.

48. Liljeberg HG, Bjorck IM. Delayed gastric emptying rate as a potential mechanism for lowered glycaemia after eating sourdough bread: studies in humans and rats using test products with added organic acids or an organic salt. Am J Clin Nutr 1996;64:886–93.

49. Lee B, Wolever T. Effect of glucose, sucrose and fructose on plasma glucose and insulin responses in normal humans: comparison with white bread. Eur J Clin Nutr 1998;52:924–8.

50. Bagdade J, Bierman EL, Porte D. The significance of basal insulin levels in the evaluation of the insulin response to glucose in diabetic and nondiabetic subjects. J Clin Invest 1967;46:1549–57.

51. Barrett-Connor E, Schrott H, Greendale G, et al. Factors associated with glucose and insulin levels in healthy postmenopausal women. Diabetes Care 1996;19:333–40.

52. Roberts SB. High-glycemic index foods, hunger; and obesity: is there a connection? Nutr Rev 2000;58:163–9.

53. Frost G, Leeds A, Trew G, Margara R, Dornhorst A. Insulin sensitivity in women at risk of coronary heart disease and the effect of a low glycemic diet. Metabolism 1998;47:1245–51.

54. Salmeron J, Ascherio A, Rimm E, et al. Dietary fiber, glycemic load, and risk of NIDDM in men. Diabetes Care 1997;20:545–50.

55. Liu S, Manson J, Stampfer MJ, et al. Dietary glycemic load assessed by food-frequency questionnaire in relation to plasma high-density-lipoprotein choles-terol and fasting plasma triacyglycerols in postmenopausal women. Am J Clin Nutr 2001;73:560–6.

56. Holt S, Brand J, Soveny C, Hansky J. Relationship of satiety to postprandial gly-caemic, insulin and cholecystokinin responses. Appetite 1992;18:129–41.

57. Chapman I, Goble EA, Wittert GA, et al. Effect of intravenous glucose and eug-lycemic insulin infusions on short-term appetite and food intake. Am J Physiol 1998;274:596–603.

58. Gielkins HAJ, Verkijk M, Lam WF, et al. Effects of hyperglycemia and hyperinsu-linemia on satiety in humans. Metabolism 1998;47: 321–4.

59. Lavin JH, Wittert GA, Andrews J, et al. Interaction of insulin, glucagon-like pep-tide 1, gastric inhibitory peptide, and appetite in response to intraduodenal car-bohydrate. Am J Clin Nutr 1998;68: 591–8.

60. Woo R, Kissileff H, Pi-Sunyer FX. Elevated postprandial insulin levels do not in-duce satiety in normal-weight humans. Am J Physiol 1984;247:R745.

61. Raben A, Tagliabue A, Christensen NJ, Madsen J, Holst JJ, Astrup A. Resistant starch: the effect on postprandial glycemia, hormonal response, and satiety. Am J Clin Nutr 1994;60:544–51.

62. Heini AF, Kirk KA, Lara-Castro C, Weinsier RL. Relationship between hunger-satiety feelings and various metabolic parameters in women with obesity during controlled weight-loss. Obes Res 1998;6:225–30.

63. Hospers J, van Amelsvoort J, Weststrate J. Amylose-to-amylopectin ratio in pas-tas affects postprandial glucose and insulin responses and satiety in males. Int Food Sci Nutr 1994;59:1144–9.

64. Holt S, Miller J. Increased insulin responses to ingested foods are associated with lessened satiety. Appetite 1995;24:43–54.

65. Ludwig D, Majzoub J, Al-Zahrani A, et al. High glycemic index foods, overeating and obesity. Pediatrics 1999;103:E261–6.

66. Holm J, Bjorck I. Bioavailability of starch in various wheat-based bread products: evaluation of metabolic responses in healthy subjects and rate and extent of in vitro starch digestion. Am J Clin Nutr 1992;55:420–9.

67. Granfelt Y, Liljeberg H, Drews A, Newman R, Bjorck I. Glucose and insulin responses to barley products: influence of food structure and amylose-amylopectin ratio. Am J Clin Nutr 1994;59:1075–82.

68. Guss J, Kissileff H, Pi-Sunyer FX. Effects of glucose and fructose solutions on food intake and gastric emptying in nonobese women. Am J Physiol 1994; 267:R1537–44.

69. Rodin J. Effects of pure sugar vs. mixed starch fructose loads on food intake. Appetite 1991;17:213–9.

70. Spitzer L, Rodin J. Effects of fructose and glucose preloads on subsequent food intake. Appetite 1987;8:135–45.

71. Barkeling B, Granfelt Y, Bjorck I, Rossner S. Effects of carbohydrates in the form of pasta and bread on food intake and satiety in man. Nutr Res 1995;15:467–76.

72. Kiens B, Richter EA. Types of carbohydrate in an ordinary diet affect insulin ac-tion and muscle substrates in humans. Am J Clin Nutr 1996;63:47–53.

73. Schwartz M. Staying slim with insulin in mind. Science 2000;289: 2066–7.

74. Woods S, Porte D. Relationship between plasma and cerebrospinal fluid insulin levels of dogs. Am J Physiol 1977;233:E331–4.

75. Porte D, Seeley R, Woods S, Baskin D, Figlewicz D, Schwartz M. Obesity, diabetes and the central nervous system. Diabetologia 1998; 8:863–81.

76. Woods S, Stein L, McKay L, Porte D. Chronic intracerebroventricular infusion of insulin reduces food intake and body weight of baboons. Nature 1979; 282:503–5.

77. Brüning J, et al. Role of brain insulin receptor in control of body weight and re-production. Science 2000;289:2125.

78. Vanderweele D, Pi-Sunyer FX, Novin D, Bush M. Chronic insulin infusion suppresses food ingestion and body weight gain in rats. Brain Res Bull 1980;5:7–11.

79. Vanderweele D, Haraczkiewicz E, Vasselli J. Tolbutamide affects food ingestion in a manner consistent with its glycemic effects in the rat. Physiol Behav 1988;44:679–83.

80. Schwartz M, Boyko E, Kahn S, Ravussin E, Bogardus C. Reduced insulin secretion: an independent predictor of body weight gain. J Clin Endocrinal Metab 1995;80:1571–6.

81. Daly ME, Vale C, Walker M, Alberti KG, Mathers JC. Dietary carbohydrates and insulin sensitivity: a review of the evidence and clinical implications. Am J Clin Nutr 1997;66:1072–85.

82. Thompson R, Hayford J, Darney M. Glucose and insulin responses to diet: effect of variations in source and amount of carbohydrate. Diabetes 1978;27:1020–6.

83. Fukagawa NK, Anderson JW, Hageman G, Young VR, Minaker KL. High-carbohydrate, high-fiber diets increase peripheral insulin sensitivity in healthy young and old adults. Am J Clin Nutr 1990;52:524–8.

84. Chen M, Bergman R, Porte D. Insulin resistance and beta-cell dysfunction in aging: the importance of dietary carbohydrate. J Clin Endocrinol Metab 1988; 67:951–7.

85. Borkman M, Campbell L, Chisholm D, Storlien L. Comparison of the effects on insulin sensitivity of high carbohydrate and high fat diets in normal subjects. J Clin Endocrinol Metab 1991;72:432–7.

86. Ferrannini E. Insulin resistance versus insulin deficiency in non-insulin dependent diabetes mellitus: problems and prospects. Endocr Rev 1998;19:477–90.

87. Martin B, Warram J, Krowleski A, Bergman R, Soeldner J, Kahn C. Role of glucose and insulin resistance in development of type 2 diabetes. Results of a 25-year follow-up study. Lancet 1992;340:925–9.

88. Lillioja S, Mott D, Spraul M, et al. Insulin resistance and insulin secretory dysfunction as precursors of non-insulin dependent diabetes mellitus. Prospective studies of Pima Indians. N Engl J Med 1993;329: 1988–92.

89. Weyer C, Bogardus C, Mott DM, Pratley R. The natural history of insulin secretory dysfunction and insulin resistance in the pathogenesis of type 2 diabetes mellitus. J Clin Invest 1999;104:787–94.

90. Rimm EB, Giovannucci E, Willett WC, et al. Prospective study of alcohol consumption and risk of coronary disease in men. Lancet 1991;2:464–8.

91. Willett WC, Sampson L, Stampfer M, et al. Reproducibility and validity of a semiquantitative food frequency questionnaire. Am J Epidemiol 1985;122:51–65.

92. Willett W. The use of a self-administered questionnaire to assess diet four years in the past. Am J Epidemiol 2001;127:188–99.

93. Austin MA, Breslow JL, Hennekens CH, et al. Low density lipoprotein subclass patterns and risk of myocardial infarction. JAMA 1988;260:1917–21.

94. Rimm E. Reproducibility and validity of an expanded self-administered semiquantitative food frequency questionnaire among male health professionals. Am J Epidemiol 1992;135:1114–26.

95. Hu FB, Rimm E, Smith-Warner SA, et al. Reproducibility and validity of dietary patterns assessed with a food-frequency questionnaire. Am J Clin Nutr 1999;69:243–9.

96. Hu F, Stampfer M, Manson J, et al. Trends in the incidence of coronary heart disease and changes in diet and lifestyle in women. N Engl J Med 2000;343:530–7.

97. Tseng M. Validation of dietary patterns assessed with a food-frequency questionnaire. Am J Clin Nutr 1999;70:422 (letter).

98. Marshall J. High-fat, low-carbohydrate diet and the etiology of non insulin-dependent diabetes mellitus: the San Luis Valley Diabetes Study. Am J Epidemiol 1991;134:590–603.

99. Meyer KA, Kushi LH, Jacobs DR Jr, Slavin J, Sellers TA, Folsom AR. Carbohydrates, dietary fiber, and incident type 2 diabetes in older women. Am J Clin Nutr 2000; 71:921–30.

100. Himsworth H. Diet and the incidence of diabetes mellitus. Clin Sci 1935; 2:117–47.

101. West KM, Kalbfleisch JM. Influence of nutritional factors on prevalence of diabetes. Diabetes 1971;20:99–108.

102. Kawate R, Yamakido M, Nishimoto Y, et al. Diabetes mellitus and its vascular complications in Japanese migrants on the island of Hawaii. Diabetes Care 1979;2:161–70.

103. Ringrose H, Mollard C, Taylor R, et al. Energy intakes and diabetes prevalence of rural and urban Melanesia and Indian populations in Fiji. Proceedings of the XII International Congress of Nutrition. San Diego: International Congress of Nutrition, 1981.

104. Tsunehara CH, Leonetti DL, Fujimoto WY. Diet of second generation Japanese-American men with and without non-insulin dependent diabetes. Am J Clin Nutr 1990;52:731–8.

105. Himsworth H, Marshall E. The diet of diabetics prior to the onset of the disease. Clin Sci 1935;2:95–115.

106. Medalie JH, Papier C, Herman JB, et al. Diabetes mellitus among 10,000 adult men. I. Five-year incidence and associated variables. Isr J Med Sci 1974; 10:681–97.

107. Bennett PH, Knowler WC, Baird H, et al. Diet and development of non-insulin-dependent diabetes mellitus: an epidemiological perspective. In: Pozza Ge, ed. Diet, diabetes, and atherosclerosis. New York: Raven Press 1984:109–19.

108. Lundgren H, Bengtsson C, Blohme G, Lapidus L, Sjöström. Adiposity and adipose tissue distribution in relation to incidence of diabetes in women: results from a prospective population study in Gothenburg, Sweden. Int J Obes 1989;13:413–23.

109. García-Palmieri MB, Sorlie P, Tillotson J, Costas R, Cordero E, Rodriguez M. Relationship of dietary intake to subsequent coronary heart disease incidence: the Puerto Rico Heart Health Program. Am J Clin Nutr 1980;33:1818–27.

110. Grundy SM. The optimal ratio of fat-to-carbohydrate in the diet. Annu Rev Nutr 1999;19:325–41.

111. Harris M, Flegal K, Cowie C, et al. Prevalence of diabetes: impaired fasting glucose and impaired glucose tolerance in U.S. adults. Diabetes Care 1998; 21:519–24.

112. Mokdad A, Ford E, Bowman B, et al. Diabetes trends in the U.S. Diabetes Care 2000;23:1278–83.

113. Kuczmarski RJ, Flegal KM, Campbell SM, Johnson CL. Increasing prevalence of overweight among U.S. adults. JAMA 1994;272:205–11.

114. National Heart Lung and Blood Institute. Clinical guidelines on the identification, evaluation, and treatment of overweight and obesity in adults—The Evidence Report. Obes Res 1998;6(suppl):51S–209S.

115. NCEP. Executive Summary of the Third Report of the National Cholesterol Education Program (NCEP) Expert Panel on Detection, Evaluation, and Treatment of High Blood Cholesterol in Adults (Adult Treatment Panel III). JAMA 2001;285:2486–97.

POSTSCRIPT

Do Foods With a High Glycemic Index Increase Disease Risk?

According to Ludwig, foods of high glycemic index like potatoes, rice, and pasta so disrupt normal metabolism and promote weight gain that people should avoid eating them. Pi-Sunyer disagrees. He says that nearly everything about the glycemic index is so uncertain that it cannot be used to classify foods as good or bad. The glycemic index is, in fact, increasingly used to judge foods. Popular diet books with titles like *Good Carbs, Bad Carbs; The Insulin Resistance Diet;* or *Syndrome X* list foods to avoid on the basis of their glycemic index. Among these, *The New Glucose Revolution* (Marlowe & Company, 2003) gives a particularly clear account of the rationale for this dietary approach. In *Nutrition Today* (March/April 1999), the lead author of this book, Australian nutritionist Jennie Brand-Miller and her colleague Kaye Foster-Powell, state that the benefits of consuming low glycemic index foods are so well supported by research that "it is difficult to understand how nutrition advice can be given today *without* incorporating it." In 2002 these authors provided a table of nearly 1300 glycemic index values derived from a wide variety of sources in the *American Journal of Clinical Nutrition* (vol. 76, pp. 5–56). However, Marion Franz, a nutritionist who specializes in education about diabetes, agrees that the glycemic index has some use in diabetes prevention, but suggests *"how much* a person eats is more important than *what* he or she eats" (*Nutrition Today,* March/April 1999).

This last point is worth further consideration. One reason why nutrition research is so subject to interpretation is the difficulty of disentangling cause and effect. Epidemiologic studies, for example, identify associations between a dietary factor and a disease risk but do not prove that the factor causes the disease. Similar considerations might apply to the glycemic index. Perhaps obesity itself is a cause—rather than an effect—of the excessive increase in blood glucose and insulin that occurs in response to high glycemic index foods.

These discussions often fail to emphasize the difference between glycemic *index* (which rates the rapidity with which carbohydrates are absorbed) and what is sometimes called glycemic *load* (which accounts for the total amount of carbohydrate). Carrots, for example, are a high glycemic index food because their carbohydrates are absorbed rapidly. They are, however, low in glycemic load because a single carrot contains only a few grams of absorbable carbohydrates, and people would need an unusually large portion to raise blood sugar levels significantly.

Thus, as with most other matters pertaining to nutrition and health, it may be too simplistic to attribute risk factors for chronic disease to just one cause. The Japanese population, for example, has long subsisted on rice (and white rice at that) as a principal source of calories, yet this nation's men and women display the longest life expectancies in the world. Mediterranean groups subsisting on bread and pasta also display unusually low rates of chronic disease. Both populations, however, habitually consume largely plant-based diets, generally consume fewer calories, and engage in more physical activity than is typical of the U.S. population. Today, as the diet and activity patterns of these countries are changing and increasingly resemble U.S. patterns, so do their patterns of chronic disease. Overall lifestyles may be equally or more important than the glycemic index, especially when people use the index as the *sole* criterion of dietary choice.

Although Ludwig and Pi-Sunyer may appear to hold irreconcilable opinions, they agree on several key points. Both say or imply that whole grains are more healthful than "refined" sugars and starches from which nutrients and fiber have been removed in processing; they distinguish between good and bad carbohydrates. Both emphasize the need to balance energy intake with physical activity. Although Pi-Sunyer believes that the evidence does not warrant public health campaigns against widely consumed carbohydrates, he is not at all an advocate of diets high in sugars. Similarly, Ludwig would not suggest that people substitute potato chips for boiled potatoes just because the chips have a lower glycemic index. Overall, the opinions of these two distinguished scientists may agree more than they disagree.

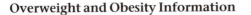

Overweight and Obesity Information

Overweight and obesity information from the Centers for Disease Control and Prevention (CDC) is provided on this Web site. The CDC is a federal agency that provides statistical information and dietary advice about obesity prevention and control. Maps on this site document dramatic increases in statewide levels of obesity from the late 1980s to the present. Click on the "Obesity Trends" button to see these maps.

http://www.cdc.gov/nccdphp/dnpa/obesity/index.htm

The Fat Acceptance Movement on the Web

The Fat Acceptance Movement on the Web site lists organizations and resources devoted to promoting the human and civil rights of "people of size."

http://www.seafattle.org/falinks.html

The National Academies Press: Dietary Reference Intakes

The Food and Nutrition Board of the Institute of Medicine (IOM) is responsible for developing the national standards for intake of essential nutrients, the Dietary Reference Intakes. This site provides the entire report, which includes sections on energy intake and expenditure.

http://www.nap.edu/books/0309085373/html/

President's Council on Physical Fitness and Sports

The President's Council on Physical Fitness and Sports promotes research and education about the benefits of physical activity. This Web site provides information and reports, but also offers links to physical activity resources of federal agencies and private health organizations.

http://www.fitness.gov

PART 3

Diet, Physical Activity, and Health

*T*he issues in this part debate critical problems that affect the nutritional health of the public. Today, overweight and obesity are the principal public health nutrition problems facing people in industrialized countries such as the United States. How serious a health problem is the obesity epidemic, and what, if anything, should be done about it? In recent years, experts have challenged government dietary advice to reduce fat intake as a means to prevent weight gain. Instead, they say, high-carbohydrate diets promote obesity. Others believe that the key to weight maintenance is adequate physical activity, with little agreement about the meaning of "adequate." Given what we do know about the need to improve diet and activity patterns, what is the best way to encourage the public to follow current recommendations? The selections in this part debate such questions.

- Is Body Weight a Reliable Measure of Overall Health?

- Can Low-Carbohydrate, Higher-Fat Diets Promote Health and Weight Loss?

- Must Exercise Be Daily and Intense to Prevent Chronic Disease?

- Do Education Campaigns Induce Communities to Change Their Diets and Improve Health?

ISSUE 6

Is Body Weight a Reliable Measure of Overall Health?

YES: Alison E. Field et al., from "Impact of Overweight on the Risk of Developing Common Chronic Diseases During a 10-Year Period," *Archives of Internal Medicine* (July 9, 2001)

NO: Annemarie Jutel, from "Does Size Really Matter? Weight and Values in Public Health," *Perspectives in Biology and Medicine* (Spring 2001)

ISSUE SUMMARY

YES: Epidemiologist Alison E. Field and her team of investigators say that overweight adults are at increased risk of chronic disease, even if they are not obese.

NO: Health sociologist Annemarie Jutel says that the risks of overweight are exaggerated and that its cure—dieting—is a greater hazard.

By the turn of the twenty-first century, more than half of all Americans were considered overweight. For this reason alone, the question of whether or not body weight over and above certain cut points increases health risks is a matter of intense public and professional interest. Advocates of equal rights for overweight individuals (the fat liberation or size acceptance movement) insist that obesity does not necessarily doom one to increased health risks and that an obese person who is physically fit is healthier—sometimes *much* healthier—than someone who is thinner but unfit. Furthermore, chronic disease risk factors such as high blood pressure, high blood cholesterol, or high blood sugar are prevalent in thin as well as fat people. They view the health risks of dieting and eating disorders as far more serious than those of overweight. The idea that obesity is a health problem, they explain, is "socially constructed" (meaning a matter of social prejudices) rather than based on science.

Is obesity a health risk and, if so, at what level of overweight? Scientists define overweight and obesity in terms of the Body Mass Index (BMI), a single number derived from a person's weight for height: body weight in kilograms divided by height in meters, squared (kg/m^2). Health officials used to say that a BMI of 27 was the cut point for healthy weights. Today, they define *healthy weights* as those of BMIs of 18.5 to 24.9. *Overweight* is a BMI range from 25.0 to 29.9. *Obesity* is a BMI above 30.0. The precision of these numbers gives the appearance of great accuracy, yet it should be obvious that the cut points are necessarily arbitrary. Someone with a BMI of 25.0 will not have a noticeably higher risk than someone with a BMI of 24.9, but someone with a BMI of 33 is quite likely to have a higher risk. Whether or not the BMI adequately distinguishes the risks of people with differing proportions of body muscle and fat also is a point of contention.

Alison E. Field and her colleagues used epidemiologic data from two large, prospective clinical investigations to examine the effect of body weight on health risks over a 10-year period. These investigators collected information about body weight and height from participants at the beginning of the studies. Ten years later, they determined whether or not the participants had developed high blood cholesterol, gallstones, diabetes, high blood pressure, colon cancer, heart disease, or stroke. Using standard statistical tests, they computed relative risks (RR) for those conditions by BMI category. Although Field et al. observed RRs above 1.0 for most overweight categories and risk factors, some of these results did not reach statistical significance and could have occurred by chance alone (high blood cholesterol and stroke in women, for example). Because RRs increased even for BMIs now considered "healthy," these investigators say that the ideal BMI range is really 18.5 to 21.9—numbers so low that they are achieved by few Americans. [Hint: In this study, a RR of 1.0 means that a weight category is *not* associated with any increase in risk. An RR above 1.0 indicates a statistical increase in risk, and the higher the RR, the higher the risk. For participants in the overweight category, for example, an RR of 3.5 means that even slight overweight is associated with 3.5 times the increase in the risk of diabetes.]

Such conclusions, according to Annemarie Jutel, derive from mistaken attempts to quantify wellness, define overweight as statistical deviance, and apply health judgments to appearance. Why, Jutel asks, are not other factors—diet, physical activity, and use of medications—considered equally important as measures of health? The focus on measurement of body weight rather than on other determinants encourages dieting, eating disorders, excessive exercising, and feelings of inadequacy—all of which may be worse for health than the small increase in risk sometimes posed by plumpness. Health, she says, is more than a number, especially one based on an "unsuitable screening tool."

If, as Field et al. argue, even mild overweight raises health risks, then should public health officials advise everyone to strive for an even lower BMI—perhaps 22 or less? Or, as Jutel claims, should people not worry about BMI but instead focus on other measures of fitness as a way to measure health? In examining this argument, it is also useful to ask: How suitable are epidemiologic studies for deciding such questions? Similarly, how valid are qualitative arguments derived from social science in comparison to those derived from quantitative science? Why might one or the other seem more compelling?

In the following selections, Field and her colleagues say that even small increments in body weight increase health risks, but Jutel says that that body weight has little effect on health in the absence of other risk factors.

Alison E. Field et al.

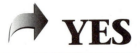

YES

Impact of Overweight on the Risk of Developing Common Chronic Diseases During a 10-Year Period

In the United States, obesity has become a serious public health problem. According to the third National Health and Nutrition Examination Survey, 32% of adults in the United States are overweight and an additional 22.5% are obese. Moreover, the prevalence of obesity has been increasing sharply among children and adults during the past 3 decades, and the trend is expected to continue.

Overweight and obesity are risk factors for cardiovascular disease, certain cancers, diabetes, and mortality. In addition, overweight also exacerbates many other chronic diseases, such as hypertension, osteoarthritis, gallstones, dyslipidemia, and musculoskeletal problems. Unfortunately, comparison of results across epidemiologic studies has been difficult because of the lack of consensus on weight categories. Further complicating the issue is that the new US dietary guidelines and the World Health Organization now define overweight as a body mass index (BMI) (calculated as weight in kilograms divided by the square of height in meters) of 25 or more, a major shift downward from the old US cutoffs of 27.3 for women and 27.8 for men. The US dietary guidelines classify BMI as follows: less than 18.5 is underweight, 18.5 to 24.9 is the healthy weight range, 25.0 to 29.9 is moderately overweight, and 30.0 or more is severely overweight or obese. Since a relatively large proportion of the population has a BMI between 25.0 and 27.0, the change in cutoff for overweight has resulted in a substantial increase in the prevalence of overweight. Moreover, the change has resulted in some confusion regarding the health risks associated with overweight (ie, BMI of 25.0–29.9), since a sizable proportion of this group was previously considered to have a healthy weight.

The majority of articles with original data, as opposed to review articles, on the health risks of obesity have limited themselves to a few health outcomes. Although this is the standard approach for epidemiologic articles, providing data on multiple outcomes is the most efficient way to illustrate the impact of overweight on physical health. To assess the adverse impact of overweight, we

From A. E. Field, E. H. Coakley, A. Must, J. L. Spadano, N. Laird, W. H. Dietz, E. Rimm, and G. A. Colditz, "Impact of Overweight on the Risk of Developing Common Chronic Diseases During a 10-Year Period," *Archives of Internal Medicine,* vol. 161 (July 9, 2001), pp. 1581–1586. Copyright © 2001 by The American Medical Association. Reprinted by permission. References omitted.

have analyzed the 10-year associated risks of developing high cholesterol level, hypertension, gallstones, type 2 diabetes, heart disease, stroke, and colon cancer among women in the Nurses' Health Study and men in the Health Professionals Follow-up Study, 2 large ongoing prospective cohort studies.

METHODS

The Nurses' Health Study

The Nurses' Health Study was established in 1976, when 121 701 female registered nurses from across the United States, aged 30 to 55 years, answered a mailed questionnaire on risk factors for cancer and heart disease. Questionnaires, mailed to these women every other year since 1976, ask about diagnosis during the past 2 years, as well as a wide variety of lifestyle factors including diet, physical activity, smoking, and contraception.

For diseases of particular interest, we write to the nurse to obtain permission to review the medical records pertaining to the diagnosis. In addition, all women reporting diabetes are sent a supplementary questionnaire to obtain additional information regarding the symptoms and diagnosis. Several repeated mailings are sent to nonrespondents, and these are followed by telephone interviews. In instances where we cannot obtain the medical records, we attempt to acquire as much information as possible to code a disease as probable, even if definite confirmation cannot be achieved. For deceased participants, we write to the next of kin to obtain permission to review the medical records. The records are reviewed by medically trained personnel according to established criteria.

Health Professionals Follow-Up Study

The Health Professionals Follow-up Study is a prospective study of 51 529 men, aged 40 to 75 years when the study began in 1986. Follow-up questionnaires are sent biennially to update information on exposure and disease. The follow-up has been greater than 90% through the 1994 questionnaire cycle. The follow-up procedures for medical diagnoses are similar to those used in the Nurses' Health Study. . . .

Results

The mean age in the 2 cohorts was similar (52.9 vs 54.5 years for women and men, respectively), and both cohorts were predominantly white (≥93%); however, the prevalences of obesity (BMI in 1986, ≥30.0) (14.8% vs 8.2%) and current smoking (21.1% vs 9.9%) were higher among the women than the men.

During 10 years of follow-up, more than half of the men and women were diagnosed as having high blood pressure (16% of women and 19% of men) or

Table 1

Distribution of Disease Incidence by Period Among 77 690 Women in the Nurses' Health Study and 46 060 Men in the Health Professionals Follow-up Study

	Women				Men			
Disease	Never, No.	Before 1986, No.	After 1986, No.	Cumulative Incidence, 1986–1996, %	Never, No.	Before 1986, No.	After 1986, No.	Cumulative Incidence, 1986–1996, %
Diabetes	74 578	1730	1382	1.9	43 313	1540	1207	2.8
Gallstones	67 491	4966	5233	7.8	42 782	1769	1509	3.5
Hypertension	51 301	17 909	8480	16.5	29 650	10 721	5689	19.2
High cholesterol level	47 037	7800	22 853	48.6	26 357	7136	12 567	47.7
Colon cancer	75 739	1430	521	0.7	45 673	346*	387	0.8
Heart disease	72 754	2449	2487	3.4	40 417	3524	2119	5.2
Stroke	76 674	378	638	0.8	45 183	393	484	1.1

*These 346 men had been diagnosed as having colon cancer when they enrolled in the study. All people with cancer at baseline were excluded from the sample eligible for analysis; thus, the numbers in this cell sum to greater than the size of the sample for analysis.

high cholesterol level (49% of women and 48% of men) (Table 1). In addition, approximately 2% of the women and 3% of the men developed diabetes. Gallstones were diagnosed more often during a 10-year period among the women (7.8% vs 3.5%), whereas heart disease was more common among the men (5.2% vs 3.4%).

In both cohorts, the risk of developing diabetes, gallstones, hypertension, heart disease, and stroke increased with severity of overweight. Among both women and men, those with a BMI of 35.0 or more were approximately 20 times more likely to develop diabetes . . . than their same-sex peers with a BMI between 18.5 and 24.9. Moreover, adults who were overweight but not obese (ie, BMI between 25.0 and 29.9) were more than 3 times as likely as their leaner peers to develop diabetes during 10 years (Table 2).

Women who were overweight but not obese were also significantly more likely than their leaner peers to develop gallstones, . . . hypertension, . . . high cholesterol level, . . . and heart disease. . . . The associations with the development of colon cancer and stroke were elevated but not significant. The results were similar in men, with the exception that obese men were significantly more likely to have a stroke . . . during the 10 years of follow-up. Among both women and men, the risks of developing diabetes, gallstones, hypertension, and heart disease increased with severity of overweight. . . .

Not only did the risk of developing diabetes, gallstones, hypertension, colon cancer, heart disease, and stroke increase with degree of overweight (Table 2), but also the risk of developing more than 1 outcome increased with weight category. Among women and men with a diagnosis of hypertension or high cholesterol level, the risk of developing additional morbidities increased across categories of BMI. . . .

Table 2

Ten-Year Risk (1986–1996) of Developing an Obesity-Related Morbidity Among 77 690 Female Nurses and 46 060 Male Health Professionals in the United States

	Diabetes	Gallstones	Hypertension	High Cholesterol Level	Colon Cancer	Heart Disease	Stroke
				Adjusted Odds Ratios (95% CI)*			
			Women				
10-y risk of developing disease, %†	5	6	14	58	0.6	3	0.5
Body mass index, kg/m²							
<25.0	Referent	Referent	Referent	Referent	Referent	Referent	Referent
25.0–29.9	4.6 (3.9–5.4)	1.9 (1.7–2.0)	1.7 (1.6–1.8)	1.1 (1.1–1.2)	1.2 (1.0–1.5)	1.4 (1.2–1.5)	1.2 (1.0–1.4)
30.0–34.9	10.0 (8.4–11.8)	2.5 (2.3–2.7)	2.1 (1.9–2.2)	0.9 (0.9–1.0)	1.3 (1.0–1.7)	1.5 (1.3–1.7)	1.0 (0.8–1.4)
≥35.0	17.0 (14.2–20.5)	3.0 (2.7–3.3)	2.3 (2.1–2.6)	0.7 (0.6–0.7)	1.8 (1.3–2.6)	1.5 (1.3–1.8)	1.1 (0.8–1.7)
			Men				
10-y risk of developing disease, %†	8	13	13	46	0.5	4	1
Body mass index, kg/m²							
<25.0	Referent	Referent	Referent	Referent	Referent	Referent	Referent
25.0–29.9	3.5 (2.9–4.1)	1.4 (1.3–1.6)	1.7 (1.6–1.8)	1.3 (1.2–1.3)	1.2 (1.0–1.5)	1.5 (1.4–1.7)	1.2 (1.0–1.5)
30.0–34.9	11.2 (9.3–13.6)	2.3 (1.9–2.7)	2.7 (2.4–3.0)	1.2 (1.1–1.3)	1.7 (1.2–2.4)	2.0 (1.7–2.3)	2.0 (1.5–2.7)
≥35.0	23.4 (19.4–33.2)	2.9 (2.1–4.1)	3.0 (2.3–3.9)	1.3 (1.1–1.6)	1.3 (0.5–3.2)	2.2 (1.5–3.1)	2.3 (1.2–4.4)

*Adjusted for age, smoking status, and race. CI indicates confidence interval.

†Risk, estimated from a logistic regression model, for a 50- to 59-year-old woman or man who is white, never smoked, and has a body mass index less than 25.

Comment

During 10 years of follow-up, the incidence of diabetes, gallstones, hypertension, and heart disease in both men and women, and of colon cancer (women only) and stroke (men only), increased with BMI in 1986. Even adults who were overweight but not obese (ie, $25.0 \leq BMI \leq 29.9$) were significantly more likely than their leaner peers to develop 1 or more of these diseases.

Although there has been debate about whether the relationship between weight and risk of death is linear, J-shaped, or U-shaped, the results have consistently shown that adults with BMI greater than 30.0 are at increased risk of death. Among 45- to 75-year-old men and women in the American Cancer Society's Cancer Prevention Study I, the risk of death increased linearly with BMI among the never smokers. The risk was particularly pronounced for death from cardiovascular disease and among men. Manson et al also observed a linear association between BMI and mortality during 16 years of follow-up among 15 195 women who were never smokers in the Nurses' Health Study. However, several other studies have observed that the risk was elevated in low-weight, as well as in overweight, adults or did not increase significantly until BMI was greater than 27.0.

Although mortality is a clearly defined outcome, the results of mortality analyses can be difficult to interpret. Except for diseases that are almost always fatal regardless of treatment, mortality is a function of incidence of disease, stage of illness at diagnosis, and effectiveness of treatment. Many forms of cancer and cardiovascular disease are treatable by either pharmacotherapy or intervention (ie, angioplasty [repair of blood vessel] or surgery); thus, the relationship between excess weight and death from cancer or cardiovascular disease does not necessarily translate to the same relationship with the development of cancer or cardiovascular disease. Moreover, several chronic diseases, such as hypertension and hypercholesterolemia, increase the risk of cardiovascular disease, but these conditions rarely are the direct cause of death. Nevertheless, both conditions have substantial economic and emotional costs because of their high prevalence. Because of the focus on mortality rather than morbidity as the outcome, less lethal diseases that may have important costs associated with them have a minimal impact on the results, thus highlighting why morbidity is an important outcome when the effects of obesity are studied.

Our group previously reported on the health consequences of obesity observed in the Nurses' Health Study and the Health Professionals Follow-up Study. Other investigators have also observed that overweight is predictive of developing type 2 diabetes, hypertension, dyslipidemia, coronary heart disease, stroke, gallbladder disease, osteoarthritis, sleep apnea and respiratory problems, and certain cancers. Although an increase in risk is found across studies, the magnitude of the risk is difficult to compare because it has been classified in a variety of ways. Because there is a near-linear relationship between BMI and risk of developing type 2 diabetes, hypertension, and gallstones, the choice of how the reference group is defined can have a large impact on the results. The higher the BMI cutoff is for the reference group, the lower the risks will appear to be in the higher weight groups because people at increased risk have been placed in the reference group. One strength of our study is that the same BMI cutoffs were used as predictors of 7 morbidities. Moreover, the weight classification we used was that espoused by the US dietary guidelines, so the categories have inherent meaning.

Our observation that women and men who have a BMI between 25.0 and 29.9 are at significantly increased risk of developing numerous health conditions offers support for lowering the overweight cutoff from a BMI of 27.0 to that of 25.0 in the recent weight guidelines from the US Department of Agriculture. Moreover, our finding that men and women in the upper half of the healthy weight category (ie, BMI between 22.0 and 24.9) are significantly more likely than their leaner peers to develop health problems highlights the necessity of counseling patients who are in the healthy weight range to maintain their weight or increase their physical activity levels. Because few people are able to lose weight and maintain the weight loss, it is important to intervene early, before the person has developed a serious weight problem. Although treatment for obesity is recommended only for overweight individuals with a BMI of 30.0 or more, or of 27.0 or more if they have other risk factors for disease, it may be prudent to counsel slightly leaner patients if they are gaining weight, as well as patients who are overweight but do not meet the treatment cutoffs (ie, BMI of 25.0–26.9), on how to modify their diet and physical activity to control their weight.

Annemarie Jutel ← **NO**

Does Size Really Matter?
Weight and Values in Public Health

Overview

Preoccupation with body weight and obesity dominates many health promotion strategies. In the United States, *Healthy People 2000* places the prevention of obesity as one of its highest priorities. Australia, Great Britain, France, the United States, Canada, and New Zealand have an array of position papers, clinical guidelines, and expert task force reports on the prevention and treatment of overweight and obesity. Many researchers have argued, however, that the risks of obesity are exaggerated and ill-defined. Other lifestyle factors such as exercise and diet may be more important than weight itself in health maintenance. While these factors may covary with weight, they are more difficult to quantify. Furthermore, weight loss is often a futile exercise that may have more serious negative consequences than positive benefits on health.

Paradoxically, both policy and popular belief neglect these arguments. Few women are willing to give away their scales, and few doctors are willing to put more credence in a patient's report of activity than in the weight on the scale. Doctors are less likely to investigate lifestyle choices or even to provide health advice to slender patients than they are to heavy ones, and heavy women are more likely to cancel or postpone medical appointments for fear of being reprimanded by health care professionals. Obsessive exercise, crash diets, and cigarettes keep many women artificially slim, despite the risks to health presented by this pursuit of slenderness.

Notwithstanding the growing scientific and popular debate about whether weight loss is healthy, even for the obese, there remains an intense focus on body weight as an indicator of health, in official policy as well as in cultural practices. Historically grounded values about quantification and aesthetics infuse the policies underpinning medical and popular fascination with weight as a reflection of health. In addition, different national policies contribute to crystallizing social beliefs about body fat and its nefarious qualities, and these policies promulgate some contradictions.

The focus on weight in contemporary health care is buttressed upon a desire to quantify wellness and to locate health in a model of precise normalcy. In the 19th century, Adolphe Quetelet devoted his work to measuring body sizes of vast populations. His last work, published in 1871, describes this anthropometric project as an attempt to discover evidence of a Supreme Being, of God's rules on earth. . . . Many 19th-century anthropologists relied on measurement of the body to identify racial groups and to confirm the superiority of the white man, "gifted with the powers of knowing and ruling which give them sway over the world."

This desire to capture the average man as well as the deviant, in measurement and proportion, led to the emergence of a new disease concept by the early 20th century. Being overweight became a clinical "condition," carrying with it a corresponding set of rules for diagnosis, treatment, and prognosis. It might seem surprising to think of being overweight as a new clinical entity. Previous concern with body size, however, was based not on weight or measurement but rather on fatness, an important distinction.

Excess body fatness had been a concern in both medical and lay circles for centuries. Hippocrates prescribed taking exercise on an empty stomach, then sitting down to eat, out of breath, for reducing. He noted that fat people were much more likely to die suddenly than thin people. The semantic distinction, however, between fatness and overweight supports an entire approach to the body, which influences contemporary practices regarding weight. The words *fatness* and *obesity* are qualitative descriptors suggesting corpulence, largeness, and probably heaviness. They are not linguistically charged, as *overweight* is, with the notion of measurable excess or statistical deviance. . . .

A focus on weight became prominent at the end of 19th century and gathered steam during the early 20th. Scales were marketed as finally being affordable for doctors' offices. The "Reliance Personal Weighing Machine," sold by Messrs. Arnold and Sons for 21 shillings, graced the pages of the *Lancet* in 1897. The Medico-Actuarial society carefully pored over 812,221 "build cards," or client records, to determine which body weights were most likely to predict mortality amongst their policy owners. The Metropolitan Life Insurance Company's assessment of financial risk led its writers to define overweight as an illness: "The practice [of being reluctant to insure people who are overweight] shows that [the insurance company] consider overweight as a very serious disability, and, indeed, treat it as though it were a disease," explains the Metropolitan Life's booklet, *Overweight: Its Cause and Treatment.*

The height–weight charts, designed to reply to the economic motive of insurance selection, were assimilated by the medical community, though initially with resistance. "No weight table is sufficient by itself to base an estimate of the ideal state," wrote William Christie in 1927. "Standard tables which show the average for men and women of our race at any given age and height are fallacious, because no allowance is made for the distinctions of personal physique, nor consideration given to obvious rolls of fat." On the other hand, Royal Copeland, a prolific writer on the subject of obesity, made no qualms about using the 1913 Medico-Actuarial tables, and neither did many of his contemporaries. Height and weight charts became standard fixtures in medical textbooks, and as late as 1940, Dr. Hugo Rony's medical textbook *Obesity and Leanness* still relied upon these earlier actuarial studies.

The importance accorded to weight in the health assessment is evidence of what Barbara Stafford, John La Puma, and David Schiedermayer describe as an uncritical medical focus on patient appearance that is framed by an expectation of aesthetic perfection. Mirroring early beliefs that physical imperfections reflect inner shortcomings, contemporary physicians unconsciously use visual and perceptual judgments in their evaluation of health, drawing their patients into an aesthetic of normality. As a result, geometrical concepts, numbers, and proportions support definitions of health. "Capturing" normality in a formula, or proportion, such as a height-weight chart, reflects moral and aesthetic judgments about how one ought to look. These views play an important role in the management of the "problem" of overweight. In Western society, values of homogeneity and visual aesthetics guide our judgments of what is good and healthy, and imprint themselves firmly on our approach to weight management.

These values are borne out in policy documents that serve as the base for both population and individual health strategies. In the campaign for weight loss, they reproduce and institutionalize many moral beliefs about the body. As other enterprises rely on the "truths" produced in these documents, there is reproduction ad infinitum of beliefs that individuals should reduce weight if they are large and should monitor their weight vigilantly if they are not. The brief review of policies that follows highlights the many ways in which values enter into the discussion of health and normality, and how these values reinforce discourses about body size.

Policy Approaches

United States

The U.S. National Institutes of Health (NIH) *Clinical Guidelines on the Identification, Evaluation and Treatment of Overweight and Obesity in Adults: The Evidence Report* provides a vivid illustration of the kinds of issues that place weight management before health management in the eyes of many lay and medical people. This document relies on an interpretation of evidence that prioritizes the hard measurement of the physical body over assessment of lifestyle and behavior. To justify the development of the guidelines, the authors cite, among others, a paper by McGinnis and Foege entitled "Actual Causes of Death in the United States." However, this article reports that 300,000 deaths a year are attributable to "activity and diet patterns": it does not establish the relationship between obesity and mortality that the developers of the *Clinical Guidelines* presume. And yet the NIH's misreading of the literature provides strong foundation for the recommendations that ensue.

The *Clinical Guidelines* propose a treatment strategy for the diagnosis and management of overweight and obese patients. The suggested protocol reinforces the view of the body as an object for medical observation and measurement, rather than as individuals' primary vehicle for contact with the world, a vehicle that reflects their experiences; bears the inscription of their unique social, physiological, and cultural situation; and defies, in many instances, precise measurement or categorization. The content of the recommended examination overlooks these experiences or, at best, subordinates them to a trivial position, and is reminiscent of Foucault's description of the 18th-century medical gaze that considers the patient an impediment to understanding the nature of pathology:

> In order to know the truth of the pathological fact, the doctor must abstract the patient . . . Here, the strange nature of the medical gaze: it is taken up in an indefinite spiral, addressing all that which is visible in illness, but starting from the patient, who hides that which is visible by showing it.

Here is a fear that the patient will distort the diagnosis by contributing to its construction. The fear may be augmented the common assumption, held even by health care workers, that fat people are less likely to be reliable than others. As in Foucault's description, the notion that the physician, as a sort of agent of authority, will better detect the truth than the patient pervades the NIH document. Underpinning this search for truth is the absolute confidence in quantification and numbers, which the patient can only offer by standing on the scales.

Prior to implementing a treatment protocol for the overweight patient, the report advises the physician to obtain certain information through examination. The examination relies upon measurement: history of body mass index (BMI),[1] height, weight, waist circumference, and assessment of risk factors. With the possible exception of the assessment of risk factors, the patient does not participate in the examination beyond offering his or her body for measurement.

But risk factor assessment, as described in this document, requires only minimal patient input and could be obtained, if one followed the guidelines, by measuring techniques alone—lipid profiles, ECG, blood electrolytes, blood glucose, sedimentation rates, radiological imaging—or by history of surgical or medical intervention (contained in medical charts and usually considered more reliable than a patient's nonspecific and non-medicalized reports of "chest pain" or "I had an operation on my heart"). Physical inactivity is last in the five categories of risk factors, arranged in order of priority—despite its being associated with the highest cause of premature death, and potentially being contributory to the other factors. I surmise that this disregard for physical activity is related to the difficulty with which the medical and scientific communities receive non-quantified information that cannot be easily and objectively confirmed.

In explanatory text, the *Clinical Guidelines* do discuss interaction with the patient, but in a limited and subordinate role. They indicate that "questions directed towards weight history, dietary habits, physical activities, and medications may provide useful information." The conditional *may* implies that this information is only a possible adjunct, just potentially useful. In fact, information about physical activity and/or nutrition is not even included in the accompanying schematic representation, implying that such information is indeed secondary to quantitative measurement. Similarly, the *Clinical Guidelines* only suggest that "a nutrition assessment will also *help* to assess the diet and physical activity habits of overweight patients." The patient's words do little more than contribute to a truer picture which is obtained through the measurement of body dimensions. Furthermore, there is a logical flaw in these explanatory words, because a nutrition assessment can, in no way, assess physical activity.

The NIH *Clinical Guidelines* concentrate on "useful tools readily available in a physician's office" as diagnostic tools. These tools are weight, height, and BMI; notably, they do not include patient input. To diagnose potentially problematic body weight, measurement alone suffices. The report advises clinicians to assess risk factors but do not prioritize physical inactivity or dietary problems. The absence of prioritization supports my argument that these policies focus on the viewed, measurable body and trivialize the input that the patient can contribute to the understanding of his or her condition. Measurement underpins the positivistic need to track and investigate all the aberrations of the body. In this case, the simple quantitative nature of its underlying premises *creates* the problem of overweight.

Australia

In Australia, the National Health and Medical Research Council (NHMRC) has prepared a similar document, *Acting on Australia's Weight: A Strategic Plan for the Prevention of Overweight and Obesity*. This document is firmly anchored in an economic rationale. The report states that overweight Australians are a financial burden on the health system. Not only does the impact on the national health budget concern the panel: "It is estimated," they write, "that 300,000 consumers spend . . . $500 million for weight control programs," and this, they believe, is alarming. They rely, for their illustration of the cost of commercial weight loss programs, on a telephone survey to various weight loss centers to determine the price of *hypothetical* weight loss. The authors calculated the cost of a 12-week weight-loss program and divided it by the number of kilograms of *expected* weight loss on the particular diet. Using this study as a rational for Australian healthy policy is problematic. The prices charged by weight loss centers are arbitrary, can increase on the whim of the industry, and importantly, do not reflect efficacy of treatment.

More alarming, however, is that *Acting on Australia's Weight* uses the weight-loss industry as a key player in the education for the prevention of overweight, which it identifies as an area for strategic action. The panel identifies a number of potential leaders in this area of action, but actually hands a portion of the responsibility for the prevention of overweight directly to this private industry player who stands to make significant financial gains from suggesting that weights should be monitored, controlled, and possibly reduced.

Evaluating what the Australian weight-loss industry considers to be overweight reveals considerations that are not based on health or medical evidence. *The Weight Management Industry Code of Practice* is the guiding document for the self-regulating weight-loss industry in Australia. According to this code, the only time weight should be a contraindication to participation in a weight loss program is if a prospective client's body mass index (BMI) is below 20. However, health professionals in the United States, Canada, France, New Zealand, and, ironically, Australia generally accept the range of 20 to 25 as being a healthy height to weight ratio. The code of practice thus invites individuals who are not overweight to lose weight for reasons that have nothing to do with health. Thus, an individual who is 1.7m tall (5'7") would be eligible for enrollment in a weight reduction program at a weight of just 57.8kg (127 lbs.).

Wooley and Garner point out that demand for treatment is not a justification: "Desperate consumers are willing to bear the burden of responsibility for failure in exchange for continuing access to treatment." The immense popular demand sustains the industry, which in turn fosters even greater demand, especially when vested with the responsibility for educating the public on the dangers of overweight. Wooley and Garner explain that self-referring for treatment of other generic problems is generally perceived as a positive thing. The onus is then upon a therapist to explore the reasons for her seeking assistance. However, they write:

> Such an exploration is rarely undertaken with patients who seek obesity treatment. Often they are seen in specialised treatment centres and their mere arrival is considered evidence of appropriate self-screening. To the extent that obesity is defined as a medical problem, such questions may seem less pressing. The benefits of weight loss are so universally prized that it may seem absurd to ask why a patient is seeking treatment at this or any time.

The weight-loss management code of practice refuses to acknowledge that demand does not constitute need, and the Australian public policy document reinforces this. The expert panel also reminds us that "overweight and obese people experience . . . social problems, such as discrimination" and recommends that urgent steps be taken to prevent people becoming overweight and obese. Interestingly, they do not advise anti-discrimination measures to enhance the experience of obese individuals; they shift the responsibility to the obese.

Negativity toward the obese exists even within the medical community. Obese patients become symbols of inadequacy; failure to lose weight fuels their personal feelings of inadequacy and reinforces beliefs of the both medical community and the community at large about the ineptitude of heavy people. Wooley and Garner write:

> patients' attempts to describe the difficulties they are encountering have often been discredited as evidence of their inability to face the truth about themselves . . . Many obese individuals are poised to accept psychologic interpretations for their condition or even to provide their own psychogenic explanation; they, like others, assume that they could not have become obese unless they possessed some fundamental character deficit.

The overweight victims become the perpetrators of the belief as much as those who discriminate against them by fully internalizing the oppressive beliefs about how the body should look if one is to be healthy.

France

The Australian and American approaches to overweight and obesity are not typical of all national attitudes towards the large body. Although other countries may rely heavily on statistical, quantitative, and economic views of the ideal body, they do not necessarily emphasize weight in the same manner as health policy makers in the United States and Australia.

For example, overweight and obesity take a back seat in the French framework for public health action, *Santé 2010*. The issue of weight loss occupies fewer than five paragraphs in an almost 400-page book on the state of health in France. Furthermore, weight loss is first mentioned 123 pages into the work. In contrast, the American *Healthy People 2000* lists "reduce overweight to a prevalence of no more than 20 percent among people aged 20 and older" as no less than the second priority in their health status objectives.

Perhaps this is simply because the French aren't as overweight as the Americans. According to data collected by the National Institute for Statistics and Economic Studies, only 8.5 percent of men and 8.3 percent of women in France are obese (BMI $\geq$ 30), while in the United States, 19.9 percent of men and 25.1 percent of women have a BMI greater than 30. The National Institute statistics show that although the height of both males and females in France increased between 1970 and 1980, the weight of the males stayed the same, and the weight of the females decreased by approximately one kilogram. The authors of *Santé 2010* (1993) applaud the fact that French women gain less weight between the ages of 20 and 50 than women from any other European country. On the other side of the coin, they report that eating disorders affect a growing percentage of the vulnerable age groups.

Santé 2010 expresses pride in the thin French populace while acknowledging, practically in the same breath, the risks involved with a too-acute focus on weight loss. But French documents on obesity and its clinical management also shift the blame away from the overweight person and instead emphasize individual circumstances. Though similar to the Australian and American documents in its quantitative perspective, the *Guide to Diagnosis, Prevention and Treatment of Obesity in France* contains some distinct differences. Notably, though France compliments itself on its slender populace, it does not assume that obesity is the invariable result of personal inadequacy or proof of the inseparable "sins" of gluttony and sloth, which are integral to the discussion in Anglophone literature.

The French paper de-emphasizes measurement and instead stresses the participation of the individual in health assessment. The suggested clinical encounter includes three points: evaluation of the patient request, clinical assessment, and family history. The clinical assessment relies heavily on input from the patient, and puts evaluation of nutritional habits and physical activity on par with, if not before, biological variables. The authors warn against relying on measurements alone, pointing out that "major obesity may be well tolerated by some, while even mild overweight can have a devastating effect on health in other cases, particularly in an individual who is susceptible to metabolic illness, or associated disease."

Despite its title, this document focuses on health promotion strategy rather than on weight in and of itself. As the authors write, "the issue here is to reduce the factors which favor weight gain rather than to defend the notion of an 'ideal weight.' The zone of desirable weights for good health is great. Encouraging thinness to avoid obesity would be an unrealistic and ungrounded proposition which risks producing alarming behavioural and nutritional side-effects." The authors suggest that weight may be more helpful for evaluating population trends than for monitoring the success of individual diet or lifestyle changes, and they believe that "ideal" weights of less than 25 kg/m² are often unrealistic and unjustifiable. Furthermore, the French document mentions the problem of social rejection and personal malaise of the obese in a way that contrasts strikingly with the Australian approach. "For a certain number of individuals for whom obesity does not constitute a vital risk, but is essentially a source of psychological pain," write Basdevant and his colleagues, "the priority should be given to restoring self-esteem, encouraging quality of life, and fighting against social rejection," rather than castigating the heavy.

The French document addresses "obesity"; notably, it does not address "overweight," an important distinction from other approaches. The very word *overweight* does not exist in adjectival form in the French language—its most widely used form in the English language. Description of high body fat is qualitative rather than quantitative, and might include being *bien en chair* (fleshy), *fort* (stocky), *potelé* (chubby), or *grasouillet* (plump). There is no reference in these terms to a measuring standard which one has exceeded. Yet while the report generally encourages lifestyle changes over weight loss, it still remains locked into the weight-loss discourse, and at several important junctures it emphasizes weight loss rather than health gains. For example, the section on "advice to obese subjects to increase physical activity in daily life" starts with the decree that "Walking is vital to control your weight." Overall, however, this document considers individual circumstances and minimizes normative measurements in its definition of health.

Canada

Canadian health guidelines also reject the notion that there is a hard-and-fast "perfect" weight. The *Canadian Guidelines for Healthy Weights* (Health and Welfare Canada 1988) serve as an explanatory document in the face of increasing social preoccupation with weight and the potential exploitation of this concern by the weight management industry. These *Canadian Guidelines* do not focus on "overweight" or on "obesity," but rather on the non-evaluative notion of "weight." This reflects an individual-centered approach that hesitates to group people in categories of "unhealthy" or "irresponsible" on the basis of weight. This report does not assume a definitive and generalized view on the desirability of weight loss but rather emphasizes that there is a wide range of acceptable weights, that even normal weight can fluctuate, and that health care professionals must focus on realistic weights that relate to positive body image. The report pays heed to the lower weight groups as well, indicating that a BMI less than 20 should trigger concern and lead a health care professional to seek an underlying cause of the low weight.

The *Canadian Guidelines* note that professionals, policy makers, and individual citizens use weight as an assessment tool. The *Guidelines* attempt to ensure that this tool is properly utilized, resulting in the establishment of "realistic, practical and meaningful body weights or images of healthy body weight." The *Guidelines* maintain, for example, that population data cannot be used on an individual basis, and they decry the exploitation of weight problems by private industry. A companion publication, T*he Report of the Task Force on the Treatment of Obesity* is devoted to preventing such exploitation by underlining the risks associated with weight loss, the prevalence of social pressures on women to be too thin, and finally, the financial benefits of these social pressures for the weight loss industry.

The authors of the Canadian report review much of the same evidence that underpins the NIH *Clinical Guidelines.* However, they also scrutinize benefits associated with obesity and adverse effects of weight reduction, and conclude that while weight reduction may improve the health of some overweight/obese people, it is neither easy nor innocuous. "The decision to treat obesity," they caution, "is one that should be carefully considered beforehand." They emphasize that BMI alone, though helpful, is inadequate for determining a patient's need for weight reduction; an individual may have an optimal BMI that is above the average range. Furthermore, they point out, as other evidence-based guidelines fail to do, that many individual circumstances—age, muscularity, health status—can render the BMI an unsuitable screening tool. They do not see self-referral as diagnostic, and, in fact, underline the fact that many healthy individuals may expose themselves to significant risk by pursuing weight loss for cosmetic purposes.

The Canadian Health and Welfare Department focuses on health, rather than on normative measurements. As with their French counterparts, weight remains the point of reference, but the content of their discussions rapidly illustrates their health-centered perspective. The word *overweight,* with its linguistic implication of excess, does not appear in the title and is rarely used in the text of either document. The BMI guidelines used by the Canadian task force do not use the term *over-* (or for that matter, *under-*) weight without qualification, specifying "possibly overweight." They suggest that the BMI scale should be "used as a 'continuum' where the risk of developing health problems increases with shifts away from the 'generally acceptable range.'" But they emphasize that a very lean athletic individual may be healthy at a BMI below the acceptable range, just as a short stocky and muscular individual may also have a BMI above this range without risk to his/her health. They write: "body weight partly reflects eating and physical activity habits; however, no two individuals are alike."

James Douketis and William Feldman report in *Prevention of Obesity in Adults,* as part of the Canadian Task Force on the Periodic Health Examination, that BMI need not even be part of routine physical examination:

> There is inadequate evidence at this time to recommend the inclusion or exclusion of BMI in a routine physical examination . . . given the lack of long-term effectiveness of weight reduction therapy in the large majority of obese persons. Weight reduction can be cautiously recommended in obese persons with coexistent diseases who may benefit from weight loss, after taking into account the high recidivism rate and adverse effects of weight loss.

The Canadian documents provide evidence of a very different approach to looking at weight. They recognize that people are concerned about weight but they also acknowledge that these concerns may not necessarily warrant action. By assuming such a position, Canadian health experts lay the groundwork for defining health as an individual state of which measurement may be a component, but certainly not a defining characteristic.

Redefining Health

Preoccupation with weight can be a crippling problem, especially for women, even women of "normal" weight (though men are certainly not immune to them either). Feminist scholars have written extensively about the social and culture emphasis placed on the lean body and about the issues facing women in this domain. As Susan Bordo argues, the practices of femininity, and particularly of dietary restriction and body modeling, reinforce the "feel and conviction of lack, of insufficiency, of never being good enough. At the farthest extremes, the practices of femininity may lead us to utter demoralization, debilitation, and death." Obsessive exercise, eating disorders, and feelings of inadequacy that may accompany an inability to achieve "ideal" weights are great impediments to health maintenance. The fear of being weighed was shown in one study to be the most important factor in women postponing or canceling medical appointments; another study noted a correlation between increased BMI and decreased preventive health care services (Fontaine et al. 1998). Not only are physical activity and diet patterns significant factors in premature death, they are also potentially easier to change than body shape, as they are based on behavior rather than on metabolism, genetics, or bone structure.

However, to emphasize behavior rather than body size, clinicians must learn to view health and the body in different terms. Instead of considering the patient's body as an object for assessment, to be measured and categorized with respect to accepted normative standards, the clinician must see it as an integral part of the individual's identity. Individuals are active beings whose words and accounts, rather than being subordinate, are often more valuable than measurement. Recognizing the values that have, for more than a century, infused clinical practice, may help lead to an understanding of health not as a static condition but rather an active state, one which often defies precise measurement and categorization.

Note

1. The Body Mass Index (BMI, sometimes referred to as the Quetelet Index) is calculated as weight in kilograms divided by height in meters squared. The NIH *Critical Guidelines* consider individuals whose BMI exceeds 25 "overweight," and those whose BMI is 30 or greater "obese."

POSTSCRIPT

Is Body Weight a Reliable Measure of Overall Health?

In these selections, Field and her colleagues use quantitative methods to demonstrate increasing risk for chronic disease with increasing body weight. Jutel argues that using the BMI to define health reduces a complex human condition to one number and, therefore, is inherently misleading and inadequate.

The implications of this argument are extraordinarily important for personal as well as public decisions about diet and activity practices. Using current BMI standards and the latest national data (Flegal et al., *Journal of the American Medical Association*, October 9, 2002), nearly 65 percent of the U.S. population is defined as overweight and in need of dietary advice, drug therapy, or more extreme kinds of medical intervention such as stomach stapling or intestinal bypass surgery. If Field et al. are correct, people now considered at the upper end of the healthy weight range are, in fact, overweight and in need of such medical intervention. As Dutch investigators point out in the 2001 *Annual Review of Public Health,* obesity is now a global problem and one already associated with astronomical personal and monetary costs to society. If more people are defined as overweight, the costs will rise even further.

Thus, the arguments presented here demand careful examination. The Field et al. study is not the only one to find a strong association between BMI and disease risk. June Stevens and her colleagues at the University of North Carolina, Chapel Hill, for example, specifically examined the relationship between fitness and fatness in 2,500 women and 2,900 men (see *American Journal of Epidemiology,* September 2002). Her group observed increases in the hazard ratios (a term similar to relative risk) for deaths from all causes—especially from heart disease—among those who were overweight. The hazard ratios were a bit lower for those who were fit but not a great deal lower. Her study concluded that overweight increases disease risk and that fitness does not entirely overcome such increases. A study by scientists at the Rand Corporation (*Public Health,* May 2001) compared obesity to other risk factors for poor health such as poverty, cigarette smoking, and problem drinking. The Rand study found obesity to be a stronger predictor of poor health and of poor quality of life than any other risk factor except poverty. Indeed, such quantitative studies invariably find obesity to be associated with an increase in risk to health.

The cut point for concern about obesity and health continues to be a matter of debate. The body weights in the study by Field et al. were self-reported. Because of the tendency to underreport overweight, these weights actually could be higher than given in the paper. Also at issue is the size of the increased risk: at what point does an increase in body weight begin to make a *significant* difference in risk? An RR of 2.0 is a 100 percent increase in risk, a percentage that sounds quite high but could mean that two people out of 1,000 have a high cholesterol level instead of just one.

In thinking about this question, one more issue requires consideration: the difference between population recommendations and those for individuals. An increase in risk in a population does not necessarily mean that someone with a BMI of 26 needs to lose weight. As advocates for size acceptance correctly maintain, other factors become critically important when assessing the health risks of individuals. It is essential to keep the distinction between populations and individuals firmly in mind when making personal health choices or advising others about dietary choices. At the same time, all experts agree that weight loss is the first line of defense against syndrome X problems such as high cholesterol, blood pressure, and diabetes, and overweight people who have such risk factors would be well advised to try to reduce their BMI to healthier levels.

ISSUE 7

Can Low-Carbohydrate, Higher-Fat Diets Promote Health and Weight Loss?

YES: Gary Taubes, from "What If It's All Been a Big Fat Lie?" *The New York Times Magazine* (July 7, 2002)

NO: Bonnie Liebman, from "Big Fat Lies: The Truth About the Atkins Diet," *Nutrition Action Health Letter* (November 2002)

ISSUE SUMMARY

YES: Freelance science journalist Gary Taubes says that government advice to eat less fat produces the opposite of its intended effect; it makes Americans fatter. Instead, high-fat diets help people to lose weight and reduce chronic disease risk factors.

NO: Science journalist Bonnie Liebman, director of nutrition at the Center for Science in the Public Interest (CSPI), a consumer advocacy organization in Washington, D.C., counters that high-fat diets raise risks for heart disease and cancer and, when excessive in calories, induce weight gain.

Government agencies spend little money on public education about nutrition, and few Americans are aware of the *Dietary Guidelines for Americans* or of the information booklet that accompanies the U.S. Department of Agriculture (USDA) Food Guide Pyramid. Most Americans learn about nutrition from the media. Because food is a very large business, and because everyone eats every day, the public is fascinated by stories about diet and health, and newspapers, magazines, and television produce such stories almost daily. Consequently, the ways in which the media handles nutrition issues is a matter of great public and professional interest.

In the following selections, two science journalists argue about the implications of government advice to eat less fat. The article by Gary Taubes caused a furor when it appeared in *The New York Times Magazine* in July 2002. In it, Taubes uses research on the glycemic index to make three especially contentious arguments: (1) carbohydrates make us fat; fat does not, (2) low-carbohydrate, high-fat diets like the one developed by the late Dr. Robert Atkins help people lose weight and reduce chronic disease risk factors, and (3) government advice to eat more carbohydrates, such as that given in the Food Guide Pyramid, promotes obesity and the chronic diseases for which obesity is a risk factor. The Atkins diet, he says, makes sense because it avoids the problems caused by eating carbohydrates— overproduction of insulin and consequent hypoglycemia, insulin resistance, and hunger. Taubes charges government agencies and some scientists with suppressing or ignoring the fact that "20 years of low-fat recommendations have not managed to lower the incidence of heart disease in this country and may have led instead to the steep increase in obesity and type 2 diabetes." This failure of public policy, he suggests, deserves nothing less than an apology.

As might be expected, so strong an attack on conventional dietary wisdom stimulated other journalists to enter the debate. One is Bonnie Liebman, who has long been devoted to educating the public about diet and health. Liebman's point-by-point rebuttal suggests that Taubes's arguments are based on a biased and distorted selection of facts and information given to him by experts. Health authorities have never promoted low-fat diets as the key to weight loss (they actually were promoting caloric restriction); Americans as a population have never eaten a low-fat diet, so low-fat diets cannot be responsible for obesity; and the Atkins diet is too high in saturated fat to be considered healthful. Instead, she says, Americans should continue to follow advice to restrict intake of saturated fat, should avoid overeating carbohydrates because of their calories, should reduce overall calories in order to lose weight, and should choose healthier fats (from vegetables rather than from animals) and healthier carbohydrates (whole grains rather than refined grains).

The implications of this debate are worth careful thought. If Taubes is correct, health authorities should reverse the Pyramid to emphasize consumption of high-fat, high-protein foods and to deemphasize consumption of processed grains—a design closer to the Healthy Eating Pyramid developed by Dr. Walter C. Willett than to the USDA's Food Guide Pyramid. Furthermore, people who wish to lose weight should be encouraged to go on Atkins-like diets, high in animal fat and protein and low in carbohydrate. If, as Liebman charges, this interpretation of the science is incorrect, health authorities should continue to promote largely plant-based diets—though those emphasizing good carbohydrates—as a means to promote health.

In the following selections, Taubes argues that lower-carbohydrate, higher-fat diets are better for health and control of body weight, but Liebman says that such diets raise risks for heart disease and cancer and have no particular benefit for weight loss.

Gary Taubes

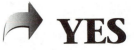

What If It's All Been a Big Fat Lie?

When Atkins first published his "Diet Revolution" in 1972, Americans were just coming to terms with the proposition that fat—particularly the saturated fat of meat and dairy products—was the primary nutritional evil in the American diet. Atkins managed to sell millions of copies of a book promising that we would lose weight eating steak, eggs and butter to our heart's desire, because it was the carbohydrates, the pasta, rice, bagels and sugar, that caused obesity and even heart disease. Fat, he said, was harmless.

Atkins allowed his readers to eat "truly luxurious foods without limit," as he put it, "lobster with butter sauce, steak with béarnaise sauce . . . *bacon* cheeseburgers," but allowed no starches or refined carbohydrates, which means no sugars or anything made from flour. Atkins banned even fruit juices, and permitted only a modicum of vegetables, although the latter were negotiable as the diet progressed. . . .

Thirty years later, America has become weirdly polarized on the subject of weight. On the one hand, we've been told with almost religious certainty by everyone from the surgeon general on down, and we have come to believe with almost religious certainty, that obesity is caused by the excessive consumption of fat, and that if we eat less fat we will lose weight and live longer. On the other, we have the ever-resilient message of Atkins and decades' worth of best-selling diet books, including "The Zone," "Sugar Busters" and "Protein Power" to name a few. All push some variation of what scientists would call the alternative hypothesis: it's not the fat that makes us fat, but the carbohydrates, and if we eat less carbohydrates we will lose weight and live longer.

The perversity of this alternative hypothesis is that it identifies the cause of obesity as precisely those refined carbohydrates at the base of the famous Food Guide Pyramid—the pasta, rice and bread—that we are told should be the staple of our healthy low-fat diet, and then on the sugar or corn syrup in the soft drinks, fruit juices and sports drinks that we have taken to consuming in quantity if for no other reason than that they are fat free and so appear intrinsically healthy. While the low-fat-is-good-health dogma represents reality as we have come to know it, and the government has spent hundreds of millions of dollars in research trying to prove its worth, the low-carbohydrate message has been relegated to the realm of unscientific fantasy.

Over the past five years, however, there has been a subtle shift in the scientific consensus. It used to be that even considering the possibility of the alternative hypothesis, let alone researching it, was tantamount to quackery by association. Now a small but growing minority of establishment researchers have come to take seriously what the low-carb-diet doctors have been saying all along. Walter Willett, chairman of the department of nutrition at the Harvard School of Public Health, may be the most visible proponent of testing this heretic hypothesis. Willett is the de facto spokesman of the longest-running, most comprehensive diet and health studies ever performed, which have already cost upward of $100 million and include data on nearly 300,000 individuals. Those data, says Willett, clearly contradict the low-fat-is-good-health message "and the idea that all fat is bad for you; the exclusive focus on adverse effects of fat may have contributed to the obesity epidemic."

These researchers point out that there are plenty of reasons to suggest that the low-fat-is-good-health hypothesis has now effectively failed the test of time. In particular, that we are in the midst of an obesity epidemic that started around the early 1980's, and that this was coincident with the rise of the low-fat dogma. (Type 2 diabetes, the most common form of the disease, also rose significantly through this period.) They say that low-fat weight-loss diets have proved in clinical trials and real life to be dismal failures, and that on top of it all, the percentage of fat in the American diet has been decreasing for two decades. Our cholesterol levels have been declining, and we have been smoking less, and yet the incidence of heart disease has not declined as would be expected. "That is very disconcerting," Willett says. "It suggests that something else bad is happening."

The science behind the alternative hypothesis can be called Endocrinology 101, which is how it's referred to by David Ludwig, a researcher at Harvard Medical School who runs the pediatric obesity clinic at Children's Hospital Boston, and who prescribes his own version of a carbohydrate-restricted diet to his patients. Endocrinology 101 requires an understanding of how carbohydrates affect insulin and blood sugar and in turn fat metabolism and appetite. This is basic endocrinology, Ludwig says, which is the study of hormones, and it is still considered radical because the low-fat dietary wisdom emerged in the 1960's from researchers almost exclusively concerned with the effect of fat on cholesterol and heart disease. At the time, Endocrinology 101 was still underdeveloped, and so it was ignored. Now that this science is becoming clear, it has to fight a quarter century of anti-fat prejudice.

The alternative hypothesis also comes with an implication that is worth considering for a moment, because it's a whopper, and it may indeed be an obstacle to its acceptance. If the alternative hypothesis is right—still a big "if"—then it strongly suggests that the ongoing epidemic of obesity in America and elsewhere is not, as we are constantly told, due simply to a collective lack of will power and a failure to exercise. Rather it occurred, as Atkins has been saying (along with Barry Sears, author of "The Zone"), because the public health authorities told us unwittingly, but with the best of intentions, to eat precisely those foods that would make us fat, and we did. We ate more fat-free carbohydrates, which, in turn, made us hungrier and then heavier. Put simply, if the alternative hypothesis is right, then a low-fat diet is not by definition a healthy diet. In practice, such a diet cannot help being high in carbohydrates, and that can lead to obesity, and perhaps even heart disease. . . .

⌘

Scientists are still arguing about fat, despite a century of research, because the regulation of appetite and weight in the human body happens to be almost inconceivably complex, and the experimental tools we have to study it are still remarkably inadequate. This combination leaves researchers in an awkward position. To study the entire physiological system involves feeding real food to real human subjects for months or years on end, which is prohibitively expensive, ethically questionable (if you're trying to measure the effects of foods that might cause heart disease) and virtually impossible to do in any kind of rigorously controlled scientific manner. But if researchers seek to study something less costly and more controllable, they end up studying experimental situations so oversimplified that their results may have nothing to do with reality. This then leads to a research literature so vast that it's possible to find at least some published research to support virtually any theory. The result is a balkanized community—"splintered, very opinionated and in many instances, intransigent," says Kurt Isselbacher, a former chairman of the Food and Nutrition Board of the National Academy of Science—in which researchers seem easily convinced that their preconceived notions are correct and thoroughly uninterested in testing any other hypotheses but their own. . . .

With these caveats, one of the few reasonably reliable facts about the obesity epidemic is that it started around the early 1980's. According to Katherine Flegal, an epidemiologist at the National Center for Health Statistics, the percentage of obese Americans stayed relatively constant through the 1960's and 1970's at 13 percent to 14 percent and then shot up by 8 percentage points in the 1980's. By the end of that decade, nearly one in four Americans was obese. That steep rise, which is consistent through all segments of American society and which continued unabated through the 1990's, is the singular feature of the epidemic. Any theory that tries to explain obesity in America has to account for that. Meanwhile, overweight children nearly tripled in number. And for the first time, physicians began diagnosing Type 2 diabetes in adolescents. Type 2 diabetes often accompanies obesity. It used to be called adult-onset diabetes and now, for the obvious reason, is not.

So how did this happen? The orthodox and ubiquitous explanation is that we live in what Kelly Brownell, a Yale psychologist, has called a "toxic food environment" of cheap fatty food, large portions, pervasive food advertising and sedentary lives. By this theory, we are at the Pavlovian mercy of the food industry, which spends nearly $10 billion a year advertising unwholesome junk food and fast food. And because these foods, especially fast food, are so filled with fat, they are both irresistible and uniquely fattening. On top of this, so the theory goes, our modern society has successfully eliminated physical activity from our daily lives. We no longer exercise or walk up stairs, nor do our children bike to school or play outside, because they would prefer to play video games and watch television. And because some of us are obviously predisposed to gain weight while others are not, this explanation also has a genetic component—the thrifty gene. It suggests that storing extra calories as fat was an evolutionary advantage to our Paleolithic ancestors, who had to survive frequent famine. We then inherited these "thrifty" genes, despite their liability in today's toxic environment.

This theory makes perfect sense and plays to our puritanical prejudice that fat, fast food and television are innately damaging to our humanity. . . . Fast-food consumption, for example, continued to grow steadily through the 70's and 80's, but it did not take a sudden leap, as obesity did.

As far as exercise and physical activity go, there are no reliable data before the mid-80's, according to William Dietz, who runs the division of nutrition and physical activity at the Centers for Disease Control; the 1990's data show obesity rates continuing to climb, while exercise activity remained unchanged. This suggests the two have little in common. Dietz also acknowledged that a culture of physical exercise began in the United States in the 70's—the "leisure exercise mania," as Robert Levy, director of the National Heart, Lung and Blood Institute, described it in 1981—and has continued through the present day.

As for the thrifty gene, it provides the kind of evolutionary rationale for human behavior that scientists find comforting but that simply cannot be tested. In other words, if we were living through an anorexia epidemic, the experts would be discussing the equally untestable "spendthrift gene" theory, touting evolutionary advantages of losing weight effortlessly. An overweight homo erectus, they'd say, would have been easy prey for predators.

It is also undeniable, note students of Endocrinology 101, that mankind never evolved to eat a diet high in starches or sugars. "Grain products and concentrated sugars were essentially absent from human nutrition until the invention of agriculture," Ludwig says, "which was only 10,000 years ago." This is discussed frequently in the anthropology texts but is mostly absent from the obesity literature, with the prominent exception of the low-carbohydrate-diet books.

. . . Ancel Keys . . . introduced the low-fat-is-good-health dogma in the 50's with his theory that dietary fat raises cholesterol levels and gives you heart disease. Over the next two decades, however, the scientific evidence supporting this theory remained stubbornly ambiguous. The case was eventually settled not by new science but by politics. It began in January 1977, when a Senate committee led by George McGovern published its "Dietary Goals for the United States," advising that Americans significantly curb their fat intake to abate an epidemic of "killer diseases" supposedly sweeping the country. It peaked in late 1984, when the National Institutes of Health officially recommended that all Americans over the age of 2 eat less fat. . . .

In the intervening years, the N.I.H. spent several hundred million dollars trying to demonstrate a connection between eating fat and getting heart disease and, despite what we might think, it failed. Five major studies revealed no such link. A sixth, however, costing well over $100 million alone, concluded that reducing cholesterol by drug therapy could prevent heart disease. The N.I.H.

administrators then made a leap of faith. Basil Rifkind, who oversaw the relevant trials for the N.I.H., described their logic this way: they had failed to demonstrate at great expense that eating less fat had any health benefits. But if a cholesterol-lowering drug could prevent heart attacks, then a low-fat, cholesterol-lowering diet should do the same. "It's an imperfect world," Rifkind told me. "The data that would be definitive is ungettable, so you do your best with what is available."

Some of the best scientists disagreed with this low-fat logic, suggesting that good science was incompatible with such leaps of faith, but they were effectively ignored. . . .

Nonetheless, once the N.I.H. signed off on the low-fat doctrine, societal forces took over. The food industry quickly began producing thousands of reduced-fat food products to meet the new recommendations. Fat was removed from foods like cookies, chips and yogurt. The problem was, it had to be replaced with something as tasty and pleasurable to the palate, which meant some form of sugar, often high-fructose corn syrup. Meanwhile, an entire industry emerged to create fat substitutes, of which Procter & Gamble's olestra was first. And because these reduced-fat meats, cheeses, snacks and cookies had to compete with a few hundred thousand other food products marketed in America, the industry dedicated considerable advertising effort to reinforcing the less-fat-is-good-health message. Helping the cause was what Walter Willett calls the "huge forces" of dietitians, health organizations, consumer groups, health reporters and even cookbook writers, all well-intended missionaries of healthful eating.

***

Few experts now deny that the low-fat message is radically oversimplified. If nothing else, it effectively ignores the fact that unsaturated fats, like olive oil, are relatively good for you: they tend to elevate your good cholesterol, high-density lipoprotein (H.D.L.), and lower your bad cholesterol, low-density lipoprotein (L.D.L.), at least in comparison to the effect of carbohydrates. While higher L.D.L. raises your heart-disease risk, higher H.D.L. reduces it.

What this means is that even saturated fats—a k a, the bad fats—are not nearly as deleterious as you would think. True, they will elevate your bad cholesterol, but they will also elevate your good cholesterol. In other words, it's a virtual wash. As Willett explained to me, you will gain little to no health benefit by giving up milk, butter and cheese and eating bagels instead. . . .

The crucial example of how the low-fat recommendations were oversimplified is shown by the impact—potentially lethal, in fact—of low-fat diets on triglycerides, which are the component molecules of fat. By the late 60's, researchers had shown that high triglyceride levels were at least as common in heart-disease patients as high L.D.L. cholesterol, and that eating a low-fat, high-carbohydrate diet would, for many people, raise their triglyceride levels, lower their H.D.L. levels and accentuate what Gerry Reaven, an endocrinologist at Stanford University, called Syndrome X. This is a cluster of conditions that can lead to heart disease and Type 2 diabetes. . . .

Nutrition researchers also played a role by trying to feed science into the idea that carbohydrates are the ideal nutrient. It had been known, for almost a century, and considered mostly irrelevant to the etiology of obesity, that fat has nine calories per gram compared with four for carbohydrates and protein. Now it became the fail-safe position of the low-fat recommendations: reduce the densest source of calories in the diet and you will lose weight. Then in 1982, J. P. Flatt, a University of Massachusetts biochemist, published his research demonstrating that, in any normal diet, it is extremely rare for the human body to convert carbohydrates into body fat. This was then misinterpreted by the media and quite a few scientists to mean that eating carbohydrates, even to excess, could not make you fat—which is not the case, Flatt says. But the misinterpretation developed a vigorous life of its own because it resonated with the notion that fat makes you fat and carbohydrates are harmless.

As a result, the major trends in American diets since the late 70's, according to the U.S.D.A. agricultural economist Judith Putnam, have been a decrease in the percentage of fat calories and a "greatly increased consumption of carbohydrates." To be precise, annual grain consumption has increased almost 60 pounds per person, and caloric sweeteners (primarily high-fructose corn syrup) by 30 pounds. At the same time, we suddenly began consuming more total calories: now up to 400 more each day since the government started recommending low-fat diets.

If these trends are correct, then the obesity epidemic can certainly be explained by Americans' eating more calories than ever—excess calories, after all, are what causes us to gain weight—and, specifically, more carbohydrates. The question is why?

The answer provided by Endocrinology 101 is that we are simply hungrier than we were in the 70's, and the reason is physiological more than psychological. In this case, the salient factor—ignored in the pursuit of fat and its effect on cholesterol—is how carbohydrates affect blood sugar and insulin. In fact, these were obvious culprits all along, which is why Atkins and the low-carb-diet doctors pounced on them early.

. . . The fatter you are, the more insulin your pancreas will pump out per meal, and the more likely you'll develop what's called "insulin resistance," which is the underlying cause of Syndrome X. In effect, your cells become insensitive to the action of insulin, and so you need ever greater amounts to keep your blood sugar in check. So as you gain weight, insulin makes it easier to store fat and harder to lose it. But the insulin resistance in turn may make it harder to store fat—your weight is being kept in check, as it should be. But now the insulin resistance might prompt your pancreas to produce even more insulin, potentially starting a vicious cycle. . . .

David Ludwig, the Harvard endocrinologist, . . . notes that when diabetics get too much insulin, their blood sugar drops and they get ravenously hungry. They gain weight because they eat more, and the insulin promotes fat deposition. The same happens with lab animals. This, he says, is effectively what happens when we eat carbohydrates—in particular sugar and starches like potatoes and rice, or anything made from flour, like a slice of white bread. These are known in the jargon as high-glycemic-index carbohydrates, which means they are absorbed quickly into the blood. As a result, they cause a spike of blood sugar and a surge of insulin within minutes. The resulting rush of insulin stores the blood sugar away and a few hours later, your blood sugar is lower than it was before you ate. As Ludwig explains, your body effectively thinks it has run out of fuel, but the insulin is still high enough to prevent you from burning your own fat. The result is hunger and a craving for more carbohydrates. It's another vicious circle, and another situation ripe for obesity. . . .

Sugar and corn syrup from soft drinks, juices and the copious teas and sports drinks now supply more than 10 percent of our total calories; the 80's saw the introduction of Big Gulps and 32-ounce cups of Coca-Cola, blasted through with sugar, but 100 percent fat free. When it comes to insulin and blood sugar, these soft drinks and fruit juices—what the scientists call "wet carbohydrates"—might indeed be worst of all. (Diet soda accounts for less than a quarter of the soda market.)

The gist of the glycemic-index idea is that the longer it takes the carbohydrates to be digested, the lesser the impact on blood sugar and insulin and the healthier the food. Those foods with the highest rating on the glycemic index are some simple sugars, starches and anything made from flour. Green vegetables, beans and whole grains cause a much slower rise in blood sugar because they have fiber, a nondigestible carbohydrate, which slows down digestion and lowers the glycemic index. Protein and fat serve the same purpose, which implies that eating fat can be beneficial, a notion that is still unacceptable. And the glycemic-index concept implies that a primary cause of Syndrome X, heart disease, Type 2 diabetes and obesity is the long-term damage caused by the repeated surges of insulin that come from eating starches and refined carbohydrates. This suggests a kind of unified field theory for these chronic diseases, but not one that coexists easily with the low-fat doctrine. . . .

The 71-year-old Atkins, a graduate of Cornell medical school, says he first tried a very low carbohydrate diet in 1963 after reading about one in the Journal of the American Medical Association. He lost weight effortlessly, had his epiphany and turned a fledgling Manhattan cardiology practice into a thriving obesity clinic. He then alienated the entire medical community by telling his readers to eat as much fat and protein as they wanted, as long as they ate little to no carbohydrates. They would lose weight, he said, because they would keep their insulin down; they wouldn't be hungry; and they would have less resistance to burning their own fat. Atkins also noted that starches and sugar were harmful in any event because they raised triglyceride levels and that this was a greater risk factor for heart disease than cholesterol.

Atkins's diet is both the ultimate manifestation of the alternative hypothesis as well as the battleground on which the fat-versus-carbohydrates controversy is likely to be fought scientifically over the next few years. After insisting Atkins was a quack for three decades, obesity experts are now finding it difficult to ignore the copious anecdotal evidence that his diet does just what he has claimed.

. . . [One question is] why such a low-calorie regimen would also suppress hunger, which Atkins insisted was the signature characteristic of the diet. One possibility was Endocrinology 101: that fat and protein make you sated and, lacking carbohydrates and the ensuing swings of blood sugar and insulin, you stay sated. The other possibility arose from the fact that Atkins's diet is "keto-genic." This means that insulin falls so low that you enter a state called ketosis, which is what happens during fasting and starvation. Your muscles and tissues burn body fat for energy, as does your brain in the form of fat molecules produced by the liver called ketones. Atkins saw ketosis as the obvious way to kick-start weight loss. He also liked to say that ketosis was so energizing that it was better than sex, which set him up for some ridicule. An inevitable criticism of Atkins's diet has been that ketosis is dangerous and to be avoided at all costs.

When I interviewed ketosis experts, however, they universally sided with Atkins, and suggested that maybe the medical community and the media confuse ketosis with ketoacidosis, a variant of ketosis that occurs in untreated diabetics and can be fatal. "Doctors are scared of ketosis," says Richard Veech, an N.I.H. researcher who studied medicine at Harvard and then got his doctorate at Oxford University with the Nobel Laureate Hans Krebs. "They're always worried about diabetic ketoacidosis. But ketosis is a normal physiologic state. I would argue it is the normal state of man. It's not normal to have McDonald's and a deli-catessen around every corner. It's normal to starve."

Simply put, ketosis is evolution's answer to the thrifty gene. We may have evolved to efficiently store fat for times of famine, says Veech, but we also evolved ketosis to efficiently live off that fat when necessary. Rather than being poison, which is how the press often refers to ketones, they make the body run more efficiently and provide a backup fuel source for the brain. . . .

The bottom line is that for the better part of 30 years Atkins insisted his diet worked and was safe, Americans apparently tried it by the tens of millions, while nutritionists, physicians, public-health authorities and anyone concerned with heart disease insisted it could kill them, and expressed little or no desire to find out who was right. During that period, only two groups of U.S. researchers tested the diet, or at least published their results. In the early 70's, J.P. Flatt and Harvard's George Blackburn pioneered the "protein-sparing modified fast" to treat postsurgical patients, and they tested it on obese volunteers. Black-burn, who later became president of the American Society of Clinical Nutrition, describes his regime as "an Atkins diet without excess fat" and says he had to give it a fancy name or nobody would take him seriously. The diet was "lean meat, fish and fowl" supplemented by vitamins and minerals. "People loved it," Blackburn recalls. "Great weight loss. We couldn't run them off with a baseball bat." Blackburn successfully treated hundreds of obese patients over the next decade and published a series of papers that were ignored. When obese New Englanders turned to appetite-control drugs in the mid-80's, he says, he let it drop. He then applied to the N.I.H. for a grant to do a clinical trial of popular diets but was rejected.

The second trial, published in September 1980, was done at the George Washington University Medical Center. Two dozen obese volunteers agreed to follow Atkins's diet for eight weeks and lost an average of 17 pounds each, with no apparent ill effects, although their L.D.L. cholesterol did go up. The researchers, led by John LaRosa, now president of the State University of New York Downstate Medical Center in Brooklyn, concluded that the 17-pound weight loss in eight weeks would likely have happened with any diet under "the novelty of trying something under experimental conditions" and never pursued it further.

. . . And then there's the study by Gary Foster at the University of Pennsylvania, Sam Klein, director of the Center for Human Nutrition at Washington University in St. Louis, and Jim Hill, who runs the University of Colorado Center for Human Nutrition in Denver. The results . . . of these studies are remarkably consistent. Subjects on some form of the Atkins diet— . . . as at the Philadelphia V.A.—lost twice the weight as the subjects on the low-fat, low-calorie diets.

. . . For the first time, the N.I.H. is now actually financing comparative studies of popular diets. Foster, Klein and Hill, for instance, have now received more than $2.5 million from N.I.H. to do a five-year trial of the Atkins diet with 360 obese individuals. At Harvard, Willett, Blackburn and Penelope Greene have money, albeit from Atkins's nonprofit foundation, to do a comparative trial as well.

Should these clinical trials also find for Atkins and his high-fat, low-carbohydrate diet, then the public-health authorities may indeed have a problem on their hands. Once they took their leap of faith and settled on the low-fat dietary dogma 25 years ago, they left little room for contradictory evidence or a change of opinion, should such a change be necessary to keep up with the science. . . .

After 20 years steeped in a low-fat paradigm, I find it hard to see the nutritional world any other way. I have learned that low-fat diets fail in clinical trials and in real life, and they certainly have failed in my life. I have read the papers suggesting that 20 years of low-fat recommendations have not managed to lower the incidence of heart disease in this country, and may have led instead to the steep increase in obesity and Type 2 diabetes. I have interviewed researchers whose computer models have calculated that cutting back on the saturated fats in my diet to the levels recommended by the American Heart Association would not add more than a few months to my life, if that. I have even lost considerable weight with relative ease by giving up carbohydrates on my test diet, and yet I can look down at my eggs and sausage and still imagine the imminent onset of heart disease and obesity. . . .

This is the state of mind I imagine that mainstream nutritionists, researchers and physicians must inevitably take to the fat-versus-carbohydrate controversy. They may come around, but the evidence will have to be exceptionally compelling. Although this kind of conversion may be happening at the moment to John Farquhar, who is a professor of health research and policy at Stanford University and has worked in this field for more than 40 years. When I interviewed Farquhar in April, he explained why low-fat diets might lead to weight gain and low-carbohydrate diets might lead to weight loss, but he made me promise not to say he believed they did. He attributed the cause of the obesity epidemic to the "force-feeding of a nation." Three weeks later, after reading an article on Endocrinology 101 by David Ludwig in the Journal of the American Medical Association, he sent me an e-mail message asking the not-entirely-rhetorical question, "Can we get the low-fat proponents to apologize?"

NO ←

Bonnie Liebman

Big Fat Lies:
The Truth About the Atkins Diet

What If It's All Been a Big Fat Lie?" asked the cover story of the July 7th *New York Times Magazine.* The article, by freelance writer Gary Taubes, argues that loading our plates with fatty meats, cheeses, cream, and butter is the key not just to weight loss, but to a long, healthy life.

"Influential researchers are beginning to embrace the medical heresy that maybe Dr. Atkins was right," writes Taubes.

Taubes claims that it's not fatty foods that make us fat and raise our risk of disease. It's carbohydrates. And to most readers his arguments sound perfectly plausible.

Here are the facts—and the fictions—in Taubes's article, which has led to a book contract with a reported $700,000 advance. And here's what the scientists he quoted—or neglected to quote—have to say about his reporting.

⋅◦⟨◦⟩◦⋅

Perhaps the most telling statement in Gary Taubes's *New York Times Magazine* article comes as he explains how difficult it is to study diet and health. "This then leads to a research literature so vast that it's possible to find at least some published research to support virtually any theory."

He got *that* right. It helps explain why Taubes's article sounds so credible.

"He knows how to spin a yarn," says Barbara Rolls, an obesity expert at Pennsylvania State University. "What frightens me is that he picks and chooses his facts."

She ought to know. Taubes interviewed her for some six hours, and she sent him "a huge bundle of papers," but he didn't quote a word of it. "If the facts don't fit in with his yarn, he ignores them," she says.

Instead, Taubes put together what sounds like convincing evidence that carbohydrates cause obesity.

"He took this weird little idea and blew it up, and people believed him," says John Farquhar, a professor emeritus of medicine at Stanford University's Center for Research in Disease Prevention. Taubes quoted Farquhar, but misrepresented his views. "What a disaster," says Farquhar.

Others agree. "It's silly to say that carbohydrates cause obesity," says George Blackburn of Harvard Medical School and the Beth Israel Deaconess Medical Center in Boston. "We're overweight because we overeat calories."

It's not clear how Taubes thought he could ignore—or distort—what researchers told him. "The article was written in bad faith," says F. Xavier Pi-Sunyer, director of the Obesity Research Center at St. Luke's-Roosevelt Hospital Center in New York. "It was irresponsible."

Here's a point-by-point response to Taubes's major claims.

Claim #1: The Experts Recommend an Atkins Diet
Truth: They Don't

An Atkins diet is loaded with meat, butter, and other foods high in saturated fat. Taubes implies that many of the experts he quotes recommend it. Here's what they say:

- "The article was incredibly misleading," says Gerald Reaven, the pioneering Stanford University researcher, now emeritus, who coined the term "Syndrome X." "My quote was correct, but the context suggested that I support eating saturated fat. I was horrified."
- According to Taubes, Harvard University's Walter Willett is one of the "small but growing minority of establishment researchers [who] have come to take seriously what the low-carb-diet doctors have been saying all along."

True, Willett is concerned about the harm that may be caused by high-carbohydrate diets (see [box entitled] "What to Eat"). But the Atkins diet? "I certainly don't recommend it," he says.

His reasons: heart disease and cancer. "There's a clear benefit for reducing cardiovascular risk from replacing unhealthy fats—saturated and trans—with healthy fats," explains Willett, who chairs Harvard's nutrition department. "And I told Taubes several times that red meat is associated with a higher risk of colon and possibly prostate cancer, but he left that out."

- "I was greatly offended at how Gary Taubes tricked us all into coming across as supporters of the Atkins diet," says Stanford's John Farquhar.

Taubes's article ends with a quote from Farquhar, asking: "Can we get the low-fat proponents to apologize?" But that quote was taken out of context.

"What I was referring to wasn't that low-fat diets would make a person gain weight and become obese," explains Farquhar. Like Willett and Reaven, he's worried that too much carbohydrate can raise the risk of heart disease.

"I meant that in susceptible individuals, a *very*-low-fat [high-carb] diet can raise triglycerides, lower HDL ['good'] cholesterol, and make harmful, small, dense LDL," says Farquhar.

Carbohydrates are not what has made us a nation of butterballs, however. "We're overfed, over-advertised, and under-exercised," he says. "It's the enormous portion sizes and sitting in front of the TV and computer all day" that are to blame. "It's so gol'darn obvious—how can anyone ignore it?"

"The *Times* editor called and tried to get me to say that low-fat diets were the cause of obesity, but I wouldn't," adds Farquhar.

Claim #2: Saturated Fat Doesn't Promote Heart Disease
Truth: It Does

If there's any advice that experts agree on, it's that people should cut back on saturated fat. They've looked not just at its effect on cholesterol levels, but on its tendency to promote blood clots, raise insulin levels, and damage blood vessels. They've issued that advice after examining animal studies, population studies, and clinical studies. Taubes dismisses them with one narrow argument.

Saturated fats, he writes, "will elevate your bad cholesterol, but they will also elevate your good cholesterol. In other words, it's a virtual wash."

Experts disagree. "Fifty years of research shows that saturated fat and cholesterol raise LDL ['bad'] cholesterol, and the higher your LDL, the higher your risk of coronary heart disease," says Farquhar. Yet Taubes has no qualms about encouraging people to eat foods that raise their LDL.

He's willing to bet that higher HDL ("good") cholesterol will protect them. No experts—at the American Heart Association; National Heart, Lung, and Blood Institute; or elsewhere—would take that risk.

"The evidence that raising HDL is protective is less solid than the evidence that raising LDL is bad," says David Gordon, a researcher at the National Heart, Lung, and Blood Institute.

Claim #3: Health Authorities Recommended a Low-Fat Diet as the Key to Weight Loss
Truth: They Didn't

"We've been told with almost religious certainty by everyone from the Surgeon General on down, and we have come to believe with almost religious certainty, that obesity is caused by the excessive consumption of fat, and that if we eat less fat we will lose weight and live longer," writes Taubes.

It's true that some diet books, notably Dean Ornish's *Eat More, Weigh Less,* have encouraged people to eat as much fat-free food as they want. (Of course, Ornish is talking about fruits, vegetables, and whole grains, not fat-free cakes, cookies, and ice cream.) But "everyone from the Surgeon General on down" is baloney.

"The Surgeon General's report doesn't say that fat causes obesity," says Marion Nestle, who was managing editor of the report and is now chair of the nutrition and food studies department at New York University. "Fat has twice the calories of either protein or carbohydrate. That's why fat is fattening unless people limit calories from everything else."

And health authorities like the American Heart Association; National Heart, Lung, and Blood Institute; and U.S. Department of Agriculture never urged people to cut way back on fat. Their advice: "Get no more than 30 percent of calories from fat." At the time that advice was issued, the average person was eating 35 percent fat.

Claim #4: We're Fat Because We Ate a Low-Fat Diet

Truth: We Never Ate a Low-Fat Diet

"At the very moment that the government started telling Americans to eat less fat, we got fatter," says Taubes. "We ate more fat-free carbohydrates, which, in turn, made us hungrier and then heavier."

It's hard to believe this claim passed the laugh test at *The Times*. If you believe Taubes, it's not the 670-calorie Cinnabons, the 900-calorie slices of Sbarro's sausage-and-pepperoni-stuffed pizza, the 1,000-calorie shakes or Double Whoppers with Cheese, the 1,600-calorie buckets of movie theater popcorn, or the 3,000-calorie orders of cheese fries that have padded our backsides. It's only the low-fat Snackwells, pasta (with fat-free sauce), and bagels (with no cream cheese).

"It's preposterous," says Samuel Klein, director of the Center for Human Nutrition at the Washington University School of Medicine in St. Louis. "There's no real evidence that low-fat diets have caused the obesity epidemic."

Taubes argues that in the late 1970s, health authorities started telling Americans to cut back on fat, and that we did. Wrong.

According to the U.S. Department of Agriculture, *added* fats (oils, shortening, lard, and beef tallow) have gone up steadily since the late 1970s (see "Hardly a Low-Fat Diet"). *Total* fats (which include the fat in meats, cheese, and other foods) have also gone up, though not as steadily.

So how can Taubes write that "the major trends in American diets, according to USDA agricultural economist Judith Putnam, have been a decrease in the percentage of fat calories and a 'greatly increased consumption of carbohydrates'"?

The key is the word "percentage." The percentage of fat calories in our diets declined because, while we ate more fat calories, we ate even more carbohydrate calories.

"We're eating roughly 500 calories a day more than we did in 1980," Putnam told us. "More than a third of the increase comes from refined grains, a fifth comes from added sugars, and a third comes from added fats."

Government surveys show no change—or a slight decrease—in fat consumption since the late 1970s. But they don't look at how much fat is produced, how much is sold, and how much is wasted. The surveys simply ask consumers what they eat. And it's possible that once people were told to eat less fat, they (consciously or unconsciously) started under-reporting how much they ate.

Says Putnam: "People don't adequately report added fats, added sugars, and refined grains."

The bottom line: Taubes blames the obesity epidemic on a low-fat diet that the nation never ate.

Claim #5: Carbs, Not Fats, Cause Obesity
Truth: The Evidence Blaming Obesity on Carbs Is Flimsy

The evidence that carbohydrates make you fat can be called "Endocrinology 101," says Taubes, implying that it's well-established fact. In a nutshell, Endocrinology 101 says that "we're hungrier than we were in the '70s" because we're eating more carbohydrates.

"Sugar and starches like potatoes and rice, or anything made from flour, like a slice of white bread," are "known in the jargon as high-glycemic-index carbohydrates, which means they are absorbed quickly into the blood," explains Taubes.

"As a result they cause a spike of blood sugar and a surge of insulin within minutes. The resulting rush of insulin stores the blood sugar away and a few hours later, your blood sugar is lower than it was before you ate. . . . The result is hunger and a craving for more carbohydrates."

It sounds convincing, but there's a problem: "It's not proven at all," says Penn State's Barbara Rolls. "We have no firm data that glycemic index affects body weight or how full people feel after eating."

Harvard's David Ludwig has done a few studies on glycemic index and weight. In the largest, he found that 64 overweight adolescents who were told to eat lower-glycemic-index foods lost an average of four pounds, while 43 overweight adolescents who were told to make modest cuts in calories and fat gained three pounds.

"It's hard to tease apart what led to the weight loss in that study," explains Rolls, "because calorie density, fiber, and glycemic index all go hand in hand."

In other words, foods with a low glycemic index—most vegetables, fruits, and whole grains—are also high in fiber and low in calorie density.

What's more, Ludwig's study didn't randomly assign children to one diet or another, so the two groups weren't comparable. "The low-glycemic-index group had fewer minorities," says Columbia's Pi-Sunyer. Whites in both groups were more likely to lose weight.

And he and others question the whole glycemic index theory. Among his criticisms: "People eat meals, where low-glycemic foods balance out high-glycemic foods."

For example, "people don't eat pasta alone," he explains. "They eat it with olive oil, clams, tomatoes, or other foods, and that dampens the differences in their effects on insulin."

And, contrary to Taubes's claims, there is no good evidence that insulin triggers weight gain. "Insulin crosses the blood-brain barrier and turns off food intake," says Pi-Sunyer. "That makes sense. You've just eaten, so you don't need to eat for a while. If anything, insulin should lower food intake."

Claim #6: The Atkins Diet Is the Best Way to Lose Weight
Truth: We Don't Know the Best Way to Lose Weight

"Until we have more research, no one has the solution to the safest and most effective weight loss," says Washington University's Samuel Klein.

"Preliminary data from several studies suggest that, at least over the short-term, the Atkins diet is superior to a low-fat diet in a free-living environment," he says. "But it's too early to say that the Atkins diet is better."

Even if ongoing studies show that the Atkins diet promotes weight loss, we won't know if other diets—ones high in unsaturated fat or protein or vegetables and whole grains, for example—would work as well or better.

"We need lots more randomized controlled trials to evaluate the different permutations," says Walter Willett. (He and Blackburn are embarking on a study testing a high-*unsaturated*-fat Mediterranean diet, not the high-*saturated*-fat Atkins diet, as Taubes implies.)

"What's important is not theories, but evidence."

Claim #7: The Atkins Diet Works Because It Cuts Carbohydrates
Truth: If the Atkins Diet Works, It's Not Clear Why

If the Atkins diet *does* work, it may have nothing to do with the glycemic index or Atkins's promises. "It's unlikely to be related to the explanation in Atkins's book," says Klein, "because that doesn't make physiological sense."

Other possibilities: In one study, the people on a low-carb diet were told to follow *Dr. Atkins' New Diet Revolution,* which could have been more persuasive than what the people on a lower-fat diet got—a manual designed by academics.

Or, says Klein, "it may simply be easier to cut carbs." Everyone knows what they are: bread, pasta, rice, potatoes, sweets, etc.

Or, the monotony of a low-carb diet could have curbed the dieters' appetites. "You lose a lot of foods when you cut out carbs," says Klein. And with less variety, says Blackburn, "people eat less, so they lose more weight."

"It's also possible that a chemical is released by a high-fat diet that suppresses the appetite," adds Klein. "We just don't know."

Claim #8: The Atkins Diet Is Safe
Truth: It Isn't

Taubes not only neglects to mention that the meat in an Atkins diet may promote cancer. He ignores some researchers' concerns about other adverse effects.

"The Atkins diet may produce more weight loss in the first three weeks, but it's not spectacular," says Harvard's George Blackburn. "Who cares if one group loses a few more pounds than the other if it can hurt your bones?"

The problem: All the protein that Atkins recommends leads to acidic urine. "And there's no dispute that an acid urine leaches calcium out of bones," says Blackburn.

"You can buffer the diet by taking a couple of Tums a day, but now we're into medical supervision of people on the diet," he adds.

Blackburn and others also want to know whether an Atkins diet makes the blood vessels less elastic. "Studies suggest that a diet high in animal fats may cause blood vessels to constrict," he says. "That's a root cause of atherosclerosis."

In preliminary studies, the LDL ("bad") cholesterol of people on the Atkins diet didn't go up. That's comforting. (Of course, LDL didn't go *down* either, as it usually does with weight loss.)

"The harm caused by saturated fat could be overcome by weight loss," Klein explains. But what happens once people stop losing weight and start trying to maintain the loss? Will their LDL climb? "We don't know."

Claim #9: Low-Fat Diets Don't Help People Lose Weight
Truth: Low-Fat Diets Work If Dieters Cut Calories

"Low-fat weight-loss diets have proved in clinical trials and real life to be dismal failures," writes Taubes.

It's not clear which clinical trials he's referring to. In 1998, the National Heart, Lung, and Blood Institute issued guidelines to help doctors treat obesity.

Its conclusion: People who are told to cut fat (but not calories) lose some weight because they inadvertently eat fewer calories. But people who cut fat *and* watch calories lose more.

"A low-fat diet helps people eat fewer calories," says Rena Wing, a professor of psychiatry and human behavior at the Brown University Medical School in Providence, Rhode Island. "Maybe people *want* to hear that if they eat a lower-fat diet they don't have to eat fewer calories, but that's not true."

What about Taubes's claim that low-fat diets are a failure "in real life"?

Wing's National Weight Loss Registry keeps track of people—so far, about 3,000—who report having lost at least 30 pounds and having kept the weight off for at least six years. The registry can't "prove" *which* diet is best because it's not a controlled experiment. But it does offer evidence of what works in the long run.

"People on low-carbohydrate diets like Atkins's are very rare in the registry," says Wing.

"The people in our registry consistently report eating around 24 percent of calories from fat," she adds. They also expend roughly 2,800 calories a week—that's like walking four miles a day.

Furthermore, a low-fat diet aided weight loss in a six-year study of 3,200 people called the Diabetes Prevention Program.

"Patients were put on a low-fat diet with about 25 percent of calories from fat and they participated in 150 minutes of physical activity a week," says Wing.

"They lost about seven percent of their body weight and kept most of it off for four years. And they reduced their risk of diabetes by 58 percent."

Of course, it was both diet *and* exercise that led to their success. But if a low-fat diet *promotes* weight gain, as Taubes argues, the exercise—only about 20 minutes a day—would have had to not only counter the fattening effects of the low-fat diet, but actually lead to weight loss. Unlikely.

Claim #10: Taubes Examined the Evidence Objectively
Truth: He Let His Biases Rule

The New York Times Magazine isn't the *National Enquirer*. Readers expect *The Times* to run articles that are honestly reported and written. Yet in August, *The*

Washington Post revealed that Taubes simply ignored research that didn't agree with his conclusions.

For example, *The Post* asked Taubes why he made no mention of a review of nearly 50 studies on weight loss in the National Heart, Lung, and Blood Institute's 1998 Clinical Guidelines on treating obesity. The panel of experts was chaired by Columbia University's Pi-Sunyer, who has served as president of both the American Society of Clinical Nutrition and the American Diabetes Association.

"Anything that Pi-Sunyer is involved with, I don't take seriously," said Taubes. "He just didn't strike me as a scientist."

If Taubes had written a news article for the front page of *The Times,* comments like those would have ended his career. But when it comes to reporting about diet, the bar is set lower. Surely, the public deserves better.

WHAT TO EAT

Judging by *The New York Times Magazine* article, you'd think that experts were in a tug-of-war over whether to endorse low-fat or low-carbohydrate diets. Not so. Here's what they agree on . . . and where they differ:

Cut saturated (and trans) fat Forget Atkins. Experts agree that people should cut back on saturated (and trans) fat. That includes burgers, french fries, pizza, ice cream, and sweets made with butter, shortening, or stick margarine.

"There's a clear benefit from replacing unhealthy fats with healthy fats," says Harvard's Walter Willett. "The fat in poultry, fish, and nuts is much better than the fat in red meat and dairy." Healthy fats also include salad dressings, mayonnaise, cooking oils, and fish oils.

But the sky's not the limit, as Atkins would argue. "We're not working in the fields and burning calories all day, so we need to pay attention to all forms of calories," says Willett. "You can't eat unlimited quantities of fats or you'll gain weight."

Don't overdo carbohydrates A high-carb diet can cause trouble for the estimated 25 percent of Americans who have the Metabolic Syndrome, also called Syndrome X or insulin resistance (see "Read My Lipids," [*Nutrition Action Health Letter*] October 2001).

"Too much carbohydrate will raise triglycerides, lower HDL cholesterol, and make LDL small and dense, all of which raises the risk of heart disease," says Stanford University's John Farquhar.

That doesn't happen to everyone. Syndrome X doesn't show up in people who are not genetically susceptible, or in people who get too few calories or too much exercise to be overweight. (In China, Japan, and other Asian nations, diets are high in carbohydrates, yet heart disease rates are rock–bottom low.) But many Americans are genetically susceptible, pudgy, couch potatoes.

"A high-carb diet is worse for overweight, underexercised people and for people from racial groups—Latino, Asian, Indian—in whom a higher proportion have a genetic disposition to Type 2 diabetes," Farquhar explains.

But will a high-carbohydrate diet make you *fat?* Most researchers say no. Even people who get higher insulin levels on a high-carb diet don't gain weight. "If anything, more studies show that insulin resistance protects against weight gain," says Stanford's Gerald Reaven.

Willett isn't sure. "It may be easier to control weight if you cut back on refined starches, sugars, and potatoes," he says. His new study is testing that theory.

In any case, it would be foolish to assume that the calories in fat-free carbohydrates will bounce off your body like Teflon. And it's clear that some carbs—like vegetables, fruits, and whole grains—are healthier than refined carbs like white bread, soft drinks, and sweets.

"The type of carbohydrate matters," says Willett, "just as the type of fat matters."

Look for a weight-loss strategy that works for you   Until more studies are done, it's too early to say *which* diet makes it easiest to lose weight. Some people may find it easier to cut back on bread, pasta, rice, potatoes, and sweets, while others find it easier to cut back on fried foods, oils, salad dressings, mayonnaise, and margarine. Just make sure that you cut calories, and that the fats and carbs you do eat are healthy. "Most everyone agrees that we need to eat more fruits and vegetables, that our grains should be whole rather than refined, that our protein foods should be lean, and that our oils should come from plants or fish," says Penn State's Barbara Rolls.

"To say that experts don't know what people should eat is deliberately misleading."

POSTSCRIPT

Can Low-Carbohydrate, Higher-Fat Diets Promote Health and Weight Loss?

In these selections, two science journalists argue about how best to interpret research on diet composition and health. Taubes says that low-fat diets are so unhealthful that they cause obesity and chronic disease. Liebman says that high-fat diets are generally high in saturated fatty acids and calories and therefore contribute to heart disease and weight gain. She also raises concerns that bear on the conduct of science journalism: Did Taubes overinterpret research that is still incompletely understood? Did he quote his sources inappropriately? In appearing to promote the Atkins diet, did he further confuse the public about the causes and consequences of obesity?

Taubes's *The New York Times Magazine* article is about half the length of a version he wrote for professionals the previous year (*Science,* March 2001). The tone of that version is quite different; in it, Taubes explains the history of government dietary advice as "a story of what can happen when the demands of public health policy—and the demands of the public for simple advice—run up against the confusing ambiguity of real science." Such scientifically cautious statements disappeared in the *Times's* editing process, perhaps explaining why Liebman wonders how some of his statements got past "the laugh test."

Regardless of his intentions, Taubes's article elicited storms of protest from his fellow journalists. First to join the debate was Sally Squires of the *Washington Post* (August 27, 2002), who interviewed Taubes himself, investigated his journalistic background, and reinterviewed several of his sources. Her lengthy article, "What if the Big Fat Story Is Wrong?" concludes that much good science contradicts his arguments. It also documents the remarkable reaction to the *Times* article: increased sales of books by Atkins, a lucrative book contract for Taubes, and a public increasingly confused about diet and health. Other journalists, however, questioned Squires's own journalistic standards in producing this piece (see Liz Cox, *Columbia Journalism Review,* November/December 2002, at ⟨http://www.cjr.org⟩).

In part, the ferocity of this debate derives from the claims made for the Atkins diet. This diet, developed decades ago, promotes "unlimited" consumption of fat and protein but restrictions on carbohydrate (see http://atkinscenter.com). Such advice inevitably means a diet high in meat and dairy foods but low in fruits and vegetables as well as sugars and grain foods. Dr. Atkins's diet books have been best-sellers, and many people claim to have lost weight following such plans. As explained by Jane Brody in *The New York Times* (September 10, 2002), the Atkins diet helps people lose weight because they consume fewer calories when they don't eat bread, cake, cookies, soft drinks, pasta, and rice. The diet seems easy, she says, because it appears to allow people to eat as much meat, fat, eggs, and cheese as they like.

How is the public to interpret journalistic debates of this type? One way to approach answering this question is to identify points of agreement. Taubes and Liebman agree that it is better to eat some fats and carbohydrates than others (the good kinds), and that calories matter in weight loss. Neither thinks that fat or carbohydrate should be eliminated from the diet. Perhaps most important, both think that testing the safety and effectiveness of the Atkins diet would be a good idea.

Others think so, too. The May 22, 2003 issue of *The New England Journal of Medicine* included two studies that compared the effects of low-carbohydrate diets to low-fat diets on weight loss in extremely overweight individuals. Study subjects on the low-carbohydrate diets lost more weight and showed better improvement in risk factors (lower triglyceride levels and lower insulin resistance) than those on the low-fat diets. Although these results might seem to support the benefits of low-carbohydrate diets, the amounts of weight lost were small, especially compared to the subjects' starting weights. Furthermore, few maintained the weight loss beyond six months. In both studies, 60 percent of the subjects stopped participating, most likely because they were not losing weight. Such results suggest that reducing caloric intake by any means will help people lose weight and reduce risk factors for chronic disease.

ISSUE 8

Must Exercise Be Daily and Intense to Prevent Chronic Disease?

YES: Institute of Medicine of the National Academies, from "Physical Activity," *Dietary Reference Intakes: Energy, Carbohydrate, Fiber, Fat, Fatty Acids, Cholesterol, Protein, and Amino Acids*, A Report of the Institute of Medicine (September 5, 2002)

NO: I-Min Lee et al., from "Physical Activity and Coronary Heart Disease in Women: Is 'No Pain, No Gain' Passé?" *Journal of the American Medical Association* (March 21, 2001)

ISSUE SUMMARY

YES: To prevent weight gain and chronic disease, the Institute of Medicine of the National Academies recommends 60 minutes of daily physical activity of moderate intensity (such as walking at a rate of 4 to 5 miles per hour) in addition to activities normally performed as part of a sedentary lifestyle.

NO: Associate professor at the Harvard School of Public Health I-Min Lee and colleagues say that even light-to-moderate activity lowers heart disease rates among women and that as little as one hour of walking per week predicts lower risk.

In 2000 the federal committee preparing the *Dietary Guidelines for Americans* recommended that adults accumulate at least 30 minutes of moderate physical activity on most days of the week, preferably daily. A moderate activity, the committee said, expends as much energy as walking 2 miles in 30 minutes (4 miles per hour). In 2002 the Food and Nutrition Board (FNB), a committee of the Institute of Medicine of the National Academies, issued *Dietary Reference Intakes* for energy and *macronutrients* (carbohydrate, fat, protein, and their constituents). In the judgment of the FNB, 30 minutes of exercise per day is not enough to help adults maintain body weights in the healthful range of the body mass index (BMI). Instead, adults require at least 60 minutes per day of moderately intense activity over and above what they do in the course of normal daily activities—a doubling of the amount recommended in the *Dietary Guidelines*.

150

The FNB defined moderate intensity as walking at a rate of 4 to 5 miles per hour. It based this definition on metabolic studies of oxygen consumption at differing levels of physical activity. Walking at that rate causes an oxygen use corresponding to an energy expenditure of 4.5 to 8.0 kilocalories (shorthand: calories) per minute. Physiologists measure oxygen use in Metabolic Equivalents (METs), which, for all practical purposes, are equivalent to calories. METs contribute to a person's daily Physical Activity Level (PAL), which in turn depends on body size, age, and the intensity of the activity. Because 30 minutes of walking at 4 miles per hour would only raise the PAL from the *sedentary* (a PAL of 1.3 or below) to the *low-active* category (a PAL between 1.4 and 1.6), the committee said that 60 minutes would be needed to raise the PAL to the *active* category (between 1.6 and 1.9)—in *addition* to the activities usually performed in the course of a day (defined as Energy Expenditures of Physical Activity, or EEPA).

In contrast, I-Min Lee and her colleagues used an epidemiological approach to assess the risk of coronary heart disease among more than 39,000 women health professionals. The investigators collected information about physical activity levels at the start of the study in the mid-1990s and associated those energy expenditures with the risk of reporting a heart attack (myocardial infarction, or MI), coronary artery bypass grafting (CABG), or "percutaneous transluminal coronary angioplasty" (PTCA—a procedure that uses a tiny balloon to open clogged arteries in the heart) during the ensuing four to seven years. The results revealed that practically *any* level of reported activity reduced the risk for coronary events. As little as one hour per week of walking reduced the risk by 32 percent, and even a walking pace of less than 3.2 miles per hour reduced the risk by 46 percent. On this basis, the investigators concluded that easily attainable levels of physical activity reduce heart disease risks, and that they do so even among women who are overweight, have high cholesterol levels, or smoke cigarettes.

In reading the following studies, pay attention to the methods (and try not to be discouraged by the many abbreviations). What could account for the sharp discrepancy in conclusions? Are studies that are based on metabolic measurements comparable to those based on questionnaires? What does each type of study contribute to our understanding of the role of physical activity in health? Perhaps most critical, what do the results of these studies suggest for public policy?

In the following selections, the Institute of Medicine of the National Academies contends that at least one hour of physical activity per *day* is required to demonstrate health benefits, whereas Lee et al. say that one hour per *week* is enough to significantly reduce heart disease risk among women.

Institute of Medicine of the National Academies

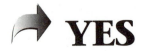 **YES**

Physical Activity

Summary

Physical activity and exercise promote health and vigor. As identified previously by other [expert] groups, some benefits can be achieved with a minimum of 30 minutes of moderate intensity physical activity most days of the week. However, 30 minutes per day of regular activity is insufficient to maintain body weight in adults in the recommended body mass index range from 18.5 up to 25 kg/m^2 and achieve all the identified health benefits fully. Hence, to prevent weight gain as well as to accrue additional, weight-independent health benefits of physical activity, 60 minutes of daily moderate intensity physical activity (e.g., walking/jogging at 4 to 5 mph) is recommended, in addition to the activities required by a sedentary lifestyle. This amount of physical activity leads to an 'active' lifestyle, corresponding to physical activity levels (PAL) greater than 1.6. . . . For children, the physical activity recommendation is also 60 minutes or more of daily activity and exercise. Increasing the energy expenditure of physical activity (EEPA) needs to be considered in determining the energy intake to achieve energy balance in weight stable adults, and adequate growth and development in children. Body weight serves as the ultimate indicator of adequate energy intake. Increasing EEPA, or maintaining an active lifestyle provides an important means for individuals to balance food energy intake with total energy expenditure.

Background Information

A distinction is made between physical activity[1] and exercise;[2] the latter is considered more vigorous and leads to improvements in physical fitness.[3] In qualitative terms, exercise can be defined as activity sufficiently vigorous to raise breathing to a level where conversation is labored and sweating is noticeable on temperate days. . . . The average physical activity level (PAL) among adults participating in the doubly-labeled water studies [a chemical method for measuring oxygen consumption and, therefore, activity levels] is about 1.7, reflecting physical activity habits equivalent to walking 5 to 7 miles/day at 3 to 4 mph in addition to the activities required by a sedentary lifestyle. Also regular physical activity may improve mood by reducing depression and anxiety, thereby enhancing the quality of life. The beneficial outcomes of regular physical activity and exercise appear to pertain to persons of all ages, and both women and men of diverse ethnic groups.

Throughout history, balancing dietary energy intake and total energy expenditure (TEE) was accomplished unconsciously by most individuals because of the large component of occupation-related energy expenditure. Today, despite common knowledge that regular exercise is healthful, more than 60 percent of Americans are not regularly physically active, and 25 percent are not active at all. It seems reasonable to anticipate continuation of the current trend for reductions in occupational activity and other activities of daily life. If this is to be offset by deliberately increasing voluntary physical exercise, it needs to be kept in mind that in previously sedentary individuals, adding periods of mild to moderate intensity exercise can unconsciously be compensated for by reducing other activities during the remainder of the day, so that total energy expenditure (TEE) may be less affected than expected. Hence, to increase physical activity and to thereby facilitate weight control, recreational activities and physical training programs need to add, and not substitute for, other physical activities of daily life.

The trend for decreased activity by adults is similar to trends for children to be less active in and out of school. As both lack of physical activity and obesity are now recognized as risk factors for several chronic diseases, logic requires that activity recommendations accompany dietary recommendations.

History

United States

In 1953, Kraus and Hirschland alerted health and fitness professionals, the general public, and President Dwight D. Eisenhower to the relatively poor physical condition of American youth. Events led to the formation of the President's Council on Youth Fitness. Under President John F. Kennedy, the council was renamed the President's Council on Physical Fitness and in 1965 established five levels of physical fitness for adult men and women. Subsequently, the word "sports" was added to the title of the organization, making it the President's Council on Physical Fitness and Sports.

. . . The recent DHHS report, *Physical Activity and Health: A Report of the Surgeon General,* offered specific recommendations for physical activity and justified those on the basis of the healthful effects of exercise. The 2000 *Dietary Guidelines for Americans* recommends that adults accumulate at least 30 minutes and children 60 minutes of moderate physical activity most days of the week, preferably daily. In addition, that report recommended combining sensible eating with regular physical activity and acknowledged that physical activity and nutrition work together for better health. The physical activity and fitness goal of *Healthy People 2010* is to increase the proportion of Americans that engage in daily physical activity to improve health, fitness, and quality of life.

Canada

In Canada, similar processes have occurred. An early initiative was the Toronto International Conference on Physical Activity and Cardiovascular Health in 1966. Toronto was also the site of the 1988 International Consensus Conference on Exercise, Fitness and Health. In 1992, coinciding with Canada's 125th birthday, the Second International Conference on Physical Activity, Fitness, and Health was held. That meeting resulted in publication of the report, *Physical Activity, Fitness, and Health.*

Most recently, in cooperation with Health Canada and the Canadian Society of Exercise Physiology, Canada's *Physical Activity Guide to Healthy Active Living* has been published. This guide describes the benefits of regular physical activity and makes specific recommendations to improve fitness and achieve particular health-related outcomes such as decreasing the risk of premature death from chronic diseases (heart disease, obesity, high blood pressure, type II diabetes, osteoporosis, stroke, colon cancer, and depression). The recommendations include 60 minutes of "light effort" exercises (e.g., light walking, easy gardening), 30–60 minutes of "moderate effort" exercises (e.g., brisk walking, biking, swimming, water aerobics, leaf raking), or 20–30 minutes of "vigorous effort" exercises (e.g., aerobics, jogging, hockey, fast swimming, fast dancing, basketball). For moderate and vigorous activities, the Canadian recommendations are for 4 or more days/week and also include participation in flexibility activities (4–7 days/week) and strength activities (4–7 days/week).

Physical Activity Level and Energy Balance

Aside from dietary energy intake, energy expenditure of physical activity (EEPA) is the variable that a person can control, in contrast to age, height, and gender. Energy expenditure can rise many times over resting rates during exercise, and the effects of an exercise bout on energy expenditure persist for hours, if not a day or longer. Thus, changing activity level can have major impacts on total energy expenditure (TEE) and on energy balance. Further, exercise does not automatically increase appetite and energy intake in direct proportion to activity-related changes in energy expenditure. In humans and other mammals, energy intake is closely related to physical activity level when body mass is in the ideal range, but too little or too much exercise may disrupt hypothalamic and other mechanisms that regulate body mass.

Impact of Physical Activity on Energy Expenditure and on PAL

Metabolic Equivalents (METs)

The impact of various physical activities is often described and compared in terms of METs (i.e., multiples of an individual's resting oxygen uptake), and one MET is defined as a rate of oxygen (O_2) consumption of 3.5 ml/kg/min in adults. . . . A rate of energy expenditure of 1.0 MET thus corresponds to 1.22 kcal/min in a man weighing 70 kg (0.0175 kcal/kg/min × 70 kg), and to 1.0 kcal/min in a woman weighing 57 kg (0.0175 kcal/kg/min^{-1} × 57 kg). . . .

Knowing the intensity of a type of physical activity in terms of METs (see Table 1 for the METs for various activities) allows a simple assessment of its impact on the energy expended while the activity is performed. . . .

Table 1

Intensity and Impact of Various Activities on Physical Activity Level (PAL) in Adults[a]

Activity	Metabolic Equivalents (METs)[b]	ΔPAL/10 min[c]	ΔPAL/h[c]
Leisure			
Mild			
Billiards	2.4	0.013	0.08
Canoeing (leisurely)	2.5	0.014	0.09
Dancing (ballroom)	2.9	0.018	0.11
Golf (with cart)	2.5	0.014	0.09
Horseback riding (walking)	2.3	0.012	0.07
Playing			
Accordion	1.8	0.008	0.05
Cello	2.3	0.012	0.07
Flute	2.0	0.010	0.06
Piano	2.3	0.012	0.07
Violin	2.5	0.014	0.09
Volleyball (noncompetitive)	2.9	0.018	0.11
Walking (2 mph)	2.5	0.014	0.09
Moderate			
Calisthenics (no weight)	4.0	0.029	0.17
Cycling (leisurely)	3.5	0.024	0.14
Golf (without cart)	4.4	0.032	0.19
Swimming (slow)	4.5	0.033	0.20
Walking (3 mph)	3.3	0.022	0.13
Walking (4 mph)	4.5	0.033	0.20
Vigorous			
Chopping wood	4.9	0.037	0.22
Climbing hills (no load)	6.9	0.056	0.34
Climbing hills (5-kg load)	7.4	0.061	0.37
Cycling (moderately)	5.7	0.045	0.27
Dancing			
Aerobic or ballet	6.0	0.048	0.29
Ballroom (fast) or square	5.5	0.043	0.26
Jogging (10-min miles)	10.2	0.088	0.53
Rope skipping	12.0	0.105	0.63

continued

Activity	Metabolic Equivalents (METs)[b]	ΔPAL/10 min[c]	ΔPAL/h[c]
Vigorous (continued)			
Skating			
Ice	5.5	0.043	0.26
Roller	6.5	0.052	0.31
Skiing (water or downhill)	6.8	0.055	0.33
Squash	12.1	0.106	0.63
Surfing	6.0	0.048	0.29
Swimming	7.0	0.057	0.34
Tennis (doubles)	5.0	0.038	0.23
Walking (5 mph)	8.0	0.067	0.40
Activities of Daily Living			
Gardening (no lifting)	4.4	0.032	0.19
Household tasks, moderate effort	3.5	0.024	0.14
Lifting items continuously	4.0	0.029	0.17
Light activity while sitting	1.5	0.005	0.03
Loading/unloading car	3.0	0.019	0.11
Lying quietly	1.0	0.000	0.00
Mopping	3.5	0.024	0.14
Mowing lawn (power mover)	4.5	0.033	0.20
Raking lawn	4.0	0.029	0.17
Riding in a vehicle	1.0	0.000	0.00
Sitting	0.0	0.000	0.00
Taking out trash	3.0	0.019	0.11
Vacuuming	3.5	0.024	0.14
Walking the dog	3.0	0.019	0.11
Walking from house to car or bus	2.5	0.014	0.09
Watering plants	2.5	0.014	0.09

[a]PAL is the physical activity level that is the ratio of the total energy expenditure to the basal energy expenditure.

[b]METs are multiples of an individual's resting oxygen uptakes, defined as the rate of oxygen (O_2) consumption of 3.5 mL of O_2/min/kg body weight in adults.

[c]In the PAL shown here, an allowance has been made to include the delayed effect of physical activity in causing excess post-exercise oxygen consumption (EPOC) and the dissipation of some of the food energy consumed through the thermic effect of food (TEF).

Source: Adapted from Fletcher et al. (2001).

Bijnen and coworkers (1998) found that activities with METs greater than 4 are more effective than less intensive activities in reducing cardiovascular mortality. A rate of energy expenditure of 4.5 METs corresponds to the upper boundary for moderate activities (Table 1). . . . A rate of exertion of 4.5 METs is reached, for example, by walking at a speed of 4 mph (Table 1).

Physical Activity Level (PAL)

While METs describe activity intensities relative to a resting metabolic rate, the PAL is defined as the ratio of total energy expenditure (TEE) to basal energy expenditure (BEE). Thus, the actual impact on PAL depends to some extent on body size and age, as these are determinants of the BEE. The impact of these factors can be judged by examining the ratio MET $= 1.0 \times 24$ hours/BEE. . . .

For a typical 30 year-old reference man and woman 1.77 m and 1.63 m in height and weighing 70 kg and 57 kg, BEEs are 1684 and 1312 kcal/day, respectively. . . .

Because it is the most significant physical activity in the life of most individuals, walking/jogging is taken as the 'reference activity,' and the impact of other activities can be considered in terms of exertions equivalent to walking/jogging, to the extent that these activities are weight bearing and hence involve costs proportional to body weight. The effect of walking/jogging on energy expenditure at various speeds is given in Table 1 in terms of METs and is also shown in the upper panel of Figure 1. The middle panel describes the energy expended in kcal/hour for walking/jogging at various speeds by individuals weighing 70 or 57 kg (the reference body weights for men and women, respectively). The lower panel describes the total cost of walking/jogging one mile at various speeds, including the increments in energy expenditure above the resting rate during and after walking/jogging. . . . The energy expended per mile walked/jogged is essentially constant at speeds ranging from 2 to 4 miles/hour (1 kcal/mile/kg for a man [70 kcal/mile/70 kg] to 1.1 kcal/mile/kg for a woman [65 kcal/mile/57 kg], or approximately 1.1 kcal/mile/kg body weight; Figure 1 lower panel), but increases progressively at higher speeds. . . . [W]alking at a speed of 4 miles/hour (4.5 METs, Figure 1 upper panel) for sixty minutes causes an increase in the daily . . . PAL of approximately 0.20. Walking/jogging instead at speeds of 4.5 miles/hour raises the metabolic rate to 6 METs (Figure 1 upper panel), increasing the impact on PAL by half to 0.30 for sixty minutes. . . . Indeed, walking/jogging to cover 4.5 miles in 60 minutes, at a cost of 107 kcal/mile (Figure 1, lower panel) in men . . . , or performing some equally demanding activity for 60 minutes, will cause an increase in PAL of approximately 0.30.

Impact of Body Weight on Energy Expenditure
The impact of body weight on energy expenditure while walking at various speeds is illustrated in Figure 2, while Figure 3 describes how body weight affects the total increase in energy expenditure caused by walking one mile at various speeds. . . .

Physical Activity for an Active Lifestyle
. . . [Thirty] minutes of moderately intensive exercise . . . would be sufficient to raise the PAL of a person doing only the activities of daily living (PAL $= 1.39$) from the sedentary category (PAL $\geq 1.0 < 1.4$), to the low active category (PAL $\geq 1.4 < 1.6$), but insufficient to raise PAL to the active category (PAL $\geq 1.6 < 1.9$), the average PAL category of normal weight adults in the DLW database with BMIs from 18.5 up to 25 kg/m^2. One hour of moderately intensive physical activity . . . would raise the PAL from 1.39 to 1.59, the upper range of the low active category (PAL $\geq 1.4 < 1.6$). Thus, over one hour of moderate activity would be required to raise the PAL from the sedentary to the active category (PAL $\geq 1.6 < 1.9$). Hence, the activity recommendation expressed here, one hour per day, is

Figure 1

Relationships of Energy Expenditure and Walking/Jogging Speeds

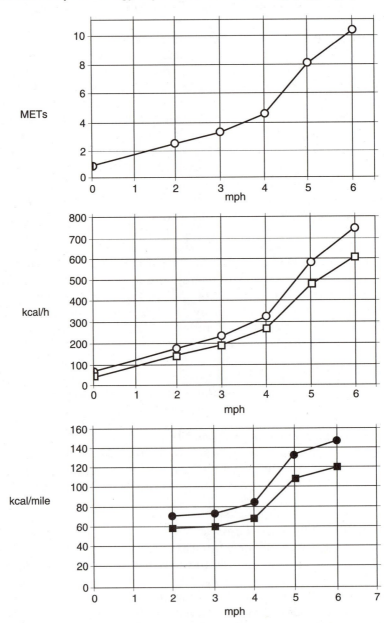

Upper panel: Rate of Energy Expenditure as a function of walking/jogging speed. Middle panel: Energy expended by a 70 kg man (○) and by a 57 kg woman (□) while walking/jogging during one hour at various speeds. Lower panel: Increase in daily energy expenditure induced by walking/jogging one mile at various speeds for a 70 kg man (●) and a 57 kg woman (■).

Figure 2

Impact of Body Weight on Energy Expenditure While Walking at Speeds of 2, 3, 4, or 5 Miles Per Hour (mph)

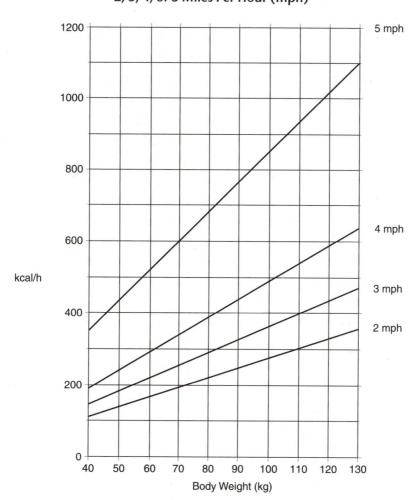

greater than in the Surgeon General's Report, but similar to that in Canada's *Physical Activity Guide* (Health Canada, 1998). For children, the recommendation of one hour or more of activity and exercise on most days is consistent with the present analysis.

In terms of making a realistic exercise recommendation for busy individuals to maintain their weight, it is important to recognize that exercise and activity recommendations consider "accumulated" physical activity. This involves consideration of EEPAs [energy expenditures of physical activity] of both low intensity activities of daily life (e.g., taking the stairs at work) as well as partici-

Figure 3

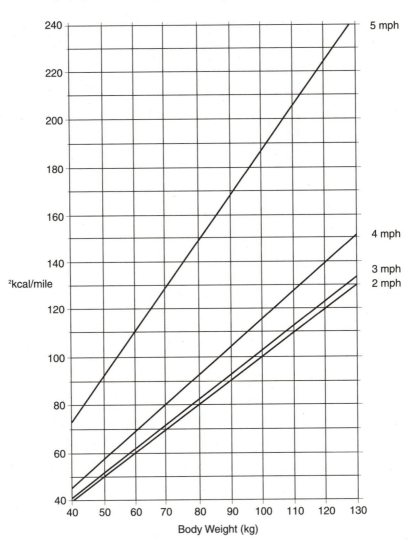

Impact of Body Weight on Cost of Walking One Mile at Speeds of 2, 3, 4, or 5 Miles Per Hour (mph) in Men and Women

pating in more vigorous exercises (e.g., taking an aerobics class at a health club). Recognition of the value of accumulated physical activity in raising TEE [total energy expenditure] makes reasonable activity patterns and sedentary occupations compatible by including significant amounts of moderate intensity activity (e.g., 60 minutes/day of brisk walking) or exercises requiring high intensities (e.g., jogging or running) performed regularly (4–7 days/week). Compared to the goal of at least 30 min/day of moderate physical activity set by the Surgeon General, a goal of one hour/day of activity also offers additional benefits in reducing risks of chronic diseases, for example, by favorably altering blood lipid profiles, changing body composition by decreasing body fat and increasing muscle mass, or both.

Healthful Effects of Activity

Men and women with moderate to high levels of physical activity or cardiorespiratory fitness have lower mortality rates than sedentary individuals with low fitness. For instance, in a study of Harvard alumni, mortality rates for men walking less than 15 km/week were 15 percent higher than in men walking more than 15 km/wk. Moreover, in the same study, men who took up vigorous sports activity lowered their risk of death by 23 percent compared to those who remained sedentary. Similar favorable effects were observed in the Aerobics Center Longitudinal Study as men in the lowest quintile of fitness who improved their fitness to a moderate level, reduced mortality risk by 44 percent an extent comparable to that achieved by men stopping to smoke. Epidemiological data on humans as well as experimental data on humans and laboratory animals provide biologically plausible explanations of how regular physical activity can favorably affect the progression of several chronic diseases. . . . In addition to the effects of physical activity in offsetting the effects of chronic diseases, regular physical exercise improves mood state.

Notes

1. Physical activity—Bodily movement that is produced by the contraction of muscle and that substantially increases energy expenditure (DHHS, 1996).
2. Exercise (exercise training)—Planned structured, and repetitive bodily movement done to promote or maintain one or more components of physical fitness.
3. Physical fitness—A set of attributes that people have that relates to the ability to perform physical activity.

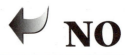
Physical Activity and Coronary Heart Disease in Women: Is "No Pain, No Gain" Passé?

Coronary heart disease (CHD) is the leading cause of mortality among women in the United States. Physical inactivity is among the risk factors for this disease. A 1990 meta-analysis concluded that physically active individuals had about half the CHD rates of those who were sedentary. However, less than one fifth of the studies in the meta-analysis included women. Since then, additional studies have been conducted in women, and the available evidence clearly indicates that active women experience lower CHD rates than inactive women.

What is less clear are the kinds and intensity of physical activities that are associated with lower risk. It is important to clarify this issue in light of a recent physical activity recommendation that calls for at least 30 minutes of moderate-intensity physical activity (eg, brisk walking at 4.8–6.4 km/h [3.0–4.0 mph]) most days of the week. This contrasts with previous recommendations that advocated vigorous-intensity exercise (eg, jogging, running) for at least 20 minutes continuously, 3 times per week. A major difference is the current emphasis on moderate instead of vigorous activity. This concession was made partly to encourage physical activity among sedentary individuals because the previous, more difficult prescription was believed to pose a barrier.

Another issue on which few data exist is whether physical activity is inversely related to risk among healthy women at high risk for CHD (eg, smokers). This has important clinical implications because if an inverse relationship exists, physicians should strongly promote physical activity in these women.

We therefore investigated the relationship between physical activity and CHD risk among women, including those at high risk, specifically exploring the association with walking.

From I-Min Lee, Kathryn M. Rexrode, Nancy R. Cook, JoAnn E. Manson, and Julie E. Buring, "Physical Activity and Coronary Heart Disease in Women: Is 'No Pain, No Gain' Passé?" *Journal of the American Medical Association,* vol. 285, no. 11 (March 21, 2001), pp. 1447–1453. Copyright © 2001 by The American Medical Association. Reprinted by permission. References omitted.

Methods

Participants

Subjects were selected from the Women's Health Study, a randomized, double-blind [the researchers and the participants do not know who is receiving which treatment], placebo-controlled [a control group of women who received pills that did nothing] trial of low-dosage aspirin and vitamin E for primary prevention of cardiovascular disease and cancer. Between September 1992 and May 1995, female health professionals throughout the United States and Puerto Rico were invited to participate. Women completed a mailed baseline questionnaire on sociodemographic characteristics, health habits, and medical history. Those who were eligible and willing to be in the trial were enrolled into a 3-month run-in phase during which women took their study pills (all placebos [sugar pills]). At the end of the run-in phase, women completed the run-in questionnaire that ascertained compliance with pill taking, health habits, and recent medical history. Women with good compliance who were still eligible and willing to participate were then randomized into the trial and started taking their randomized pill assignment.

A total of 39 876 women aged 45 years or older who were free of self-reported coronary heart disease, cerebrovascular disease, and cancer (other than nonmelanoma skin cancer) were randomly assigned to the agents tested. For this study, we excluded 504 women with missing information on physical activity or weight or who provided post-randomization reports of CHD occurring before randomization, leaving 39 372 women.

Assessment of Physical Activity

On the run-in questionnaire, we asked women to estimate the average time (0, 1–19 min/wk, 20–59 min/wk, 1 h/wk, 1.5 h/wk, 2–3 h/wk, 4–6 h/wk, or ≥7 h/wk) spent on 8 groups of recreational activities during the past year: walking or hiking; jogging (slower than 10-minute miles); running (10-minute miles or faster); bicycling, including use of stationary machines; aerobic exercise, aerobic dance, or use of exercise machines; lower-intensity exercise, including yoga, stretching, or toning; tennis, squash, or racquetball; and lap swimming. We also inquired about the usual pace of walking (do not walk regularly; <3.2 km/h [2.0 mph; easy, casual pace], 3.2–4.7 km/h [2.0–2.9 mph; normal, average pace], 4.8–6.3 km/h [3.0–3.9 mph; brisk pace], or ≥6.4 km/h [4.0 mph; very brisk/striding pace]) and the number of flights of stairs climbed daily (0, 1–2, 3–4, 5–9, 10–14, ≥15). Based on the energy cost of these activities, we assigned a multiple of resting metabolic rate (MET score) to each group of activities and stair climbing. Since resting metabolic rate (1 MET) is approximately 1 kcal/kg of body weight per hour, we estimated energy expenditure by multiplying the assigned MET score by body weight and hours per week of participation using the midpoint of time categories. We summed kilocalories per week from the 8 groups of recreational activities and stair climbing to estimate weekly energy expenditure. . . .

Assessment of Other Predictors of CHD

Information on variables that could potentially influence the association be-tween physical activity and CHD risk was ascertained from the baseline and run-in questionnaires. These variables were age, weight, height, cigarette smok-ing status, diet (including alcohol consumption), history of hypertension, his-tory of elevated cholesterol level, history of diabetes mellitus, menopausal status, use of postmenopausal hormones, and parental history of CHD. We con-sidered a history of hypertension to be positive if women reported this diagno-sis or blood pressure of higher than 140/90 mm Hg. Women were classified as having an elevated cholesterol level if they reported this diagnosis or choles-terol levels of more than 240 mg/dL (6.21 mmoI/L). A positive history of dia-betes mellitus was based on self-report.

Ascertainment of CHD

Every 6 months during the first year and then annually, women completed brief mailed questionnaires that inquired about compliance to their assigned treatment, serious adverse effects of study agents, risk factors, and end points of interest to the trial. Women reported a diagnosis of myocardial infarction (MI) or coronary revascularization procedures (coronary artery bypass grafting [CABG] or percutaneous transluminal coronary angioplasty [PTCA]) on these questionnaires, or wrote or telephoned the study staff. Deaths were reported by family members or postal authorities. Follow-up in the trial is high: at 36 months, the latest follow-up point attained by all participants, morbidity/mor-tality follow-up was more than 99% complete.

We sought medical records and other relevant information, including death certificates and autopsy reports, for women reporting MI, CABG, or PTCA, and for decedents. Reported diagnoses of CHD or death from CHD were consid-ered confirmed only after examination of all available information by an end-points committee of physicians. Myocardial infarction was confirmed using World Health Organization criteria (ie, symptoms plus either typical electrocar-diographic changes or elevated cardiac enzyme levels). Fatal CHD was docu-mented from convincing evidence of a cardiovascular mechanism from all available sources, including death certificates, hospital records, and, for deaths occurring outside the hospital, observers' impressions. CABG and PTCA were confirmed by hospital records. This report includes data as of March 1999.

Statistical Analysis

The following dimensions of physical activity were considered: (1) energy ex-pended on all activities assessed, (2) energy expended on vigorous recreational activities, and (3) walking. Recreational activities requiring at least 6 METs (ie, jogging, running, aerobic exercise, aerobic dance, use of exercise machines, tennis, squash, racquetball, and lap swimming) were categorized as vigorous.

Women were first categorized into approximate quartiles of energy ex-pended on all activities: less than 200, 200 to 599, 600 to 1499, and 1500 or more kcal/wk. . . .

For energy expended on vigorous recreational activities of at least 6 METs, women were categorized into 5 groups: no vigorous recreational activity plus less than 200 kcal/wk expended on other activities, no vigorous recreational activity plus at least 200 kcal/wk expended on other activities, and 1 to 199, 200 to 499, and 500 or more kcal/wk expended on vigorous recreational activities. The cut points were chosen so that women who participated in any vigorous recreational activities were divided into approximate thirds. Relative risks for CHD were estimated in parallel fashion to that described herein.

Because walking is the most popular leisure activity among women, this activity was specifically examined in relation to CHD risk. To prevent confounding by vigorous activities, analyses of walking were conducted among the 22 865 women (58%) who reported no vigorous recreational activity. . . .

Finally, we investigated whether the association of physical activity with CHD rates differed among women without and with the following CHD risk factors: body mass index (<25 kg/m^2 or ≥25 kg/m^2), cigarette smoking (never, past, or current), and history of hypertension or elevated cholesterol level (no or yes). . . .

Results

During the study, participants were observed for an average of 5 years, and 244 confirmed incidents of CHO occurred (nonfatal MI or fatal CHD, n = 125; CABG or PTCA, n = 199; women could have had more than 1 event). . . . More active women had a lower mean body mass index than less active women. Women with higher levels of physical activity were less likely to smoke cigarettes but more likely to consume alcohol. They also had a healthier diet, consuming less saturated fat, more fiber, and more fruits and vegetables. More active women were more likely to use postmenopausal hormones. At higher levels of physical activity, prevalences of hypertension, elevated cholesterol level, and diabetes mellitus were lower. The least active women were somewhat more likely to have had a parent with MI prior to age 60 years.

In analyses that were adjusted for age and randomized treatment assignment, there was a strong inverse association (P for linear trend $< .001$) with energy expended on all activities in relation to CHD rates (TABLE 1). The inverse association persisted after further adjustment for smoking status, diet, alcohol use, menopausal status, postmenopausal hormone use, and parental history of MI before age 60 years (P for linear trend = .03). Women who expended 600 to 1499 kcal/wk were at significantly lower risk of subsequently developing CHD than less active women (RR, 0.55; 95% confidence interval [CI], 0.37–0.82). At higher levels of energy expenditure, no additional risk reduction was observed.

When biological intermediates (body mass index, hypertension, elevated cholesterol level, and diabetes mellitus) were controlled for in secondary analyses, the inverse relationship was attenuated. The RRs associated with the 4 categories of energy expended on all activities were 1.00 (referent), 0.79, 0.62, and 0.84, respectively (P for linear trend = .14).

Nonfatal MI or fatal CHD and CABG or PTCA were then investigated separately. Significant inverse associations were observed for each end point. The

Table 1

Relative Risk (RR) of Coronary Heart Disease (CHD) According to Physical Activity

Physical Activity, kcal/wk

	Energy Expended on All Activities					Energy Expended on Vigorous Recreational Activities*					
	<200	200–599	600–1499	≥1500	P Value for Trend	0 + <200 in Other Activities	0 + ≥200 in Other Activities	1–199	200–499	≥500	P Value for Trend
No. of women	10 239	9877	10 913	8343		9329	13 536	5912	4612	5983	
No. of cases of CHD	101	56	46	41		91	69	37	24	23	
Age- and treatment-adjusted RR (95% confidence interval)	1.00 (Referent)	0.59 (0.42–0.81)	0.42 (0.30–0.60)	0.51 (0.35–0.73)	<.001	1.00 (Referent)	0.49 (0.36–0.67)	0.75 (0.51–1.10)	0.60 (0.38–0.94)	0.41 (0.26–0.66)	<.001
Multivariable RR (95% confidence interval)†	1.00 (Referent)	0.79 (0.56–1.12)	0.55 (0.37–0.82)	0.75 (0.50–1.12)	.03	1.00 (Referent)	0.65 (0.46–0.91)	1.18 (0.79–1.78)	0.96 (0.60–1.55)	0.63 (0.38–1.04)	.45

*Vigorous activities requiring ≥6 METs (resting metabolic rate = 1 MET).

†Multivariable RRs are adjusted for age; randomized treatment assignment; smoking status; consumption of alcohol, saturated fat, fiber, and fruits and vegetables; menopausal status; use of postmenopausal hormones; and parental history of myocardial infarction at >60 years of age. [Note: RR = 1.0 indicates no effect on risk. RR < 1.0 suggests that physical activity reduces risk of coronary heart disease.]

multivariable RRs for nonfatal MI or fatal CHD associated with the 4 categories of energy expended on all activities were 1.00 (referent), 0.68, 0.57, and 0.65, respectively (P for linear trend = .05). For coronary revascularization procedures, they were 1.00 (referent), 0.78, 0.49, and 0.74, respectively (P linear trend = .03).

Next, the energy expended on vigorous recreational activities of at least 6 METs was examined. When highest and lowest categories of women were compared, there was a lower risk of CHD among the most active women that was of borderline significance (RR, 0.63; 95% CI, 0.38–1.04).

Whether walking is inversely related to risk of subsequent CHD among women who did not engage in vigorous activities was also assessed. Among participants, 22 865 women (58%) reported no vigorous recreational activity; any activity these women (75% of the 22 865) carried out consisted primarily of walking. In this subgroup, both time spent walking and usual walking pace were inversely related to CHD risk when analyzed separately (TABLE 2). Women who walked at least 1 hour per week or whose usual walking pace was at least 4.8 km/h (3.0 mph) experienced about half the CHD risk of women who did not walk regularly. To ascertain which of the 2 walking parameters was more important, variables for both were entered in a single multivariable model. In doing so, time spent walking (P for linear trend = .01) but not usual pace of walking (P for linear trend = .55) was significantly related to lower CHD rates, indicating that time but not pace independently predicted lower risk.

Finally, whether the association of physical activity with CHD risk differed among women without and with CHD risk factors was examined. There was no evidence that the inverse association differed between women of normal weight and overweight women (P for interaction = .95). There also was no evidence that the inverse relationship differed between women without and with elevated cholesterol level (P for interaction = .71). However, there were significant interactions by smoking status and history of hypertension (P for interaction = .01 and .001, respectively). Physical activity was inversely associated with CHD rates in current and past smokers, but not in women who had never smoked (P for linear trend = .005, .10, and .75, respectively). Among nonhypertensive women, an inverse association with physical activity (P for linear trend = .001) was observed; among hypertensive women, a u-shaped relationship (P for quadratic trend = .07) was observed.

Comment

This study clearly indicates that physically active women have lower CHD rates. It is encouraging to observe that vigorous activities were not necessary for lower CHD rates. Among women who did not engage in vigorous activities, walking (a light- to moderate-intensity activity, depending on pace) was associated with lower risk. These data suggest that walking need not be fast-paced for benefit; time spent walking was more important than walking pace. Additionally, we observed inverse associations between physical activity and CHD risk among those who were overweight, smokers, and women with elevated cholesterol levels. Among hypertensive women, there was a u-shaped association between physical activity and CHD risk.

Table 2

Relative Risks (RRs) of Coronary Heart Disease (CHD) According to Walking Parameters*

| | Walking Parameter | | | | | | | | | |
| | Time Spent Walking per wk | | | | | Usual Walking Pace, km/h† | | | | |
	Do Not Walk Regularly	1–59 min	1.0–1.5 h	≥2 h	P Value for Trend	Do Not Walk Regularly	<3.2	3.2–4.7	≥4.8	P Value for Trend
No. of women	5826	6034	4406	6599		5826	2958	8356	5725	
No. of cases of CHD	68	45	19	28		68	21	50	21	
Age- and treatment-adjusted RR (95% confidence interval)	1.00 (Referent)	0.68 (0.46–0.99)	0.37 (0.22–0.62)	0.33 (0.21–0.52)	<.001	1.00 (Referent)	0.57 (0.35–0.93)	0.50 (0.35–0.72)	0.33 (0.20–0.54)	<.0001
Multivariable RR (95% confidence interval)‡	1.00 (Referent)	0.86 (0.57–1.29)	0.49 (0.28–0.86)	0.48 (0.29–0.78)	<.001	1.00 (Referent)	0.56 (0.32–0.97)	0.71 (0.47–1.05)	0.52 (0.30–0.90)	.02

*Data are shown for women who reported no vigorous recreational activities requiring ≥6 METs (resting metabolic rate = 1 MET).

†To convert kilometers to miles, divide by 1.6.

‡Multivariable RRs are adjusted for age; randomized treatment assignment; smoking status; consumption of alcohol, saturated fat, fiber, and fruits and vegetables; menopausal status; use of postmenopausal hormones; and parental history of myocardial infarction at <60 years of age.

These findings support recent guidelines recommending moderate-intensity physical activity for at least 30 minutes most days of the week (generating energy expenditure of about 1000 kcal/wk). Moreover, they raise the possibility that even lesser degrees of activity may decrease CHD risk. We found that time spent walking but not walking pace independently predicted lower risk, implying that walking slower than 4.8 to 6.4 km/h (3–4 mph; ie, a light-intensity activity) may be beneficial. Women who walked at least 1 h/wk had about half the CHD rates of women who did not walk regularly. Assuming that walking 5 d/wk satisfies the definition of "most days of the week," the recent guidelines recommend brisk walking for at least 2.5 h/wk.

Limitations in the assessment of walking should be considered when interpreting our findings. Based on data from another study, women probably reported walking pace validly; when asked to walk at a pace they gauged to be of at least moderate intensity, both unfit and fit participants correctly walked more than 4.8 km/h (3 mph; Isabelle M. T. Bohlmann, MSc, written communication, August 2000). Time spent walking may be less validly reported. The questionnaire used probably measured purposeful walking (for transportation or exercise) only, rather than all walking (eg, walking around the home). A recent study compared walking reported on questionnaires and measured using pedometers. Reported walking was only 0.34 times the distance measured by pedometers. It is unclear whether the recent activity guidelines refer to time spent on all walking or purposeful walking. If the former were intended, our findings probably are in accord with the recommended time. Women who reported walking at least 1 h/wk were at significantly reduced risk. If only purposeful walking was measured and was 0.34 of all walking, these women would actually have spent 2.9 h/wk on all walking.

Walking was specifically investigated in 3 previous studies of women. In the Nurses' Health Study, among women with no vigorous activities, those who expended at least 3.9 MET-hours/wk walking (approximately 1 h/wk at brisk pace) had lower CHD risk compared with those who expended no more than 0.5 MET-hours/wk. In the College Alumni Health Study, walking at least 10 blocks/d (approximately 2 h/wk at brisk pace) lowered risk of cardiovascular disease in women compared with walking less than 4 blocks/d. Among men and women aged 65 years or older, walking more than 4 h/wk reduced risk of hospitalization due to cardiovascular disease compared with walking less than 1 h/wk. The differences in the time required may be partly due to comparison with reference groups who were more active than the referent in this study (no vigorous activity and no regular walking); the reference group in the Nurses' Health Study was most similar.

Few data, either in men or women, are available regarding whether walking time or pace is more predictive of lower risk. In the Nurses' Health Study, walking pace was associated with lower CHD risk after adjustment for MET-hours of walking (a combined measure of walking pace and time). Our finding that time spent walking is more important—implying that total energy expenditure is the relevant parameter—requires confirmation. Some supporting evidence comes from an experiment in which sedentary women were randomized to a control group or 1 of 3 exercise groups that walked the same distances

(4.8 km/d [3 miles/d], 5 d/wk) at 4.8, 6.4, or 8.0 km/h (3, 4, or 5 mph) for 24 weeks. All 3 exercise groups improved in fitness (measured by maximal oxygen uptake) compared with controls, with fitness improving in a dose-response fashion among exercisers. High-density lipoprotein cholesterol levels, however, increased significantly, to the same extent, among the 3 groups.

How can our findings be reconciled with those from other studies, primarily of men, that observed only vigorous-intensity activity to be associated with decreased CHD risk? We believe the data represent a spectrum of responses to physical activity. Among persons with little activity, institution of even light-to-moderate activity is associated with benefit. Among persons who are more active and fit, vigorous activity is needed for additional health benefits. Our study participants, in whom light-to-moderate activity was associated with decreased CHD risk, were relatively inactive. The most active group (the most active 21%) expended at least 1500 kcal/wk in recreational activities and stair climbing. In contrast, in a study of men in which physical activity was assessed in similar fashion to this study, subjects were much more active; the most active 20% expended at least 3129 kcal/wk. In that study, vigorous but not nonvigorous activity was associated with greater longevity.

Few data exist regarding the role of physical activity in the primary prevention of CHD among high-risk women. As with this study, the Nurses' Health Study also observed inverse associations among overweight women and smokers. Some investigators have postulated that overweight but active individuals have lower morbidity and mortality than normal-weight but sedentary individuals. In contrast, this study and the Nurses' Health Study both indicate that inactivity and overweight adversely affect CHD risk in women to a similar extent. . . .

Strengths of this study include its large size, well-characterized participants, and careful documentation of CHD. Furthermore, strict health criteria were used for enrollment into the parent trial. Therefore, it is unlikely that underlying disease could have decreased physical activity at study entry, biasing results. It is also less likely that women who did not walk were limited by physical disability.

Limitations include self-reports of physical activity. While the questionnaire used is reliable and valid for largescale studies, it does not offer the precision of, say, electronic devices that measure movement. The latter, however, are impractical for large studies. Moreover, physical activity data were gathered in this study prior to CHD occurrence; thus, any misclassification is likely random, diluting the true association. While we did adjust for a large number of potential confounders, confounding by unmeasured factors is a concern in any observational study. Participants also were not representative of the general population. The proportions of women who were overweight or had elevated blood pressure or cholesterol levels were similar to the general population, but fewer smoked and more used postmenopausal hormones. However, it is unlikely that the biologic effects of physical activity would differ in the general population.

In conclusion, this study indicates that physical activity, easily within the ability of almost all women, is associated with lower CHD rates. At least 1 hour of walking per week, regardless of pace, was associated with lower CHD rates among relatively sedentary women. Because this is less than what current guidelines suggest, confirmation of these findings is desirable. Meanwhile, a conservative approach is to endorse current guidelines recommending moderate-intensity physical activity for 30 min/d most days of the week. In the present study, this level of physical activity was associated with lower CHD rates, even among women who were overweight, smoked, or had elevated cholesterol levels.

POSTSCRIPT

Must Exercise Be Daily and Intense to Prevent Chronic Disease?

Rising levels of obesity in a population reveal that people are consuming more energy from food than the amount they expend in physical activity. To maintain healthy weights, people must balance energy intake with energy expenditure. These selections address the question of how much physical activity is necessary to maintain healthy weight and reduce risks for chronic disease. The Food and Nutrition Board (FNB) of the Institute of Medicine says that at least one hour per day of physical activity at an expenditure rate of 4.5 to 8 calories per minute is required to achieve these goals. In contrast, a group of Harvard epidemiologists concludes that women health professionals can substantially reduce their risk of coronary heart disease simply by spending one hour per week in activities at even lower rates of caloric expenditure (e.g., walking). Another group of Harvard epidemiologists reports that just one-half hour of daily brisk walking is associated with an 18 percent reduction in coronary risk (Tanasescu et al., *Journal of the American Medical Association,* October 23/30, 2002).

The studies differ in design. The FNB report was a scientific review of studies that related oxygen consumption to caloric expenditure for men and women of different ages, body weights, and metabolic rates. The FNB committee focused particularly on the amount of activity that would be needed to maintain body weight. In contrast, Lee et al. collected data on physical activity from self-reported questionnaires among 39,372 women health professionals. These women, however, may not represent the entire population of women in the United States. In addition, people tend to exaggerate their activity levels on questionnaires. If the data here were exaggerated, perhaps even less activity is required to show health benefits.

Although Lee et al. did not specifically examine the association between moderate activity and body weight, other investigators have shown that similar activity levels result in reductions in body weight and body fat in overweight and obese women (see *Journal of the American Medical Association,* January 15, 2003). Other studies have yielded more inconsistent results, largely because of difficulties in obtaining reliable information about physical activity, let alone weight change (see *Obesity Research,* October 2000).

One remarkable feature of this debate is what it means for public policy. The *Dietary Reference Intakes* are meant to establish standards of nutrient intakes adequate to prevent deficiencies but also appropriate for prevention of chronic diseases among healthy people in the United States and Canada. As such, they are used to establish policies on matters such as food assistance, food labeling, and, in this case, exercise recommendations for the public. The Institute of Medicine of the National Academies based its recommendation on scientific studies and did not consider whether one hour per day of brisk walking might or might not be realistic for most people. Lee et al. argue that their observations mean that levels of activity readily achievable by practically anyone can help reduce the risk of heart disease—the leading killer of American women as well as men.

Lee et al. explain the discrepancy in results as a matter of increments. For people who are largely sedentary, even light exercise confers benefit. For those who are already active, more intensity is needed to confer further benefit. It seems clear that both groups would agree that some activity is better than none, and more activity is better than less.

ISSUE 9

Do Education Campaigns Induce Communities to Change Their Diets and Improve Health?

YES: Bill Reger, Margo G. Wootan, and Steven Booth-Butterfield, from "A Comparison of Different Approaches to Promote Community-Wide Dietary Change," *American Journal of Preventive Medicine* (April 2000)

NO: Stephen P. Fortmann and Ann N. Varady, from "Effects of a Community-Wide Health Education Program on Cardiovascular Disease Morbidity and Mortality: The Stanford Five-City Project," *American Journal of Epidemiology* (April 2000)

ISSUE SUMMARY

YES: West Virginia University researchers Bill Reger and Steven Booth-Butterfield and Center for Science in the Public Interest researcher Margo G. Wootan say that advertising and public relations campaigns can induce the public to make more healthful dietary choices.

NO: Researchers Stephen P. Fortmann and Ann N. Varady say that even long-term educational interventions in communities have little effect on overall trends in chronic disease risk.

$\mathbf{F}$ood companies spend about \$30 billion annually on advertising and other marketing techniques to promote sales of their products. Advertising increases awareness of products, induces brand loyalty, causes children to request products, and, as might be expected, increases sales. A single nationally advertised fast food chain, soft drink, or candy bar might use an annual advertising budget of \$500 million, \$100 million, or \$50 million, respectively, just for direct media: television, radio, and print. Other kinds of marketing (coupons, samples, trade shows, and supermarket placement fees, for example) add \$2 for every dollar spent on media advertising. Most food marketing is designed to sell high-profit foods—those high in fats, sugars, and corn sweeteners at the top of the U.S. Department of Agriculture (USDA) Food Guide Pyramid. No professional

174

health organization or government agency has anywhere near that level of funding for public education campaigns to promote more healthful food choices. For example, the most funding ever contributed in any one year by the National Cancer Institute and its food industry partners to the public education component of the 5 A Day for Better Health campaign (which encourages Americans to increase consumption of fruits and vegetables) was about $2 million.

In thinking about how to encourage the public to eat more healthfully (or to generally eat less), health officials and researchers have wondered whether or not the techniques used by the food industry to sell products—advertising, marketing, and public relations—could be used to improve the dietary choices of populations. In Finland, a major educational campaign among communities in North Karelia, where rates of heart disease were among the highest in the world, proved remarkably successful in improving dietary patterns, reducing heart disease risk factors, and lowering disease and death rates from that condition. Could that type of campaign succeed in the United States? The following selections address that question.

Bill Reger et al. examined whether or not a campaign involving paid advertising, public relations, and community education could influence people to switch from high-fat to low-fat milk. Their results convince them that these techniques can change food choices, that the changes are sustained, and that these methods are effective at very low cost.

In contrast, Stephen P. Fortmann and Ann N. Varady, researchers in the Stanford Five-City Project, conducted a six-year, comprehensive educational intervention focused on reducing major cardiovascular disease risk factors—high blood cholesterol, high blood pressure, and obesity—by encouraging people to stop smoking cigarettes, to become more active, and to eat less fat (which is high in calories), meat (a source of saturated fat), and salt (which can raise blood pressure). They argue that this kind of intervention has only modest effects on heart disease risk factors and no significant effect on the number of deaths and nonfatal events from heart disease and stroke. The investigators found that rates of heart disease were declining in cities that did not receive the intervention just as much as in the cities that did. They concluded that the observed reduction in heart disease must have been due to ongoing changes in society—"secular trends"—rather than to the educational intervention itself.

What might account for the differences in these conclusions? Both groups of investigators ran their health education campaigns in selected cities and used comparable cities as controls, but were they using similar methods and looking for similar outcomes? What features of their interventions seemed most effective? What were the limitations of their approaches? Are the outcomes of these studies truly comparable? What do these studies tell us about the role of food advertising and public health campaigns in influencing dietary practices?

In these selections, Reger et al. state that low-cost educational campaigns can be remarkably effective in improving specific dietary practices. Fortmann and Varady, however, maintain that changes in the societal environment rather than education are more likely to be responsible for declines in diet-related disease risk.

Bill Reger, Margo G. Wootan, and
Steven Booth-Butterfield

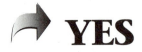 **YES**

A Comparison of Different Approaches to Promote Community-Wide Dietary Change

Introduction

Saturated fat consumption significantly impacts heart disease, the number one cause of death for American men and women. Although many foods make up the American diet, six types of food (cheese, beef, milk, baked goods, margarine, and butter) contribute half of all dietary saturated fat. Changing the consumption of those few foods could go a long way toward improving Americans' diets and health. For example, if the average American who consumes the average quantities of calories, saturated fat, and milk switched from drinking whole milk to fat-free milk, he or she could decrease saturated fat intake from 12% of calories to 10% of calories, the level recommended by the federal government.

The Center for Science in the Public Interest developed the 1% Or Less campaign to target one of the top sources of saturated fat in Americans' diets. The campaign encourages adults and children over the age of 2 years to switch from high-fat (whole or 2%) to low-fat (1% or fat-free) milk. The 1% Or Less campaign targets the reduction of a major source of saturated fat in Americans' diets, while preserving the benefits of consuming milk.

Because public health education funds are limited, it is important to determine which methods are most effective for promoting healthy lifestyles to communities. The pilot 1% Or Less campaign, which used paid advertising, public relations (PR), and community educational activities in supermarkets, schools, and work-sites, was shown to be effective in influencing many members of one community to switch from high-fat to low-fat milk. A follow-up study demonstrated that the approach also was effective when the message was delivered by combining paid advertising and PR in the absence of community educational activities. The studies described in this work assessed the effectiveness of two additional approaches to promoting healthy eating. Two community demonstration projects with similar budgets examined the effects of

From Bill Reger, Margo G. Wootan, and Steven Booth-Butterfield, "A Comparison of Different Approaches to Promote Community-Wide Dietary Change," *American Journal of Preventive Medicine*, vol. 18, no. 4 (April 2000), pp. 271–275. Copyright © 2000 by *American Journal of Preventive Medicine*. Reprinted by permission of Elsevier. References omitted.

combining PR and community educational activities with paid advertising in the absence of additional programming.

Methods

In the winter of 1997, we studied three rural West Virginia communities. In Parkersburg, population 34,000, the campaign consisted of PR and community-based educational activities. In Beckley, population 18,000, only paid advertising conveyed the campaign message. Martinsburg, population 14,000, served as the comparison city. At least 135 miles separate the three cities. Each of the communities is located in a different media market (they have separate newspapers, television, and radio stations) and none is exposed to the media of any of the other study communities. We chose the three cities, in part, because of the similarity of their demographic characteristics to one another and to Clarksburg/Bridgeport and Wheeling, West Virginia, the sites of two previous 1% Or Less campaigns.

Public relations and community-based education The Parkersburg campaign ran for 8 weeks and cost approximately $51,000. A full-time health educator trained approximately 150 community volunteers to conduct educational activities in supermarkets, schools, worksites, churches, synagogues, shopping malls, and meetings of civic organizations. The educational activities resembled those conducted in the pilot 1% Or Less campaign in Clarksburg and Bridgeport, West Virginia. More than 1300 people participated in milk taste tests in which participants tasted whole, 2%, 1%, and fat-free milk while wearing dark sunglasses to mask the appearance of the milk. Taste tests were conducted in supermarkets, schools, worksites, a shopping mall, and other community locations.

Ten out of the eleven supermarkets in the Parkersburg area displayed signs in their dairy cases encouraging customers to choose low-fat milk. Health professionals trained by campaign staff gave presentations to approximately 1100 people (at worksites, clinics of The Special Supplemental Nutrition Program for Women, Infants & Children (WIC), hospitals, and meetings of civic groups) about the importance of nutrition and drinking low-fat milk. Educational activities, such as milk taste tests, speaker presentations, newsletter articles, and displays that compared the amount of fat in whole, 2%, 1%, and fat-free milk, were conducted at 16 worksites (27 large worksites were targeted as sites for campaign activities), both area hospitals, the local WIC office, and 14 civic organizations (out of approximately 40 local civic groups). All 13 primary schools, all four middle schools, and two of the three area high schools participated in the campaign. Schools used peer education, conducted milk taste tests, and taught interdisciplinary lessons to promote low-fat milk consumption to students.

The PR strategy used in Parkersburg was similar to that of the previous 1% Or Less campaigns in West Virginia. Public relations activities included the following: (1) a kick-off press conference, (2) a joint press conference held by the two area hospitals at which prominent local physicians encouraged the community to switch to low-fat milk, (3) an announcement of changes in low-fat milk consumption at the midpoint of the campaign, (4) two radio broadcasts from supermarkets while milk taste tests were being conducted, and (5) a press conference at the end of the campaign.

Paid advertising   The 1% Or Less campaign in Beckley consisted of 6 weeks of paid advertising and cost $50,000. The campaign used the same two 30-second television and two 60-second radio advertisements used in the pilot 1% Or Less campaign and the follow-up study conducted in Wheeling, West Virginia. The advertisements were designed for broad appeal but targeted primarily middle-aged women. The placement plan for the advertising, developed by a professional agency, included 281 broadcast television, 366 cable television, and 160 radio advertisements. The television advertising resulted in 670 household gross rating points per week, suggesting that 85% of households were exposed to the commercials approximately 8 times per week for 4 weeks.

Telephone surveys   We conducted baseline telephone interviews with approximately 400 people in each community (1232 total for the three communities) to assess demographic characteristics and milk-usage patterns. Postcampaign questionnaires in the intervention cities also evaluated exposure to the 1% Or Less messages and programs. The survey instruments were very similar to those used in the two previous West Virginia campaigns. We purchased random telephone numbers from Scientific Telephone Samples (Santa Ana, California). The adult in the household with the most recent birthday was interviewed for the precampaign survey. After the campaign ended, precampaign survey respondents were called again to complete the postcampaign survey. All telephone interviews required 5 to 8 minutes to complete.

Supermarket milk sales   We collected milk sales data for the month before, for the month after, and for the month 6 months after the campaign from all 21 supermarkets in the three communities. Because data were missing for 1 month for one store in Beckley and for 1 month for one store in Martinsburg, we used no data from those two stores in any of the computations. We collected sales data for whole, 2%, 1%, 1/2%, and fat-free unflavored milk, which make up 94% of the beverage milk consumed nationally. We did not collect data on flavored milk, buttermilk, cream, or lactose-reduced milk. . . .

Results

The PR strategies in Parkersburg helped establish the 1% Or Less campaign as newsworthy. The Parkersburg campaign generated 27 news stories on television, radio, and in newspapers. No Beckley or Martinsburg television stations, radio stations, or newspapers covered the 1% Or Less campaign.

Telephone Survey

Immediately after the campaigns, 826 of the 1232 precampaign respondents completed a postintervention telephone survey (33% dropout rate). We found no statistically significant differences between those respondents lost to follow-up and those who completed both the precampaign and postcampaign surveys in any of the three communities on any of the survey variables (including the type of milk consumed at baseline, gender, age, education, household income, or employment status).

Using only the respondents who completed both the pre-intervention and postintervention surveys, we compared the demographic characteristics of the three communities. We found no differences for baseline milk drinking, age, education level, employment status, or household income. However, we found that Parkersburg had more Caucasian respondents, . . . Martinsburg had more male respondents, . . . and Martinsburg had a more transient population . . . compared with the other cities.

After the campaign of community–based educational programs and PR activities in Parkersburg, a significant shift occurred from high-fat to low-fat milk compared with the comparison city (Table 1). The proportion of high-fat milk drinkers who reported drinking low-fat milk after the campaign was 19.6% compared with 6.8% for the comparison city. . . . In Beckley, where the campaign included only paid advertising, 12.8% of high-fat milk drinkers reported drinking low-fat milk after the campaign, which was significantly greater than the 6.8% reported for the comparison city. . . . In addition, the campaign of community-based programs and PR activities in Parkersburg resulted in a greater switch from high-fat to low-fat milk (19.6%) than did the advertising-only campaign in Beckley (12.8%). . . .

Table 1

Campaign Effects on Low-Fat Milk Consumption

City	Campaign type	Self-reported switching to low-fat milk	Low-fat milk sales in supermarkets, market share (%)		
			pre-campaign	post-campaign	6-month follow-up
Parkersburg	community programming and public relations	19.6%*	23%	28%^{ns}	29%^{ns}
Beckley	paid advertising	12.8%**	28%	34%^{ns}	27%^{ns}
Martinsburg	none	6.8%	23%	22%	21%

The percent of high-fat milk drinkers who reported drinking low-fat milk after the campaign was determined from the telephone surveys. Low-fat milk sales in supermarkets are reported as a percent of all milk sold for the month before, the month after, and 6 months after the 1% Or Less campaigns in West Virginia in 1997.

*$p < 0.0001$

**$p < 0.01$

^{ns}not statistically significant.

Supermarket Milk Sales

Sales of low-fat milk in Parkersburg, which had the campaign of community-based educational programs and PR, made up 23% of overall milk sales during the month before the campaign (2114 gallons per supermarket per month), 28% of milk sales after the campaign (2243 gallons per supermarket per month), and 29% of milk sales at the 6-month follow-up (2640 gallons per supermarket per month) (Table 1). In Beckley, which had the paid advertising campaign, low-fat milk sales made up 28% of overall milk sales before the campaign (2095 gallons per supermarket per month), 34% of milk sales after the campaign (2137 gallons per supermarket per month), and 27% of milk sales at the 6-month follow-up (2143 gallons per supermarket per month). In the comparison city, low-fat milk sales made up 23% of total milk sales before the campaign (2853 gallons per supermarket per month), 22% of milk sales after the campaign (2597 gallons per supermarket per month), and 21% of milk sales at the 6-month follow-up (2428 gallons per supermarket per month). For both Parkersburg and Beckley, the differences in low-fat milk sales after their campaigns were not statistically significant compared with sales in the comparison city. In addition, over the course of the study period, no significant differences were observed in overall milk sales (whole, 2%, 1%, 1/2%, and fat-free milk combined) in either Parkersburg or Beckley.

Discussion

Only 3% of the health care dollars in the United States are spent on preventive measures, yet half of all deaths relate to lifestyle and other preventable factors. Because funds for prevention, including those for public health education, are limited, they must be used wisely. The studies described in this work provide further information about key components (paid advertising, PR, and community educational activities) of one effective nutrition education campaign: the 1% Or Less campaign.

The telephone survey results suggest that the 1% Or Less campaign in Parkersburg, which included community−based educational programs and PR, was effective in encouraging high-fat milk drinkers to switch to low-fat milk. Although the milk sales data show a similar trend after the campaign, the observed increase in low-fat milk sales was not statistically significant.

The community programs plus PR approach used in Parkersburg resembled the approach used in many other health promotion campaigns. Such an approach relies heavily on the availability of health-promotion staff. The program design likely is popular because many community-based organizations and health departments have staff available to conduct health-promotion programs but have limited funds for program implementation. Although this approach may seem inexpensive, the true cost of community−based educational programming is great if staff cost is included. In Parkersburg, staff cost represented 60% of the campaign's $51,000 budget.

In contrast, our previous 1% Or Less campaign in Wheeling, West Virginia, did not use any community−based educational activities. That campaign used a combination of paid advertising and PR. The ads plus PR campaign had a slightly smaller budget, $43,000, yet it resulted in 34% of high-fat milk drinkers switching to low-fat milk compared with approximately 20% in the community programs plus PR campaign in Parkersburg. The pilot 1% Or Less campaign in Clarksburg/Bridgeport, which used a combination of all three approaches (paid advertising, PR, and community programs), had a $61,000 budget and resulted in 38% of high-fat milk drinkers switching to low-fat milk.

The telephone survey results also suggest that a significant number of high-fat milk drinkers switched to low-fat milk after the advertising-only campaign in Beckley. Although the milk sales data show a similar trend, the difference between baseline (28%) and postcampaign (34%) low-fat milk market shares was not statistically significant. However, in the long term, the proportion of low-fat milk sold was virtually the same at the 6-month follow-up (27%) as at baseline (28%).

In comparison, the 1% Or Less campaign in Wheeling, which used paid advertising supported by PR activities, resulted in 34% of high-fat milk drinkers switching to low-fat milk compared with 13% in the advertising-only campaign in Beckley. In addition, low-fat milk sales increased significantly after the ads plus PR campaign, and sales remained significantly higher than baseline up to 2 years after the campaign ended (B.W., unpublished data). Because consumers are bombarded with more than $73 billion of advertising each year, PR activities may be needed to draw attention to the advertising to make it more effective. News coverage that results from PR activities adds credibility to the advertising, allows a campaign to communicate its message in more detail, and increases the number of times people hear the message.

Although the observed trends were consistent with the self-report data, the increases in low-fat milk sales observed after the two campaigns described in this work were not statistically significant. It may have been more difficult to detect the effects achieved by these campaigns because they were smaller than those produced by the previous ads plus PR, and ads plus PR plus community programs campaigns. In addition, the sample size was smaller for the two campaigns described in this work: only five supermarkets in Martinsburg (comparison city) and six supermarkets in Beckley (advertising-only campaign), and two of those supermarkets could not be used in our analysis because of missing data. The variation in overall milk sales between time points and between stores also may have affected the ability to achieve statistical significance.

Available funding restricted this investigation to three communities, two treatment and one comparison, limiting the generalizability of the findings. Ideally, community intervention research should be conducted in a cluster of randomly assigned treatment and control communities. Although the data are suggestive and consistent with previous findings, uncontrolled and unidentified variables may have accounted for the observed changes.

Our previous study demonstrates that paid advertising combined with PR activities can be an effective means to promote low-fat milk consumption. In contrast, we found that paid advertising alone was not an effective long-term strategy for promoting this dietary change. In addition, the community programs plus PR campaign seemed to be effective. However, the combination of

PR and community programs was not as effective as the combination of PR and paid advertising, even though the funding level for the community programs plus PR campaign was higher. These comparisons suggest that PR was an important component of our health-education campaigns. The 1% Or Less campaigns provide another example of how well-designed PR activities can attract news coverage and provide an inexpensive means of reinforcing and strengthening other program components.

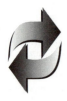

NO ⬅

**Stephen P. Fortmann
and Ann N. Varady**

Effects of a Community-Wide Health Education Program on Cardiovascular Disease Morbidity and Mortality: The Stanford Five-City Project

Epidemic cardiovascular disease (CVD), the major cause of death and disability in industrialized countries, is largely attributable to lifestyle behaviors, including diet, exercise, and cigarette smoking, both directly and as mediated by blood pressure and plasma lipoprotein levels. The importance of CVD to public health and its link with lifestyle behaviors led pioneers in CVD control to address the problem on a community level. The two earliest community-based CVD studies were the Stanford Three-Community Study in California and the North Karelia Project in Finland, both initiated in 1972. The Three-Community Study targeted CVD risk factors through a health promotion program that used mass media supplemented by individual and group education for high-risk persons in one town and mass media alone in a second town; a third town served as a control. Findings showed a significant reduction in overall cardiovascular risk in the two treatment towns, compared with the control town, in cohorts that were surveyed annually in each town at baseline and for three follow-up visits.

The Three-Community Study generated the Stanford Five-City Project, a larger-scale and longer California field trial designed to test whether a comprehensive program of community organization and health education could produce favorable changes in CVD risk factor prevalence, morbidity, and mortality. A 6-year education intervention (1980–1986) targeted all residents in two treatment communities and involved a multiple risk factor strategy delivered through multiple educational methods. The overall changes in risk factors (knowledge about CVD, blood pressure, smoking, cholesterol) have been reported elsewhere and were positive in both treatment and control towns, with the exception of obesity. The changes in knowledge about CVD and in systolic and diastolic blood pressure in the treatment cities significantly exceeded those in control cities in the cross-sectional surveys. . . .

As the North Karelia Project did, the Five-City Project included monitoring of trends in CVD rates and risk factors. The hypothesis was that the Five-City

Adapted from Stephen P. Fortmann and Ann N. Varady, "Effects of a Community-Wide Health Education Program on Cardiovascular Disease Morbidity and Mortality: The Stanford Five-City Project," *American Journal of Epidemiology,* vol. 152, no. 4 (April 2000). Copyright © 2000 by The Johns Hopkins University School of Hygiene and Public Health. Reprinted by permission of Oxford University Press and Stephen P. Fortmann. References omitted.

Project education program would significantly reduce myocardial infarction and stroke rates in the two treatment cities relative to the three control cities. CVD endpoint results have been reported for the North Karelia Project and another major US community CVD trial, the Minnesota Heart Health Project; the purpose of this [selection] is to report these results for the Five-City Project.

Materials and Methods

The design and methods of the Five-City Project and the morbidity and mortality surveillance system have been described previously and are summarized here. The two treatment cities (1980 total population) were Monterey (43,400) and Salinas (80,500), and the three control cities were Modesto (132,400), San Luis Obispo (34,300), and Santa Maria (39,700) . . . No population risk factor surveys were conducted in Santa Maria. Treatment and control cities were selected from all northern California cities by using criteria for size, distance from Stanford, and media markets. Random assignment of communities to treatment and control conditions was precluded by constraints on city selection, particularly the requirement that the broadcast media in treatment cities not reach control cities. The originally planned duration of morbidity and mortality monitoring (1979–1986) was extended to 1992 when it became apparent that the impact of the gradual risk factor changes induced by the intervention would not occur, if at all, until after the intervention ended (1986).

When this study was conducted, Salinas, Modesto, and Santa Maria were agricultural service communities with few large, nonagricultural employers (with the exception of a large winery in Modesto and of Vandenberg Air Force Base near Santa Maria). Monterey and San Luis Obispo were smaller cities, and tourism was a larger component of the local economy. About 20 percent of the Salinas and Santa Maria populations was Mexican American in 1980, and this proportion increased (absolutely and relatively) during the decade. Most other residents were White and non-Hispanic.

Morbidity and Mortality Surveillance System

Although mortality rates can be obtained directly from routine vital statistics, their precision and accuracy may not be sufficient to test the impact of community intervention, particularly over a short time and in moderate-sized cities. Also, routine vital statistics might be biased by the intervention program, for example, by altering physician reporting on death certificates. . . . The Five-City Project therefore included a community surveillance system designed to validate fatal CVD events and count nonfatal events. . . . Events occurring in residents of the five cities who were aged 30–74 years at the time of the event were included.

Selection of events and criteria.   Only nonfatal events for which residents were hospitalized (myocardial infarction [heart attack] and acute stroke) were deemed practical for inclusion; total mortality, fatal myocardial infarction and stroke, and other fatal coronary heart disease (mainly out-of-hospital sudden death) were included as fatal events. We recognized that a substantial but unknown proportion of nonfatal myocardial infarctions would be clinically unrecognized and therefore uncounted, but we assumed that this proportion would be similar for all cities. Likewise, nonfatal events occurring away from home would be missed but were also likely to be similar between cities. Fatal events that occur in travelers are reported to the county of residence and therefore were included. The criteria were designed to maximize reliability by minimizing the need for clinical judgment, manual calculations, or the use of implicit assumptions and to rely on data usually found in a hospital chart. . . .

Case identification and investigation.   Fatal events were located by regularly reviewing county vital statistics records; deaths were not investigated further if the death certificate diagnoses clearly indicated a noncardiovascular cause. All other deaths were investigated by collecting additional medical information. Information on events for which residents were hospitalized came from the medical record; for out-of-hospital deaths, the staff interviewed the next of kin and obtained a completed one-page questionnaire from the decedent's regular physician. Coroner records and autopsy results were copied for all deaths. Nonfatal events were identified through a regular review of computerized hospital discharge data, which were searched for relevant diagnoses. . . .

Validation.   Information on each event was returned to Stanford, where individual and city identifiers were removed and all data were entered into a database. Electrocardiograms [test used to evaluate health of heart] were sent to the Division of Epidemiology at the University of Minnesota (Minneapolis), where they were interpreted according to the Minnesota electrocardiogram code. These masked clinical data, including the electrocardiogram codes, were then reviewed independently by two research nurses, who determined the presence or absence of each component of the criteria by using their judgment when needed (e.g., whether or not the physical findings were sufficient to document a stroke). When the two analyses produced different endpoints, the case was reviewed and adjudicated by a panel of physicians. . . .

Quality control.   Research staff performance was monitored through biennial review of a standard set of 20 charts circulated to all investigators, plus re-review of a randomly selected 5 percent of charts reviewed previously. In addition, validators were monitored annually through blind resubmission of events validated previously.

Population estimates.   The geographic areas included in the study were defined by census tracts rather than city boundaries. Census data were obtained for 1980 and 1990, and the intercensal midyear population by 5-year age groups was estimated by linear interpolation. The 1991 and 1992 population data were estimated by linear extrapolation from the previous 10 years.

Education Program

The intervention conducted in the treatment cities was a 6-year multifactor risk reduction education program that was coordinated, comprehensive, and community-wide. Risk factor interventions had multiple target audiences and used multiple communication channels and settings (including newspapers, television and radio, mass-distributed print media, classes, contests, and correspondence courses). The program promoted reducing plasma cholesterol levels through a change in diet; reducing blood pressure through regular blood pressure checks, reduced salt intake, reduced weight, increased exercise, and full adherence to antihypertensive medication regimens; reducing cigarette smoking; reducing obesity through increased exercise and reduced dietary energy intake; and increasing both moderate and vigorous physical activity. Program planning included setting general and specific goals for each year of the campaign (e.g., reducing meat intake, promoting the adoption of one new low-fat recipe per month, reaching 50 percent of smokers with a self-help quit kit). Data from baseline population surveys in the treatment communities were used to develop an overview of knowledge, attitudes, and behavior for the target audience. This audience was segmented by age, ethnicity, socioeconomic status, overall cardiovascular risk, media use, organization membership, and motivation to change behavior (including diet). . . .

On average, each adult in the two treatment cities was exposed to about 5 hours per year of Five-City Project educational messages. About 7 percent of this exposure was provided by classes, lectures, or workshops; 34 percent by television and radio; 41 percent by booklets and kits; and 18 percent by newspapers and newsletters. . . .

Results

. . . Of this total, 9,479 first definite events occurred in different persons (i.e., only the first event for each person was counted). About twice as many events occurred in men as in women (6,239 vs. 3,240). In subsequent analyses, we combined men and women, since the Five-City Project hypotheses were not sex specific (and there was no reason to expect the intervention to affect event rates in men and women differently). Coronary disease deaths, nonfatal myocardial infarction, and stroke each accounted for about one-third of the events.

. . . The rates were quite variable, but there were no statistically significant differences among the cities. . . .

Trends in definite event rates could be affected by changes in documentation of clinical events over time. For example, if physicians gradually order more tests and record more elements of the history of each event, events previously classified as possible could be reclassified as definite. Therefore, we next examined changes in documentation of important variables over time. The proportion of all coronary events that included a record of chest pain at baseline was high (94–99 percent) and did not change appreciably over time in any of the cities. . . . For none of these three elements of the diagnostic criteria was the change significantly different between treatment and control cities. . . . Documentation of the neurologic examination in stroke patients was also fairly high at baseline (85–95 percent) and rose only slightly over time. . . .

Figure 1

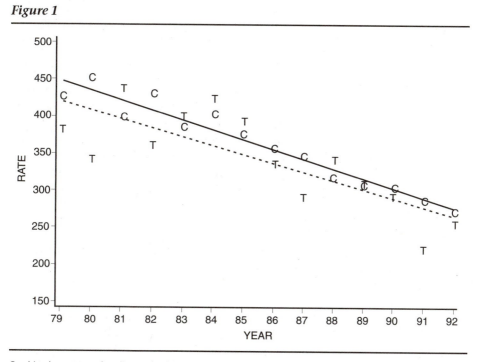

Combined-event rate of cardiovascular disease in treatment (T, solid line) and control (C, dashed line) cities, Stanford Five-City Project, northern California, 1979–1992. The lines were fitted by simple linear regression; rates per 100,000 persons.

For the remainder of the analyses, we combined all first definite events to calculate a single age- and sex-adjusted event rate for each year in each city, following the original study hypothesis. First, we examined trends over the entire 14 years of the study (figure 1). There were strong and significant declines in all five cities, and no difference in rate trends existed over time between treatment and control when the entire 14-year period was considered.

By the middle of the 1980s, it was evident to investigators that any risk reductions in the treatment cities were occurring slowly and that it would be unrealistic to expect an impact on morbidity and mortality by the end of the intervention, in 1986. Surveillance was therefore extended, and we hypothesized that trends in the late period, following the intervention (1986–1992), compared with those in the early period, during the intervention (1979–1985), would be more favorable in the treatment than the control cities. . . .

Discussion

The Stanford Five-City Project was designed to produce changes in CVD risk, morbidity, and mortality. Changes in risk factors were observed, although they were more modest than intended. Changes in blood pressure and smoking, the latter in a subset of the population, were most consistent in the data; exercise, diet, and plasma cholesterol changed little during the intervention, although plasma cholesterol levels likely fell in the late 1980s during the maintenance phase of the study.

In this paper, we have shown that the time trends in event rates appeared to change significantly in the years after the intervention was completed. In the first half of the 1980s, event rate trends were positive [rose] in the two treatment cities and negative [declined] in the three control cities, although none of the trends was statistically different from zero. After the intervention, from 1986 to 1992, the trends were uniformly downward in all cities, and the change in slope between the two periods was statistically significant. . . . [I]t is most reasonable to conclude that whatever produced the improvement acted in all five cities and that the intervention was not a cause. The conclusion that the intervention had no detectable impact on the combined-event rate trend is reinforced by the lack of any difference found in the linear component of the rate trends over the entire time period 1979–1992 (figure 1). Since some risk factor differences benefiting the treatment cities were observed, they were either insufficient to affect morbidity and mortality (given the precision of our measurement methods) or were countered by other, unmeasured factors.

Two other major community intervention studies have been conducted in the United States, in Minnesota and Rhode Island. To date, only the Minnesota Heart Health Program has reported results for morbidity and mortality, and it also failed to find compelling evidence of an intervention effect. While numerous community trials have been conducted outside the United States, only the North Karelia Project monitored morbidity and mortality trends. This study began in 1972, when the intervention area had the highest rate of coronary disease in the world, in men. Coronary disease was also highly prevalent in the control area and in Finland as a whole. There have been strong declines in coronary disease rates in Finland since 1972. Although the limited number of units precludes having great confidence in causal inference, it does appear that the intervention program was associated with an acceleration of the decline in coronary disease rates. The remarkable decline in coronary disease in Finland over the 20 years following 1972 was associated with significant declines in risk factors, which prediction models indicate largely explains the decline in disease rates.

The US community intervention studies were modeled to some extent on clinical trial experience; when these studies were designed in the mid-1970s, it was considered obligatory to include assessment of disease endpoints in addition to risk factor change. In retrospect, it was probably naive to think that these interventions could produce detectable changes in such endpoints. Even if the projected risk factor changes had been achieved during the planned 5- to 6-year interventions, they would have occurred toward the end of that time, before the full effect was in place, and there would then presumably be a delay between risk factor change and morbidity-mortality change (2 or 3 years, based on clinical trial results). In the mid-1970s, we also underestimated the strength of the secular trends in both risk factor change and coronary disease incidence in the United States as a whole and in the control cities in particular. We also clearly overestimated the ability of the education efforts to accelerate lifestyle and risk factor changes; many more sustained efforts are likely necessary. The North Karelia Project results illustrate this point.

Another unanticipated problem was the possibility that highly effective clinical therapies would be introduced widely, including in the control areas, obscuring any effect of the risk factor change. The Stanford Five-City Project never intended to alter the medical and surgical treatment of coronary disease. While it still seems unlikely that we observed any intervention effect, the data presented here are consistent with an effect from some rapidly diffusing treatment innovation occurring in the mid-1980s. . . .

Other limitations of this study include its limited generalizability because of the small number of cities selected, its quasi-experimental design, and possible confounding from differential secular trends in migration; unrecognized, non-fatal myocardial infarction; or other variables affecting the events included in the study. There are also other limitations to the accuracy and precision of the surveillance system and to the statistical modeling.

In summary, the Stanford Five-City Project documented a steepening in the decline of CVD morbidity and mortality that began relatively suddenly about the time that the education program ended in the two treatment cities, but it appears to have occurred similarly in the control cities. While the rate trends during the intervention were less favorable in both treatment cities than in the control cities, it is speculative to presume that this difference would have continued in the absence of the intervention. It is more likely that some influence affecting all cities, perhaps an innovation in the medical management of CVD, accounted for the observed change. Further exploration of this possibility is warranted. Public health policies concerning control of cardiovascular risk factors must rest on considerations other than the overall morbidity and mortality findings of US community intervention trials.

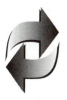

POSTSCRIPT

Do Education Campaigns Induce Communities to Change Their Diets and Improve Health?

When studying whether or not dietary factors affect disease risk, researchers often identify dietary practices in a population and attempt to relate those practices to the incidence of a particular disease in that population. In both of the studies presented here, investigators did something quite different: they actively intervened to improve dietary intake and disease rates in some communities but not in others. In West Virginia, Reger et al. used public relations and community education or advertising to encourage residents to switch from whole milk to lower-fat milk. Telephone surveys identified an impressive increase in the percentage of people in the intervention cities who said they switched to lower-fat milk (19.6 percent and 12.8 percent), as compared to that in the control city (6.8 percent) in just 6 to 8 weeks. Furthermore, the percent share of low-fat milk sold at supermarkets increased in the intervention cities but not in the control city, and that increase continued for at least two years. Although the level of increase was not statistically significant, the authors conclude that their approach—using media to influence a highly specific dietary change—was effective, and at relatively low cost.

The Stanford investigators were involved in a longer, larger, and far more complex and costly project to reduce heart disease risk factors. They used a variety of educational "channels" to encourage the populations in the intervention cities to reduce several risk factors by exposing people to about 30 hours of educational messages over a six-year period. Indeed, illnesses and deaths from heart disease fell in the intervention cities, but they also fell similarly in the control cities. The investigators concluded that the ongoing changes in society were stronger influences than education on the health behaviors of members of the communities.

A fundamental principle of health education is that education alone is hardly ever sufficient to change behavior. Improvements in health behavior almost always require several stages of change, first improvements in knowledge, then improvements in attitude, and only then improvements in behavior. It is one thing to understand that saturated fat raises blood cholesterol levels and that whole milk is a source of saturated fat (knowledge), but quite another to be willing to try lower-fat milk (attitude), and then actually start drinking it instead of whole milk (behavior). Education works best to improve knowledge, but other factors—for example, peer pressure, food availability, income, and taste—may be more important in influencing attitudes and behavior.

Food advertisers apply these principles to sell their products. They want customers not only to know about their products but also to want to buy them. They emphasize attitudes when they relate the food to fun, friends, and social acceptance. Furthermore, they know that advertising is most successful when it is highly visible, focused, and frequently repeated. A few hours watching televised food commercials readily reveal how marketers apply these principles in practice.

Both groups of investigators attempted to increase knowledge, improve attitudes, and change behavior. Both used objective measures of behavior change: sales of low-fat milk in the first study and outcomes of heart disease in the second. Both assumed that changes in behavior would be due to the intervention, not to changes in society that might lead everyone to make more healthful choices. In the West Virginia study, nearly 7 percent more people reported switching to low-fat milk, a secular trend perhaps explained by wanting to please telephone interviewers. (Sales of low-fat milk did not increase.) The Stanford intervention was particularly affected by ongoing changes in society. During the study period, rates of cigarette smoking and high blood cholesterol fell among American adults, at least in part in response to reasonably well-funded *national* public health campaigns.

That level of funding has never been applied to a campaign to improve diets, however. If, like advertising, dietary interventions were better funded, more focused, and repeated over a longer time period, they might produce more impressive results. That was certainly true of the project in North Karelia, as explained by its leader, Pekka Puska, in *Public Health Medicine* (April 2002). A systematic review of community-based interventions to increase fruit and vegetable consumption also identifies substantial gains from education programs, particularly when the messages are clear, use multiple strategies, involve the family, and continue for a long time (Donna Ciliska et al., *Journal of Nutrition Education,* volume 32, 2000). In 2003, the Robert Wood Johnson Foundation issued a *Community Action Guide* to developing and conducting such programs as part of an initiative called *The Shape We're In* (http://www.shapenews.com). But how might we generate funds for public health campaigns comparable to those for food advertising? One suggestion, published in the *American Journal of Public Health* (June 2000), is to impose small taxes on soft drinks and "junk" foods. A one-cent tax on soft drinks, for example, would generate more than one billion dollars annually, which, if spent on nutrition education, might also improve dietary attitudes and behavior and, therefore, health. Political decisions of society determine whether or not taxes of this type can be implemented.

Food and Drug Administration (FDA)

The Food and Drug Administration (FDA) Web site provides information about specific supplements as well as about rules and regulations affecting their use. Also see the section that explains the rules for health claims on the labels of foods and supplements. This site includes a link to the current list of authorized claims.

http://vm.cfsan.fda.gov/~dms/supplmnt.html

Office of Dietary Supplements at the National Institutes of Health

The Office of Dietary Supplements at the National Institutes of Health site provides ready access to the latest studies on the health effects of dietary supplements of all types, nutritional and herbal. Click on the "Health Information" and "Fact Sheets" buttons to obtain the latest information on the safety and efficacy of specific supplements of interest. This site also provides useful links to government agencies involved in supplement regulation.

http://dietary-supplements.info.nih.gov

National Center for Complementary and Alternative Medicine

The National Center for Complementary and Alternative Medicine is also part of the National Institutes of Health, and it is the government's principal agency for scientific research on complementary and alternative medicine, including herbal and nutritional therapies. This site provides information on the mission and history of the center, funding opportunities for research and training, and the results of clinical trials that test treatments or therapies, such as those involving vitamin or herbal supplements.

http://nccam.nih.gov

PART 4

Supplements and Functional Foods

*T*o increase the nutrient content of the diet in a population, nutritionists generally use three approaches: nutrition education, dietary supplements, and nutrient fortification. Fortification is the addition of nutrients to foods to replace those lost in processing. When fortification increases the nutritional value above what is normally present in a food or other healthful components are added, the food is considered "functional." Functional foods are supposed to confer health advantages beyond those conferred by the nutritional content of the food itself. The selections in this part address dietary supplements and functional foods, which are "reductionist" in the sense that they usually attribute (reduce) the benefits of healthful dietary patterns to one nutritional component. If, for example, eating fruits and vegetables is good for health, some experts believe that a particular component of those foods must be responsible for the benefit. In that case, the component might be even more beneficial if isolated, purified, and taken in larger amounts as a supplement or food additive. Because most people are genuinely interested in nutrition and health they are likely to prefer and buy foods perceived as healthful. Therefore, the use of supplements and functional foods has economic implications. Food and supplement manufacturers are eager to advertise the health benefits of their products and to minimize or ignore research studies that suggest that the products might be ineffective or harmful. The selections in this part debate the health, business, and regulatory implications of reductionist strategies to improve nutrition and health.

- Can Vitamin and Mineral Supplements Help Prevent Chronic Disease?

- Will Taking Herbal Supplements Enhance Mental Ability?

- Can Functional Foods and Nutraceuticals Benefit Health?

ISSUE 10

Can Vitamin and Mineral Supplements Help Prevent Chronic Disease?

YES: Robert H. Fletcher and Kathleen M. Fairfield, from "Vitamins for Chronic Disease Prevention in Adults: Clinical Applications," *Journal of the American Medical Association* (June 19, 2002)

NO: Demetrius Albanes, from "B-Carotene and Lung Cancer: A Case Study," *American Journal of Clinical Nutrition* (June 1999)

ISSUE SUMMARY

YES: Physicians Robert H. Fletcher and Kathleen M. Fairfield say that even in populations where deficiencies are rare, "suboptimal" vitamin intakes are common, especially among the elderly; consequently, adults should take vitamin supplements to reduce their risk for chronic diseases.

NO: Cancer prevention researcher Demetrius Albanes argues that foods—not supplements—are associated with cancer prevention and that supplemental beta-carotene, for example, may have adverse effects on health. He argues that more evidence is needed before advising adults to take nutrient supplements.

More than half the adult population of the United States regularly takes vitamin and mineral supplements, mainly in the belief that the pills will improve health by compensating for poor dietary habits, helping to increase energy or preventing and treating disease. Unquestionably, supplements are useful for overcoming deficiencies of specific nutrients. Most Americans, however, consume diets that contain enough essential nutrients to prevent signs of classic deficiency conditions such as scurvy (from lack of vitamin C), beriberi (from lack of thiamin), or pellagra (from lack of niacin). Fortification of the grain supply with iron, thiamin, niacin, riboflavin, and folate, and of dairy products with vitamins A and D, has virtually eliminated deficiencies of these nutrients in the United States, except among people whose diets are unusually deficient for a long time or who have diseases that interfere with the use of nutrients by the body.

In recent years, researchers have demonstrated additional benefits of consuming nutrient-rich fruits and vegetables beyond prevention of deficiencies. These foods also seem to help prevent heart disease and certain cancers. Because fruits and vegetables contain hundreds of nutrients and potentially protective substances commonly found in plant foods (phytochemicals), researchers are interested in identifying specific components that might be responsible for health benefits. Such studies have associated low levels of folate with heart disease, vitamin D with osteoporosis, and the antioxidant vitamins A, C, and E with heart disease and cancer. These studies suggest that supplements of these particular vitamins—and others—might improve health. The supplement industry has responded to this apparently sensible suggestion by marketing thousands of vitamin products for every conceivable health purpose. But do these supplements truly reduce the risk of heart disease and cancer in addition to preventing nutrient deficiencies?

Robert H. Fletcher and Kathleen M. Fairfield argue that many Americans exhibit subclinical levels of vitamin deficiency, meaning that although people do not display deficiency symptoms, they do have metabolic abnormalities that can be identified through biochemical laboratory tests. The authors suggest three options for correcting these minor nutrient deficiencies: dietary changes, fortification, and supplements. They argue that dietary changes, while desirable, are difficult for many people to implement, and that fortification strategies are limited by popular mistrust of chemicals added to foods. This situation, they say, leaves supplements as the preferred option.

In contrast, Demetrius Albanes urges caution before recommending vitamin supplements to anyone. He argues that the case of β (beta)-carotene makes it clear that the health effects of nutrient supplements—as compared to the foods that contain that nutrient as well as many others—are not only uncertain but potentially of considerable harm. He cites studies of the effects of this supplement on lung cancer as an example. "Observational research" (epidemiologic studies) produces consistent and convincing evidence that consuming diets high in fruits and vegetables rich in β-carotene reduces the risk of lung cancer. Intervention trials, however, show the opposite: people who take β-carotene supplements have *higher* rates of lung cancer and mortality from all causes than those who do not. In addition, study participants with low blood levels of β-carotene before the study began (at baseline) turn out to have the highest rates of lung cancer, presumably because they do not habitually consume many fruits and vegetables. Together, these findings suggest that β-carotene does not replace the benefits of the total nutrient composition of foods. Instead, β-carotene supplements seem to *increase* cancer risk, especially among smokers. While it is important to note that the amounts of the β-carotene supplements used in the clinical trials (20 to 30 milligrams) are noticeably higher than the amounts found in over-the-counter multivitamins (usually about 3 milligrams), the findings from these studies suggest that other single-nutrient supplements could also be harmful and need to be tested rigorously.

Why do so many people take supplements? How do education and income influence whether or not people take supplements? On what basis do people decide whether or not supplements are beneficial to health and well-being? What groups in society most benefit from promoting supplements as a means to improve health? Which side of this debate is more compelling, and for what reasons?

Robert H. Fletcher and
Kathleen M. Fairfield

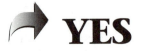 **YES**

Vitamins for Chronic Disease Prevention in Adults: Clinical Applications

In the absence of specific predisposing conditions, a usual North American diet is sufficient to prevent overt vitamin deficiency diseases such as scurvy, pellagra, and beriberi. However, insufficient vitamin intake is apparently a cause of chronic diseases. Recent evidence has shown that suboptimal levels of vitamins, even well above those causing deficiency syndromes, are risk factors for chronic diseases such as cardiovascular disease, cancer, and osteoporosis. A large proportion of the general population is apparently at increased risk for this reason.

Suboptimal Amounts of Vitamins

Suboptimal levels of a vitamin can be defined as those associated with abnormalities of metabolism that can be corrected by supplementation with that vitamin. For example, many people in the general population have serum homocysteine levels from 1.62 to 2.03 mg/L (12–15 μmol/L), which fall to baseline levels of 1.08 to 1.35 mg/L (8–10 μmol/L) after a few weeks of supplementation with folate, along with vitamins B_{12} and B_6. Similarly, in many elderly people, methylmalonic acid levels fall with vitamin B_{12} supplementation, and elevated levels of parathyroid hormone fall with vitamin D supplementation [the compounds mentioned here often increase in concentration when vitamins are deficient]. Measurements of vitamin levels in blood, serum, or red blood cells, at least with current reference points for abnormality, are not a reliable guide to this form of deficiency; in one study, supplementation substantially reduced serum homocysteine levels in elderly patients with normal serum folate concentrations.

For some vitamins, the concept of suboptimal levels is also supported by randomized trial evidence that supplementation reduces the rate of clinical events. The research evidence is conclusive that folate during the first trimester of pregnancy reduces the risk of neural tube defects in women at increased risk.

From Robert H. Fletcher and Kathleen M. Fairfield, "Vitamins for Chronic Disease Prevention in Adults: Clinical Applications," *Journal of the American Medical Association,* vol. 287, no. 23 (June 19, 2002), pp. 3127–3129. Copyright © 2002 by The American Medical Association. Reprinted by permission. References omitted.

Similarly, vitamin D supplementation, along with calcium, reduces the risk of fractures in elderly women with osteoporosis.

The high prevalence of suboptimal vitamin levels implies that the usual US diet provides an insufficient amount of these vitamins. Fruits and vegetables are the main dietary source of many vitamins, and health experts have long recommended at least 5 daily servings. A recent survey showed that only 20% to 30% of the population actually meet this goal. Although vitamin D is added to milk, many people (especially the elderly) do not consume enough dairy products to get a sufficient amount of vitamin D. Folate supplementation of cereal products is sufficient to raise folate intake only by about 100 μg, so many people do not meet the goal of 400 μg/d. Food preparation may decrease the activity for some vitamins; for example, keeping food hot longer than 2 hours results in a more than 10% loss of vitamin C, folate, and vitamin B_6. Vitamins are also lost during chilling, storage, and reheating, including more than 30% of vitamin C and folate. Alcohol consumption increases folate requirements, and aging is associated with decreased absorption of some vitamins such as B_{12}.

Correcting Suboptimal Vitamin Levels

Three options exist for correcting suboptimal vitamin intake. First, physicians could counsel patients to improve their diet. This approach would be relatively inefficient if the only goal were to increase vitamin consumption because patients would have to be counseled individually, and it is difficult to get individual patients to change their diets. Nevertheless, dietary change is a central component of an overall program of preventive care. Foods contain thousands of compounds that may be biologically active, including hundreds of natural antioxidants, carotenoids, and flavonoids. For these reasons, vitamin supplementation is not an adequate substitute for a good diet.

A second option is to add vitamins to generally consumed foods. The United States has been adding vitamin D to milk and some other dairy products since the 1930s because of the high prevalence of rickets and osteomalacia in northern climates at that time. Beginning in 1996, folate has been added to cereals to reduce the rate of neural tube defects. However, this approach is limited by popular mistrust of adding chemicals to food.

A third option is for individuals to take vitamin supplements. All major pharmacies carry their own brands of multivitamins as well as a variety of other brand name and generic multivitamins. The contents of basic multivitamins are remarkably similar across brands, with each having at least 100% of the daily value for nearly all vitamins (with the exception of vitamin K). In addition to vitamins, so-called multivitamins often contain other food supplements such as minerals and herbs. The amount of calcium in multivitamins is typically between 40 and 160 mg, well below the generally recommended dose of 1000 to 1500 mg/d, so one cannot depend on multivitamins for meeting calcium needs. Most multivitamins contain iron, whose supplementation may not be advisable for men and nonmenstruating women, given the high prevalence of the gene for hemochromatosis.

The cost for brand-name multivitamins may be around $20 to $30 annually, and some special formulations may cost a great deal more. However, one can easily buy large quantities (eg, 250–500 pills) of generic multivitamins for around $10 annually. We are aware of no evidence that the various multivitamins differ in bioavailability because of the way they are formulated. Patients can buy individual vitamins at an even lower price, which may make sense for women in the childbearing years, for whom folate supplementation might cost only $5 to $10 annually.

Special multivitamins are sold for subgroups of the population such as active men, perimenopausal women, and the elderly. The Internet and health-food stores are filled with promotions for these special-purpose multivitamins, which are often costly. The only evidence-based arguments for taking more than a common multivitamin once a day pertain to the elderly and women who might become pregnant. The recommended intake for vitamins B_{12} and D in the elderly is closer to 2 times the dietary reference intake. For women who might become pregnant, folate at 800 μg/d is appropriate.

Some vitamins, such as thiamin, riboflavin, and niacin, have received little mention in this review. Although by definition severe deficiency of these vitamins is associated with disease, they have so far not been associated with chronic diseases. The absence of evidence that these vitamins are associated with chronic diseases might be because those associations do not exist, ordinary diets provide sufficient amounts to prevent chronic disease, or the research has not yet been done to discover these relationships.

Testing

Tests for vitamin levels in blood, serum, or red blood cells are now offered by commercial laboratories, as are tests for substances such as homocysteine that mark abnormal vitamin-related metabolism. The availability of these tests raises these questions: Would this additional information lead to better preventive or therapeutic interventions than might be offered without the test? If so, what kind of patients would benefit?

It is certainly possible that some individuals, because of their diets or genetic polymorphisms, have unusual vitamin needs. Many of these people can be detected by a simple review of their medical problems, including alcoholism. The *MTHFR* polymorphism [a genetic variant of an enzyme involved in folate metabolism], which is associated with low folate levels and perhaps increased rates of cardiovascular disease, is the best studied. The abnormal *MTHFR* gene occurs in 5% to 15% of the population and might have effects on diseases related to folate deficiency. The *MTHFR* gene would be detected only by specific testing not yet commercially available. However, research into the metabolic and clinical effects of these disorders is in its infancy and not strong enough to confidently guide tailored supplementation programs. Therefore, we believe that testing individuals who do not have a well-recognized indication is premature.

Recommendations

We recommend that all adults take one multivitamin daily. This practice is justified mainly by the known and suspected benefits of supplemental folate and vitamins B_{12}, B_6, and D in preventing cardiovascular disease, cancer, and osteoporosis and because multivitamins at that dose are safe and inexpensive. It is reasonable to consider a dose of 2 ordinary multivitamins daily in the elderly, specifically because of the high prevalence of suboptimal vitamin B_{12} and D intake. However, it might be safer to supplement 1 multivitamin with additional vitamins B_{12} and D, taken separately, given the possibility that increased vitamin A intake might increase the risk of hip fracture and that the iron in most multivitamins may increase the risk of hemochromatosis in some people. The increased folate requirement in people with high alcohol intake can be met with 1 multivitamin daily or folic acid supplementation alone. For women attempting to conceive, a multivitamin plus folate at 400 μg/d is appropriate, given evidence of additional benefit with higher folate levels. We recommend multivitamins, rather than individual vitamins, because multivitamins are simpler to take and cheaper than the individual vitamins taken separately and because a large proportion of the population needs supplements of more than one vitamin. . . .

Additional Information About Vitamins

The evidence base for the clinical effects of vitamins is increasing rapidly. For physicians to keep up with new developments, there is no good alternative to electronic sources. The World Wide Web includes a vast array of information on vitamins, most of it promotional and self-serving. Physicians can find the most updated and credible information at the National Institutes of Health Web site (http://www.cc.nih.gov/ccc/supplements). In addition, Tufts University maintains an excellent nutrition Web site, as well as a Nutrition Navigator that provides quality ratings for other nutrition Web sites (http://www.navigator. tufts.edu). This site includes appropriate information for patients and health care professionals. Some textbooks and Web publications are continually updated as new research findings are published. The Institute of Medicine has published a series of books on this subject as well, with extensive review of the existing literature at the date of publication.

Demetrius Albanes

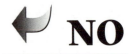

β-Carotene and Lung Cancer: A Case Study[a,b]

Abstract

The conflicting evidence of the relation between β-carotene and lung cancer in humans serves as a poignant case study with respect to what types of evidence are sufficient to support or change a nutrition recommendation. This article is a review of the available evidence of the relation between β-carotene and lung cancer, including data regarding β-carotene intake (from diet and supplements), β-carotene biochemical status, and vegetable and fruit consumption, and a discussion of the role of this evidence in making nutrition recommendations. More than 30 case-control and cohort studies were conducted over many years in various populations and indicated that people who eat more vegetables and fruit, foods rich in carotenoids, and carotenoids (β-carotene in particular), as well as those with higher blood β-carotene concentrations, have a lower risk of lung cancer than those who eat fewer such foods or have lower β-carotene concentrations. In contrast, the intervention results from large, controlled trials of β-carotene supplementation do not support the observed beneficial associations or a role for supplemental β-carotene in lung cancer prevention; instead, they provide striking evidence for adverse effects (ie, excess lung cancer incidence and overall mortality) in smokers. The findings require that caution be exercised in recommending supplemental β-carotene, particularly for smokers, and argue against changing the vegetable-fruit recommendations in the direction of greater nutrient specificity. This case study of β-carotene and lung cancer stresses the importance of having results from at least one, and preferably more, large, randomized intervention trial before public health recommendations concerning micronutrient supplementation are considered. *AM J. Clin Nutr* 1999;69(suppl);1345S−50S.

Key Words

β-Carotene, carotenoids, antioxidants, lung cancer, clinical trials, epidemiology, prevention

From Demetrius Albanes, "β-Carotene and Lung Cancer: A Case Study," *American Journal of Clinical Nutrition,* vol. 69, suppl. (June 1999), 1345S−1350S. Copyright © 1999 by The American Society for Clinical Nutrition. Reprinted by permission. The American Society for Clinical Nutrition, Inc. does not endorse any commercial enterprise.

Introduction

The conflicting evidence of the relation between β-carotene and lung cancer in humans serves as a poignant case study with respect to what types of evidence are sufficient to support or change a nutrition recommendation. The beneficial association supported by overwhelming observational epidemiologic data was abruptly challenged by the results of a few controlled trials of β-carotene supplementation. For reasons that will become clear in the course of this article, one of the central aspects of this study is highlighted by acknowledging that it would be less controversial were it titled "Vegetable consumption and lung cancer."

In this article, available evidence concerning the relation between β-carotene and lung cancer is reviewed and evaluated. To this end, relevant studies regarding β-carotene intake (including that from dietary and supplemental sources), β-carotene biochemical status, and vegetable and fruit consumption are taken into account and summarized. Randomized intervention trials are included in the definition of nutritional epidemiology in that they are among the state-of-the-science methods available to and used by chronic-disease epidemiologists to disentangle many of the myriad important diet-health associations under investigation. The term *observational epidemiology* is used to describe case-control and cohort studies.

Dietary Guidelines Relevant to β-Carotene Intake

Although dietary guidelines relevant to β-carotene intake are not discussed here in detail, they are germane as background to the case of β-carotene and lung cancer. In general, such guidelines lag behind available research and, rightfully, come after consensus building has taken place.

Two decades of dietary guidelines for Americans published jointly by the US Department of Agriculture (USDA) and the Department of Health and Human Services (DHHS) have mirrored the developing body of research concerning diet and health (1). As of 1980 and 1985, respectively, the guidelines pertaining to nutrition and cancer—and relevant to lung cancer and β-carotene in particular (albeit nonspecifically)—were "eat a variety of foods" and "eat foods with adequate starch and fiber." In 1990 "eat a variety of foods" remained a guideline but "choose a diet with plenty of vegetables, fruits, and grain products" replaced the reference to starch and fiber. This no doubt reflected, in part, the growing literature regarding the inverse association between vegetable and fruit consumption and cancer risk. By 1995, grain products were placed ahead of vegetables and fruit in the guidelines, presumably to better reflect the structure of the USDA food pyramid. Other relevant and somewhat more specific recommendations include the 1989 National Research Council *Diet and Health* report supporting consumption of ≥ 5 fruit and vegetable servings/d and the National Cancer Institute–DHHS sponsorship of the 5-A-Day Program initiated in 1991, which similarly promotes ≥ 5 servings of fruit and vegetables/d (2, 3).

Although there is no recommended dietary allowance for β-carotene, the recommendation for vitamin A of 800 and 1000 retinol equivalents (or μg retinol) for adult women and men, respectively, represents ≈4.8 and 6.0 mg β-carotene intake daily, assuming that the entire vitamin A requirement is met by provitamin A β-carotene. Therefore, current official public health guidelines are food-based and, specifically, oriented toward vegetables and fruit.

β-Carotene and Lung Cancer: What Is the Evidence?

Historical Overview

Research concerning β-carotene and lung cancer evolved for the most part similarly to that of many other questions of dietary factors and disease, such as the roles of dietary fats and fiber in human health, as follows. 1) Data from human studies bearing on the issue were accumulated, especially from observational case-control and cohort investigations published in the 1970s and 1980s. These are reviewed in detail below. 2) Abundant research was conducted on the antineoplastic [anit-cancer] effects of carotenoids and retinoids (4, 5) and the antioxidant and other biological functions of carotenoids (6). 3) Scientific discussion and debate was initiated, followed by additional research and published reviews. This occurred in the late 1980s and early 1990s. One early, widely cited paper by Peto et al (7) highlighted the potential public health significance of β-carotene and the need for controlled trials. Tacit calls for some action (ie, soft or unofficial recommendations) in this phase when the available data were highly suggestive and promising and increased scientific activity during this time may have contributed to the rising popularity of vitamin supplements during the 1980s (8, 9). 4) Randomized intervention trials to address the role of supplementation with specific micronutrients in cancer prevention were begun in the 1980s and some were completed by the mid-1990s. 5) The entire body of evidence was reinterpreted, with further discussion, debate, and consensus conferences in the mid-1990s.

Observational Epidemiologic Studies of Lung Cancer and Vegetables, Fruit, and β-Carotene

For more than a decade, overwhelming observational evidence has existed that supports an association between lower lung cancer risk and greater consumption of carotenoid-rich foods and, specifically, higher β-carotene intake. By most standards this is among the most consistent and convincing associations in the nutritional epidemiologic literature. What follows is a brief summary.

More than 30 case-control or cohort studies of relevance to the β-carotene–lung cancer association were conducted during the past 2 decades using various measures in diverse populations. Several excellent, comprehensive reviews of this research were published, including those by Ziegler (10), Willett (11), Steinmetz and Potter (12), Block et al (13), van Poppel and Goldbohm (14), and Ziegler et al (15). The observational studies link low self-reported consumption of vegetables or fruit (or both), derived from dietary histories or food-frequency or other dietary questionnaires, with increased risk of lung cancer. In many of the investigations, the inverse relation extends to the consumption of carotenoid-rich foods specifically, such as dark-green, yellow, or orange vegetables. Furthermore, in many studies a protective association was shown for β-carotene intake in particular, and several of these related lower lung cancer risk with higher biochemical status (usually serum concentration) of β-carotene. Relative risk increases of between 50% and 150% (ie, a relative risk of 1.5–2.5) were reported typically for the lowest vegetable-fruit or β-carotene categories compared with the highest. Thus, the observed associations are relatively strong and have substantial public health implications. They were shown in studies of men and women (16), in several racial groups (17), and in current smokers, former smokers, and nonsmokers (18) and therefore appear quite generalized. Taken together, these investigations of carotene-rich vegetables, β-carotene intake, and serum or plasma β-carotene concentrations in relation to lung cancer provide perhaps the most persuasive evidence for an association available in the diet-cancer epidemiologic literature today, both with respect to the magnitude and consistency of the protective association.

From the perspective of developing guidelines for the public, it is relevant and instructional to speculate about what nutrition recommendations regarding β-carotene intake might have resulted if they were based solely on the data from this body of observational research. If the β-carotene supplementation trials had not been conducted, for example, it is possible that guidelines more specific than those promoting greater consumption of vegetables and fruit might have emerged. On the basis of criteria such as consistency and strength of association, dose-response gradient, and biological plausibility, the evidence could have been considered sufficient to support additional recommendations concerning either carotenoid-rich foods or β-carotene intake in particular. Furthermore, a nutrient-specific guideline for β-carotene intake need not have specified source. A recommendation for adult daily intake of 10 mg β-carotene, for example, could be satisfied from either dietary or supplemental sources. This intake is only 67% higher than the β-carotene equivalent of the recommended dietary allowance for vitamin A for men and is well within the range of intake reported for the highest categories of β-carotene intake in the observational studies. However, such a recommendation has not been made to date, in part because of the results of the studies described below.

Randomized Intervention Trials of β-Carotene and Lung Cancer

Randomized intervention trials provide highly relevant, specific, and convincing evidence regarding supplemental nutrients (or dietary patterns) and cancer risk and have an important role in the development of related nutrition recommendations. They test specific nutrients, nutrient combinations, or dietary interventions through randomized experimental designs that avoid most of the biases inherent in observational studies. Two large randomized intervention trials of β-carotene supplementation having lung cancer as the primary study endpoint were published: the Alpha-Tocopherol, Beta-Carotene Cancer Prevention (ATBC) Study and the Beta Carotene and Retinol Efficacy Trial (CARET) (19, 20). Two other large, randomized cancer intervention trials also reported data concerning the effects of β-carotene supplementation on lung cancer: the Nutrition Intervention Trial conducted in Linxian, China, and the Physicians' Health Study (21–23).

In early 1994 the ATBC Study Group reported its initial trial intervention findings concerning β-carotene and α-tocopherol supplementation (19). This was the first report from a large (>29 000 participants), double-blind, placebo-controlled trial on the prevention of lung cancer and other cancers by supplementation with micronutrients. The results for β-carotene (20 mg in 1 capsule taken daily for 5–8 y) were surprising in that they provided no evidence for benefit in the prevention of lung cancer in older male cigarette smokers and instead suggested an adverse outcome, with more incident lung cancers diagnosed in those receiving β-carotene supplements. By the end of the study, and as reported in the final report for lung cancer, lung cancer was diagnosed in 482 men in the β-carotene–supplemented group and 412 in the group not receiving β-carotene (24). This represented relative excess of 16% for the β-carotene group. With a 95% CI of a 2–33% increase in lung cancer incidence, the finding was clearly inconsistent with the 2-fold risk reduction attributed to high β-carotene intake in so many observational studies, and it essentially ruled out a primary preventive effect on lung cancer of a 5–8-y regimen of a 20-mg β-carotene supplement in smokers. The significance of this unexpected finding was heightened by the fact that the β-carotene group also experienced increased overall mortality (ie, by 8%), including an apparent increase in ischemic heart disease mortality. The interpretation of more than a decade's worth of research on the relation between β-carotene from vegetables and fruit and lung cancer was suddenly brought into question by these findings.

A similar result for β-carotene was subsequently reported by CARET, which halted its intervention of β-carotene (30 mg) and retinyl palmitate [25 000 IU (13 664 retinol equivalents)] after an observed increase in lung cancer incidence and total mortality in the supplemented group (20). This trial studied >18 000 men and women, of whom 388 developed lung cancer, with a 28% increase in lung cancer incidence in participants who received the β-carotene–retinyl palmitate combination daily for an average of 4 y compared with participants who received placebo. Increased total mortality (17%) was also observed in the supplemented group. Until these CARET results were announced and published in early 1996, the ATBC Study findings were viewed cautiously and, by some, with skepticism. Thereafter, the concordant data from the ATBC Study and CARET created a striking apparent contradiction to the previous observational epidemiology.

Some aspects of design and findings common to both the ATBC Study and CARET are the random assignment of persons at rather high risk for lung cancer because of cigarette smoking, asbestos exposure, or both; the very high serum concentrations of β-carotene achieved; and similar relative risk increases (though somewhat greater in CARET) for lung cancer incidence and total mortality. CARET differed from the ATBC Study in that it tested a β-carotene–

vitamin A combination and included women and both current and former smokers as well as a large group of workers exposed to asbestos.

One finding in both trials that has received less attention but is highly significant for the present purposes is that the trial participants with lower baseline β-carotene intake or β-carotene serum concentrations at baseline experienced higher lung cancer incidence during the study, independent of the intervention effects (19, 24, 25). This is consistent with the previously discussed observational epidemiologic studies. In the ATBC Study this was seen in the group not supplemented with β-carotene, with 15% and 33% higher lung cancer incidence rates in subjects in the lowest quartiles of β-carotene intake and serum β-carotene, respectively, compared with those in the highest quartiles (24). Thus, within this one study both the expected beneficial relation between dietary and serum β-carotene status and lung cancer risk and the apparently adverse effect of active supplementation with 20 mg/d were observed. Results from CARET corroborated this finding (25).

The fact that the relative risk estimates for the dietary and serum β-carotene associations are not as large as in many of the prior observational studies could be easily attributed to the greater homogeneity and higher baseline risk of the ATBC Study and CARET populations. The demonstration of these protective associations, along with other established etiologic associations with lung cancer, such as risk increasing with age, number of cigarettes smoked daily, years and pack-years of cigarette smoking, degree of inhalation, and occupational asbestos exposure, added to both the validity and the generalizability of the studies' findings. It also brought to bear the question of how and why the apparently contradictory results occurred (discussed below).

In contrast with the findings from the ATBC Study and CARET, the Physicians' Health Study of 22 000 male, primarily nonsmoking physicians in the United States showed no effective difference in lung cancer incidence after 12 y of supplementation between the β-carotene group (50 mg on alternate days) and placebo group (23). This was based, however, on only 66 and 71 cases in the 2 groups, respectively, and represented a nonsignificant 7% reduction. No adverse or beneficial effects were observed in the β-carotene group, even in the small number of smoking participants (11%).

Nutrition intervention trials in the general population of Linxian, China, investigated the effects of selected micronutrients on the incidence of esophageal cancer and total mortality in nearly 30 000 men and women (primarily nonsmokers) (21). This is the only large population trial to have shown preventive effects (ie, for stomach cancer and total mortality) of a combined supplement of β-carotene, α-tocopherol, and selenium. As subsequently reported (22), there were only 31 lung cancer deaths among the 792 total cancer deaths, with slightly fewer in the group that received the supplemental β-carotene combination (11 compared with 20 deaths). Because of the nature of the combination micronutrient supplement, intervention effects from this trial could not be attributed to any 1 of the 3 agents with certainty.

In total, these trials provide solid evidence for a relatively small adverse effect of β-carotene supplementation on lung cancer in cigarette smokers. For the purposes of the present discussion, it is important to note that such an effect was detectable because of the large size and controlled experimental design of these studies, which minimized or eliminated confounding factors. Had these studies not been conducted, the observational research would likely have continued to be interpreted in favor of β-carotene being the sole beneficial substance, and the potential downside for higher-dose supplementation may never have been observed or considered possible. Investigation of the trial findings is currently underway globally and will likely lead to a greater understanding of both the role of carotenoids in human health and of carcinogenesis itself.

Although discussion of the possible biological mechanisms behind the observed adverse effects of supplemental β-carotene is beyond the scope of this article, insofar as they have potential relevance to any recommendations regarding β-carotene they are mentioned briefly. One issue in need of further investigation is whether such effects are limited to high-risk groups such as current smokers. For example, if it is corroborated through laboratory studies that such toxicity resulted from combining a high-dose β-carotene supplement with active cigarette smoking through a direct interaction between cigarette smoke and β-carotene in lung tissue, as has been discussed (26), this might suggest particular caution regarding β-carotene use by cigarette smokers. A similar logic could be used if the findings were explained by the combination of β-carotene and heavy alcohol consumption (24, 27). If the effect were dose related, then lower dosages might be considered for further study in certain populations. However, the striking lack of benefit in the Physicians' Health Study, with its primarily nonsmoking population and blood β-carotene concentrations less than half that of the ATBC Study or CARET, argues against a likely benefit in nonsmokers or from lower dosages.

Interpretation of Contradictory Study Results and Implications for Recommendations

Results from observational studies have indicated clearly that persons who report eating more vegetables and fruit, more foods rich in carotenoids, and more carotenoids and β-carotene in particular are less likely to develop lung cancer than those who eat fewer vegetables and fruit and less β-carotene. Some studies also showed that persons with higher blood β-carotene concentrations are at reduced risk for lung cancer compared with those with lower concentrations (14, 15). Recent data from some of the trials corroborate this by showing that regardless of their intervention assignment, study participants with higher intake and serum concentrations of β-carotene at baseline developed fewer subsequent lung cancers (24, 25).

From the standpoints of consistency in the literature, risk level, dose-response gradient, and temporal correctness, the reported observational associations with lung cancer are no doubt real. Indeed, the only plausible way the associations might not be real is if vegetable, fruit, and β-carotene intakes were strongly related to another truly protective (and unmeasured) exposure that is confounding their association with lung cancer; however, no such factor has yet been identified. Although some studies lacked sufficient control or adjustment for known potential confounding factors, such as smoking history, most involved adequate control.

The similarity of the associations for vegetables and fruit and β-carotene (and possibly other carotenoid) intake have been interpreted as being consistent with specific beneficial effects of this substance, the biological plausibility of which is supported by studies of several properties and functions of β-carotene, for example, antioxidation, inhibition of tumor initiation and promotion, and enhancement of immunity and cellular maturation. However, similar supportive functional research is also available for other substances found in vegetables and fruit, for example, folic acid (28) and ascorbic acid (29). Therefore, on the basis of this body of observational evidence, nutrition recommendations promoting vegetable and fruit consumption are warranted. This is strengthened by the fact that beneficial associations have also been recognized between such diets and other major chronic diseases, notably heart disease (30–33).

The trial intervention results, however, do not support the observed associations or a role for supplemental β-carotene in lung cancer prevention in the populations, dosages, and duration of supplementation tested, and they are, on the surface, at odds with the observational epidemiology. Taken together, the 4 large β-carotene trials having experimental data for >1400 lung cancer cases, and particularly the ATBC Study and the CARET, representing ≈1300 cases between them, make it highly unlikely that pharmacologic doses of supplemental β-carotene are beneficial in the prevention of most lung cancers and provide strong evidence for adverse effects (eg, increased tumor promotion or progression) in smokers. These studies raise the issue of interpretation of the cohort and case-control studies (eg, is it the β-carotene in the diet?) and have reopened the issue of the safety of β-carotene supplements, which had long been considered a nonissue. Their results require that some caution be exercised in recommendations concerning supplemental β-carotene and argue against changing related dietary recommendations in the direction of greater nutrient specificity at this time.

Additional research holds the key to providing us with a more complete understanding of these etiologic relations. In a sense, the trial results have by necessity returned the focus to observational epidemiologic studies and basic research. Observational epidemiology should again revisit carotenoids, foods, and related biochemical factors. Specifically, further evaluation of other carotenoids and phytochemicals, both in the diet and in serum, is clearly warranted because any one or more of these substances present in vegetables and fruit might be responsible for the inverse association with lung cancer. Initial studies of this kind include those of Le Marchand et al (34) and Ziegler et al (35), which further explored the role of other dietary carotenoids using newly available food-composition data. These studies identify protective associations not only for β-carotene, but for α-carotene and lutein, for example, while showing stronger relations for vegetable consumption per se. They also show that disentangling the component effects of the highly collinear dietary carotenoids is both challenging and possible.

Other investigations should further explore the issue of vegetable and fruit consumption compared with β-carotene and carotenoid intake or serology (or, where possible, both intake and serology) and evaluate associations for dietary and supplementary sources of the micronutrients. Depending on results from additional studies such as these, further testing of supplemental β-carotene (at lower dosages in lower-risk groups), other carotenoids, or other phytochemicals may be warranted once concerns about safety have been addressed. The testing of multiple nutrients, either as combinations or in factorials designs, affords the opportunity of looking at biologically based interactions and yields more information per study.

One other important issue must be considered. Any recommendation for or related to β-carotene—or for that matter any nutrient—must consider the potential effects on all important health outcomes. Each large supplementation trial has typically reported its intervention findings for most important events, such as cancer, cardiovascular disease, and total mortality. In this way, overall efficacy of β-carotene supplementation is evaluable. Although most observational (especially case-control) studies are endpoint specific, reference to the association between β-carotene and other important endpoints is also possible in cohort studies. For example, the Western Electric Study reported an inverse association between dietary carotene index and lung cancer mortality, especially in heavy smokers (36). A recent report from the study showed a similar inverse association between the carotene index and cardiovascular and overall mortality (37). Through more complete data such as these, the beneficial association between β-carotene and lung cancer can be weighed along with evidence regarding its effects on other outcomes, with more informed recommendations resulting.

Conclusions

The quantity and quality of the relevant studies, the degree of consistency among the data, the availability of a plausible mechanism or set of mechanisms, and, importantly, the beneficial (or lack of adverse) effect on other aspects of human health and disease are all highly relevant to the issue of nutrition recommendations. The case study of β-carotene and lung cancer strongly supports—if not mandates—the need for results from at least one, and preferably more, large, randomized intervention trial before the consideration of public health recommendations concerning micronutrient supplementation. Overwhelming and highly consistent observational data in favor of a beneficial association for β-carotene and carotenoids, although truly impressive, did not provide the entire picture. In the case of β-carotene and lung cancer, the trial results raised further questions that require the testing of specific hypotheses.

The β-carotene–lung cancer association is sufficient to affect recommendations only insofar as they support current guidelines concerning enhanced vegetable and fruit consumption. It is clear that persons who eat a relatively large quantity of vegetables and fruit have a substantially lower risk of developing lung cancer (12, 13), and they may experience less cardiovascular disease and delayed mortality as well. Although many available studies (14, 15) strongly implicate β-carotene and possibly other carotenoids as among the putative agents of benefit, certainty around this issue is lacking. Protective associations for greater consumption of vegetables and fruit have often been stronger than those for β-carotene (or total carotenoid) intake specifically, suggesting the possibility of an etiologic relation with lung cancer for something in such diets beyond one or a few of the micronutrients—that is, the whole being greater than the sum of its parts. Further, the supplementation trials suggest not only lack of benefit of β-carotene in lung cancer prevention, but possible harm in smokers from not only lung cancer but overall mortality as well.

Before changes are made to the current guidelines regarding foods, vegetables, and fruit, more definitive evidence is needed about specific micronutrients such as β-carotene. It is likely that neither the public nor the scientific community will be satisfied with recommendations concerned solely with foods and will remain curious about what in foods is responsible for the consistent protective association observed for cancer.

Notes

[a] From the Cancer Prevention Studies Branch, Division of Clinical Sciences, National Cancer Institute, Bethesda, MD.

[b] Address reprint requests to D Albanes, Cancer Prevention Studies Branch, Division of Clinical Sciences, National Cancer Institute, 6006 Executive Boulevard, Suite 321, Bethesda, MD, 20892-7058. E-mail: daa.nih.gov.

References

1. Kennedy E, Meyers L, Layden W. The 1995 dietary guidelines for Americans: an overview. J Am Diet Assoc 1996; 96:234–7.
2. National Research Council. Diet and health: implications for reducing chronic disease risk. Washington, DC:National Academy Press, 1989.
3. Heimendinger J, Van Duyn MA, Chapelsky D, Foerster S, Stables G. The National 5 A Day for Better Health Program: a large-scale nutrition intervention. J Public Health Manage Pract 1996; 2:27–35.
4. Sporn MB, Dunlop NM, Newton DL, Smith JM. Prevention of chemical carcinogenesis by vitamin A and its synthetic analogs (retinoids). Fed Proc 1976; 35:1332–8.
5. Mathews-Roth MM. Anti-tumor activity of β-carotene, canthaxanthine, and phytoene. Oncology 1982; 39:33–7.
6. Bendich A, Olson JA. Biological actions of carotenoids. FASEB J 1989; 3:1927–32.
7. Peto R, Doll R, Buckley JD, Sporn MB. Can dietary β-carotene materially reduce human cancer rates? Nature 1981; 290:201–8.
8. Moss AJ, Levy AS, Kim I, Park YK. Use of vitamin and mineral supplements in the United States: current users, types of products, and nutrients. Advance data no. 174. Hyattsville, MD: National Center for Health Statistics, 1989.
9. Siesinski MJ, Subar AF, Kahle LI. Trends in use of vitamin and mineral supplements in the United States: the 1987 and 1992 National Health Interview Surveys. J Am Diet Assoc 1995; 95:921–3.
10. Ziegler RG. A review of epidemiologic evidence that carotenoids reduce the risk of cancer. J Nutr 1989; 119:116–22.
11. Willett WC. Vitamin A and lung cancer. Nutr Rev 1990; 48:201–11.
12. Steinmetz KA, Potter JD. Vegetables, fruit, and cancer. I. Epidemiology. Cancer Causes Control 1991; 2:325–57.
13. Block G, Patterson B, Subar A. Fruit, vegetables, and cancer prevention: a review of the epidemiological evidence. Nutr Cancer 1992; 18:1–29.

14. van Poppel G, Goldbohm RA. Epidemiologic evidence for β-carotene and cancer prevention. Am J Clin Nutr 1995; 62(suppl):1393S–402S.
15. Ziegler RG, Mayne ST, Swanson CA. Nutrition and lung cancer. Cancer Causes Control 1996; 7:157–77.
16. Byers TE, Graham S, Hughey BP, Marshall JR, Swanson MK. Diet and lung cancer risk: findings from the Western New York Diet Study. Am J Epidemiol 1987; 125:351–63.
17. Menkes MS, Comstock GW, Vuilleumier JP, Helsing KJ, Rider AA, Brockmeyer R. Serum beta-carotene, vitamins A and E, selenium, and the risk of lung cancer. N Engl J Med 1986; 315:1250–4.
18. Knekt P, Jarvinen R, Seppanen R, et al. Dietary antioxidants and the risk of lung cancer. Am J Epidemiol 1991; 134:471–9.
19. Alpha-Tocopherol, Beta Carotene Cancer Prevention Study Group. The effect of vitamin E and beta carotene on the incidence of lung cancer and other cancers in male smokers. N Engl J Med 1994; 330:1029–35.
20. Omenn GS, Goodman GE, Thornquist, MD, et al. Effects of a combination of beta carotene and vitamin A on lung cancer and cardiovascular disease. N Engl J Med 1996; 334:1150–5.
21. Blot WJ, Li JY, Taylor PR, et al. Nutrition intervention trials in Linxian, China: supplementation with specific vitamin/mineral combinations, cancer incidence, and disease-specific mortality in the general population. J Natl Cancer Inst 1993; 85:1483–92.
22. Blot WJ, Li JY, Taylor PR, Li B. Lung cancer and vitamin supplementation. N Engl J Med 1994; 331:614 (letter).
23. Hennekens CH, Buring JE, Manson JE, et al. Lack of effect of long-term supplementation with beta carotene on the incidence of malignant neoplasms and cardiovascular disease. N Engl J Med 1996; 334:1145–9.
24. Albanes D, Heinonen OP, Taylor PR, et al. α-Tocopherol and β-carotene supplements and lung cancer incidence in the Alpha-Tocopherol, Beta-Carotene Cancer Prevention Study: effects of baseline characteristics and study compliance. J Natl Cancer Inst 1996; 88:1560–70.
25. Omenn GS, Goodman GE, Thornquist MD, et al. Risk factors for lung cancer incidence and intervention effects in CARET, the Beta-Carotene and Retinol Efficacy Trial. J Natl Cancer Inst 1996; 88:1550–9.
26. Mayne ST, Handelman GJ, Beecher G. β-Carotene and lung cancer promotion in heavy smokers—a plausible relationship? J Natl Cancer Inst 1996; 88:1513–5.
27. Leo MA, Lieber CS. Lung cancer and vitamin supplementation. N Engl J Med 1994; 331:612 (letter).
28. Glynn SA, Albanes D. Folate and cancer: a review of the literature. Nutr Cancer 1994; 22:101–19.
29. Bendich A, Machlin, LJ, Scandurra O, et al. The antioxidant role of vitamin C. Adv Free Radic Biol Med 1986; 2:419–44.
30. Gey KF, Stahelin HB, Eichholzer M. Poor plasma status of carotene and vitamin C is associated with higher mortality from ischemic heart disease and stroke: Basel Prospective Study. Clin Invest 1993; 71:3–6.
31. Knekt P, Reunanen A, Jarvinen R, Seppanen R, Heliovaara M, Aromaa A. Antioxidant vitamin intake and coronary mortality in a longitudinal population study. Am J Epidemiol 1994; 139:1180–9.
32. Morris DL, Kritchevsky DL, Davis CE. Serum carotenoids and coronary heart disease—the Lipid Research Clinics Coronary Primary Prevention Trial and Follow-Up Study. JAMA 1994; 272:1439–41.
33. Gaziano JM, Hennekens CH. Antioxidant vitamins in the prevention of coronary artery disease. Contemp Intern Med 1995; 7:9–14.
34. Le Marchand L, Hankin JH, Kolonel LN, Beecher GR, Wilkens LR, Zhao LP. Intake of specific carotenoids and lung cancer risk. Cancer Epidemiol Biomarkers Prev 1993; 2:183–7.

35. Ziegler RG, Colavito EA, Hartge P, et al. Importance of α-carotene, β-carotene, and other phytochemicals in the etiology of lung cancer risk. J Natl Cancer Inst 1996; 88:612–5.
36. Shekelle RB, Lepper M, Liu S, et al. Dietary vitamin A and risk of cancer in the Western Electric Study. Lancet 1981; 2:1185–90.
37. Pandey DK, Shekelle R, Selwyn BJ, Tangney C, Stamler J. Dietary vitamin C and β-carotene and risk of death in middle-age men. The Western Electric Study. Am J Epidemiol 1995; 142:1269–78.

POSTSCRIPT

Can Vitamin and Mineral Supplements Help Prevent Chronic Disease?

Fletcher and Fairfield promote use of vitamin supplements as an inexpensive form of nutritional insurance. On this basis, multivitamin pills that contain no more than recommended levels of constituent nutrients are unlikely to be harmful—and might do some good. But do the β-carotene trials suggest otherwise? Or do they merely reflect an isolated example in which smokers at high risk for lung cancer do worse with supplementation?

Dr. Walter C. Willett, in his book *Eat, Drink, and Be Healthy* (Simon & Schuster, 2001), recommends taking a multiple vitamin for nutritional insurance along with eating more fruits and vegetables (except potatoes). Supplement industry scientists argue even more forcefully that such products have the potential to do much good and that they do no harm when taken appropriately. In a 2001 review of research on the health effects of dietary supplements, Annette Dickenson, of the Council for Responsible Nutrition, a supplement trade association, noted that many researchers and scientists support the benefits of this approach (see http://www.fdli.org/pubs/Update/2001/Issue6/Dickinson/article.html).

Vast numbers of Americans take nutrient supplements in the belief that the pills confer benefits and are not harmful. Although many people feel better when they take supplements, it is difficult to know whether they do so because of a genuine physiological change or because they are experiencing a placebo effect and simply feel better because they are taking something, whether or not it has a physiological effect. Scientists are just beginning to address this issue. A recent randomized, double-blind, placebo-controlled trial demonstrated that older adults with type 2 diabetes who took a multivitamin and mineral supplement for one year were less likely to have an infectious illness than those taking placebos (Barringer et al., *Annals of Internal Medicine*, March 4, 2003). Such results need to be replicated in the general population before concluding that taking a multivitamin and mineral supplement reduces risk of chronic disease. Without carefully controlled clinical trials such as those conducted for β-carotene and lung cancer, it is difficult to know how to evaluate claims for protective effects of supplements against chronic disease. Resolving this debate may require much more research, and such research is exceedingly expensive. One way to approach the problem might be to suggest caution in taking supplements of single nutrients, especially in large amounts. For people who do want to take supplements, a one-a-day multivitamin is unlikely to be harmful and may sometimes help. A better way to resolve this debate might be to use the uncertainties as a basis for much more vigorous promotion of dietary choices that we know are effective: eating more fruits and vegetables.

ISSUE 11

Will Taking Herbal Supplements Enhance Mental Ability?

YES: Pierre L. Le Bars et al., from "A Placebo-Controlled, Double-Blind, Randomized Trial of an Extract of Ginkgo Biloba for Dementia," *Journal of the American Medical Association* (October 22/29, 1997)

NO: Paul R. Solomon et al., from "Ginkgo for Memory Enhancement: A Randomized Controlled Trial," *Journal of the American Medical Association* (August 21, 2002)

ISSUE SUMMARY

YES: Researcher Pierre L. Le Bars and his colleagues say that supplements of ginkgo biloba improve the cognitive and social functioning of people with Alzheimer's or other types of dementia.

NO: Researcher Paul R. Solomon and his colleagues say that ginkgo biloba has no beneficial effect on memory or cognitive function in healthy older adults.

Vitamins have well-defined functions in human physiology, and much research has focused on the health effects of taking them as dietary supplements. The effects of herbal supplements, however, are quite another matter. More than 1,500 herbal and botanical products are available as supplements in the United States. Although these products have been used for thousands of years in Chinese traditional medicine, remarkably little is known about their chemical composition or mechanism of action, and only a few have been subjected to testing in controlled clinical trials.

Despite this lack of scientific information, there might be good reasons to consider herbal supplements as a means of self-treatment. They may help people with health problems that cannot be treated successfully with conventional medicines, even if some of the benefit derives simply from placebo or other self-healing effects. Some people feel better when they take herbal supplements. Unfortunately, the makers of these products have little incentive to test them. Such research is difficult and expensive. Unless the product can be patented, which traditional herbs cannot, companies are likely to have difficulty recovering the costs of clinical trials through increased sales. Without such research, however, it is difficult to determine whether or not an herbal supplement really does improve health.

The studies here are among the few to examine whether or not herbal supplements produce scientifically measurable health benefits. Although they come to opposite conclusions, both are randomized, placebo-controlled, double-blind clinical trials. This means that investigators selected the trial subjects who would receive a supplement by a prearranged scheme (*randomization*), gave half the subjects the supplement and the other half a placebo (*placebo-controlled*), and coded the pills and study records so that neither the investigators nor the subjects knew who was taking the supplement or the placebo (*double-blind*). These precautions ensured that the trials could be conducted in as unbiased a manner as possible. Why might *not* following such precautions cause the results to be biased.

Pierre L. LeBars et al. based their work on reports from European investigators that symptoms of dementia improved among patients who took extracts of leaves of the ginkgo biloba tree. They tested the association between ginkgo and dementia by giving either supplements or placebos to demented patients in a well-controlled clinical trial that lasted 52 weeks. The results of this study revealed small but statistically significant improvements in mental performance among the group taking the ginkgo supplements. In contrast, Paul R. Solomon et al., in an equally well-controlled study lasting six weeks, found gingko supplements to have no effect whatsoever on learning and memory in older adults who were not demented.

The differences in outcome among the supplement and placebo groups in both studies were small, and investigators relied on statistical tests to decide whether differences—or the lack of differences—could have occurred by chance. Solomon et al. computed 95 percent confidence intervals (CIs) for statistical tests of differences between the groups. From a statistical standpoint, any value within the range of the 95 percent CI has a good probability of being the correct number 95 out of every 100 times the value is computed, meaning that it has a high probability of being meaningful. In statistical terms, if the range of the CI includes zero (for example, −0.2 to 0.8), any observed difference between the supplement and placebo groups could be due entirely to chance. Although the score given for the supplement group on the Stroop Test, for example, is between 1 and 2 (suggesting that those who took supplements had better mental function than those who took the placebo), the CI ranges from minus 1 (meaning that the placebo group did better) to plus 3 (meaning that the supplement group did much better). Because the CI includes zero, the results could have occurred by chance. This means that there is no statistically significant difference in mental function between the group taking supplements or the group taking placebos.

In reading these studies, it is useful to note the differences in study populations, the type of supplement, the length of the study, and the technical level of writing. Do these differences matter in interpreting the study results? LeBars et al. say gingko supplements benefit cognitive function; Solomon et al. say they do not.

Pierre L. Le Bars et al.

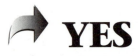 **YES**

A Placebo-Controlled, Double-Blind, Randomized Trial of an Extract of Ginkgo Biloba for Dementia

The extract of Ginkgo biloba referred to as EGb 761 is one of the most popular plant extracts used in Europe to alleviate symptoms associated with a range of cognitive disorders. It has recently been approved in Germany for the treatment of dementia. The mechanism of action of EGb in the central nervous system is only partially understood, but the main effects seem to be related to its antioxidant properties, which require the synergistic action of the flavonoids, the terpenoids (ginkgolides, bilobalide), and the organic acids, principal constituents of EGb. These compounds to varying degrees act as scavengers for free radicals, which have been considered the mediators of the excessive lipid peroxidation and cell damage observed in Alzheimer disease (AD). Although several European studies report positive results of EGb 761 in the treatment of diverse neurological disorders, few studies using standard methods have evaluated the cognitive and behavioral effects of EGb in dementia. Further, no empirical clinical trials of the extract have been conducted in the United States. Therefore, this multicenter placebo-controlled study was undertaken to assess the efficacy and safety of EGb in AD and multi-infarct dementia (MID).

Methods

Patient Population

Patients of both sexes, 45 years of age or older, with a diagnosis of uncomplicated dementia according to *Diagnostic and Statistical Manual of Mental Disorders, Third Edition, Revised (DSM-III-R)* and *International Statistical Classification of Diseases, 10th Revision (ICD-10)* criteria, either Alzheimer type (AD) or MID, were enrolled in the study. The severity of the dementia at screening was mild to moderately severe as assessed by a Mini-Mental State Examination score of 9 to 26 (inclusive) and a Global Deterioration Scale score of 3 to 6 (inclusive). To be eligible, patients had to have no other significant medical conditions includ-

From Pierre L. Le Bars, Martin M. Katz, Nancy Berman, Turan M. Itil, Alfred M. Freedman, and Alan F. Schatzberg, "A Placebo-Controlled, Double-Blind, Randomized Trial of an Extract of Ginkgo Biloba for Dementia," *Journal of the American Medical Association*, vol. 278, no. 16 (October 22/29, 1997), pp. 1327–1332. Copyright © 1997 by The American Medical Association. Reprinted by permission. References omitted.

ing cardiac disease, insulin-dependent diabetes, liver disease, chronic renal insufficiency, or another psychiatric disorder as a primary diagnosis. Patients with brain mass or intracranial hemorrhage determined by computed tomography or magnetic resonance imaging were excluded.

The use of medications for preexisting conditions was not discontinued at screening, but change in regimen or prescription of new concomitant medications known to affect cognitive function was not permitted during the study. Noncompliance was monitored by pill counts and defined by a deviation of more than 20% from the study regimen.

The study protocol and the informed consent forms were approved by the institutional review boards of the Massachusetts Mental Health Center of Harvard Medical School, Boston, and New York Institute for Medical Research, Tarrytown. Written informed consent was obtained from the patients or their legal representatives and from the caregivers.

Study Design

The study used a 52-week, double-blind, fixed-dose, placebo-controlled, parallel-group randomized design and was conducted at 6 research centers in the United States. Patients underwent a 14-day single-blind placebo run-in period. Safety assessments (adverse events and vital signs), pill counts, and drug dispensation were performed at 4-, 12-, 26-, 39-, and 52-week visits. Complete assessments of primary outcome measures were required at baseline and at 12, 26, and 52 weeks. At screening and at termination, extensive medical, neurological, and psychiatric evaluations were performed, including electroencephalogram [test of brain activity] and laboratory tests. . . . EGb . . . was supplied as a 40-mg tablet to be swallowed before each of the 3 principal daily meals, for a total daily dose of 120 mg. Patients were consecutively assigned to EGb or to placebo following a predetermined order based on separate randomization schedules for each center using balanced blocks of 10 patients. Consecutive numbers were printed on each drug study pack, and randomization codes, stored in sealed envelopes, were exclusively retained by International Drug Development Corporation independently from sponsor and investigating centers.

The EGb and the matched placebo tablets did not differ in their appearance and were film coated to ensure a similar smell and taste. EGb had the identical formulation and chemical composition as the product used in Germany. . . . The study drugs were made by a standard method and came from the same batch of Ginkgo extract. EGb is a standardized concentrated extract from the dried leaves of the Ginkgo biloba tree, specially produced by means of a multiple-step extraction procedure and consisting of 24% Ginkgo-flavoneglycosides and 6% terpenelactones (3.1% ginkgolides A, B, and C, 2.9% bilobalide).

Outcome Measures

The primary outcome measures assessed changes in 3 areas: (1) *Cognitive impairment* was assessed by the cognitive subscale of the Alzheimer's Disease Assessment Scale (ADAS-Cog), a performance-based cognitive test that objectively evaluates memory, language, praxis, and orientation. The test includes 11 items with a total score ranging from 0 to 70; the higher the score, the poorer the performance. (2) *Daily living and social behavior* was assessed by the total score of the Geriatric Evaluation by Relative's Rating Instrument (GERRI), a 49-item rating inventory completed by the caregiver. The total score is the grand mean of the following 3 subscale means: the GERRI-cognitive (21 items), the GERRI-social (18 items), and the GERRI-mood (10 items). The scores of each item, thus, of each subscale and of the grand mean, range from 1 to 5; the higher the score, the poorer the patient's functioning in the home environment. The questions are presented in an identical checklist at each visit and are answered by the caregiver who evaluates the patient's functioning during the 14 days prior to the assessment. The GERRI total score was found to be highly correlated with the overall symptom severity of the dementia, as assessed by the Global Deterioration Scale. However, longitudinal studies of annual GERRI change scores are few and its validity in this respect has yet to be rigorously tested. (3) *General psychopathology*, the changes in overall psychopathology, was assessed by the Clinical Global Impression of Change (CGIC), an interview-based global rating that quantifies the clinician's judgment of the amount of change in overall impairment compared with that at the study baseline. The CGIC does not follow a structured interview and uses a 7-point ordinal scale in which 1 is an extreme score indicating that the patient improved very much, and 7 indicates extreme worsening. . . .

Each subject was to complete 52 weeks, but if at any time a subject showed worsening of functioning or impairment, as assessed by an increase of 1 point on the CGIC, the subject could be dropped from the study and offered admission to an uncontrolled open-label humanitarian protocol. However, the investigator was encouraged to maintain the patient in the double-blind phase for at least 6 months. . . . An analysis of efficacy on an intent-to-treat (ITT) basis . . . was selected a posteriori as the primary analysis for efficacy. . . .

Results

Patient disposition during the study is summarized in Figure 1. . . . The pattern of change in group sizes during the treatment period was similar to that in the total population.

Patient characteristics at baseline were similar between treatment groups. . . .

Efficacy Analysis and ITT Analysis

. . . Although a similar ratio of subjects withdrew from each treatment group before 26 weeks (33/155 for the EGb group and 33/154 for the placebo group), 28% (44/155) of the EGb group vs. 40% (62/154) of the placebo group dropped out between 26 and 52 weeks. Consequently, 50% (78/155) of the EGb group completed the entire study compared with only 38% (59/154) of the placebo group. . . .

Figure 1

Profile of the Randomized Controlled Trial

No. of Patients Screened		549
No. of Patients Not Eligible		222
No. of Patients Randomized		327

	EGb	Placebo
Randomization	166	161
Did Not Receive Standard		
Intervention as Allocated	9	6
Excluded From Analysis	2	1
Follow Up		
4-wk Visit	155	154
12-wk Visit	142	141
26-wk Visit	122	122
39-wk Visit	93	75
52-wk Visit	78	59
Withdrawn (After Baseline)		
Intervention Ineffective	12	21
Caregiver Request	24	29
Unavailable for Follow-up	8	10
Adverse Event	10	4
Death	2	1
Concurrent Illness	4	5
Noncompliance With Protocol	13	14
Other	15	18
Completed Trial	78	59

Three patients were excluded from analysis because of protocol violations (2 because of diabetes mellitus and 1 because of unstable affective mood disorder).

Regarding the ADAS-Cog, there was no significant change observed at end point for the EGb group, whereas the placebo group showed a significant worsening of 1.5 points. . . . Considering the GERRI, mild improvement was observed for the EGb group, whereas the placebo group showed significant worsening, . . . resulting in a statistically significant difference in favor of EGb. . . . These results are depicted graphically in Figure 2. Regarding global psychopathology, a slight worsening was observed for both treatment groups on the CGIC, . . . as assessed by a deviation of 0.2 points of the rating mean (59% [183/309] of the total population were considered unchanged).

Figure 2

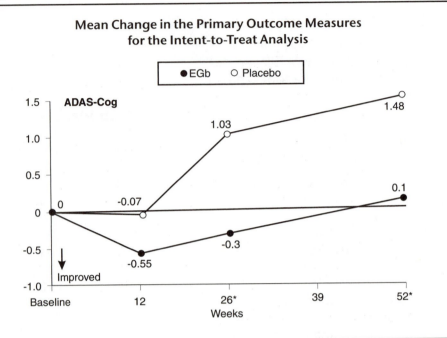

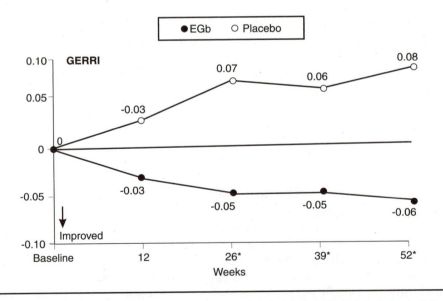

Results of Alzheimer's Disease Assessment Scale–Cognitive subscale (ADAS-Cog) and Geriatric Evaluation by Relative's Rating Instrument (GERRI) at 12-, 26-, 39-, and 52-week end points with last observation carried forward. Statistically significant differences between treatment groups are [noted with an asterisk].

When the AD subgroup was examined separately, a similar pattern of results was demonstrated across the 2 treatments. . . .

Evaluable Population

At the 26-week time point, a slight improvement was observed in the EGb group on the ADAS-Cog while the placebo group showed a significant worsening of 1.4 points. . . . The mean treatment difference was in favor of EGb ($P = .04$). On the GERRI, the EGb group showed a mean improvement (0.07 points) and the placebo group worsened by the same amount, resulting in a statistically significant treatment difference. . . .

For the evaluable 52-week end point analysis, the average timing of the end point was 46.6 weeks . . . for the EGb group and 42.3 weeks . . . for the placebo group. The difference of 4 weeks between these 2 end points followed the same pattern observed in the ITT analysis: in the EGb group, 71% (69/97) of the patients reaching 26 weeks completed the whole study compared with 51% (54/105) in the placebo group. The outcomes of the 52-week end point analysis . . . [showed] a slight improvement for the EGb group on the ADAS-Cog, while the placebo group showed continued worsening, with an increased score from 1.4 at 26 weeks to 2.1 points at end point. . . . The mean treatment difference of −2.4 points further favored the EGb group. . . . The same course of changes were observed with the care-giver assessment. The EGb group showed significant improvement . . . while the placebo counterpart deteriorated, . . . resulting in a statistically significant difference of −0.19 points for the GERRI change score. . . .

Categorical Analysis of Positive and Negative Outcomes

To compare the number of patients showing positive or negative clinical outcomes within each treatment arm of the evaluable data set, a cumulative logit analysis was conducted using the 52-week end point on the ADAS-Cog and the GERRI classification codes. . . . EGb shows a higher percentage of "improvers," while the placebo shows more "decliners," leading to highly significant differences on each assessment measure. On the ADAS-Cog, 50% of the EGb patients showed an improvement by at least 2 points compared with 29% of the placebo group; this approximately 2-fold difference was still observed when the threshold to detect an improvement in cognition was set at 4 ADAS-Cog points. On the GERRI, 37% of the EGb group were considered improved and only 19% were considered worse; the placebo group demonstrated the opposite trend with 40% worsening and 23% improving.

Safety

Five serious adverse events were reported during the study: 3 deaths (1 in the placebo group and 2 in the EGb group) due to acute intercurrent conditions not related to the study medication, and 1 stroke and 1 subdural hematoma [collection of blood under the outer membrane of the brain] (both in the placebo group) related to worsening of preexisting condition. Thirty percent (49/166) of the patients in the EGb group reported at least 1 adverse event compared with

31% (50/161) in the placebo group. . . . The adverse events . . . were equally distributed between the 2 treatment groups with the exception of the gastrointestinal tract signs and symptoms being attributed slightly more often to EGb (18 of 29 events).

Comment

This study compared the effects of EGb with a placebo in a multicenter sample of demented patients with mild to moderately severe cognitive impairment. The results . . . demonstrated the efficacy of EGb on 2 of 3 primary outcome measures: cognitive impairment and daily living and social behavior. Although the treatment effect could not be detected by the clinician's global impression of change (CGIC), it was demonstrated through objective tests of cognitive performance (ADAS-Cog) and was of sufficient magnitude for the caregiver to recognize it in the patient's behavior (GERRI).

A concern in interpreting the study outcomes, however, relates to the substantial number of patients who withdrew after the 26-week visit. To reduce the potential bias due to the attrition of the randomization sample, the efficacy analysis was primarily based on ITT methodology. The ITT analysis, however carries its own limitation. Dementia is inherently a deteriorating disease. By replacing missing data at end point with carried-forward values obtained early in the trial, the magnitude of the natural deterioration is underestimated; furthermore, different elapsed times in the study will tend to influence the effect size and possibly favor the group with the earliest end point. In the present sample, the EGb group included 50% of patients reaching the 52-week visit compared with only 38% of patients in the placebo group. Moreover, the average time of the end point occurred slightly earlier (4 weeks) for the placebo group. Despite these differences, apparently favorable to the placebo group, the ITT analysis showed that the EGb group maintained its baseline status (ADAS-Cog) or even improved slightly (GERRI), whereas both cognitive and social functioning worsened over time in the placebo group. These differences were observed even though 11% of the patients in the EGb group were not compliant with the drug regimen and 10% were treated with EGb for less than 12 weeks. The ITT and evaluable analyses showed EGb to be more effective, but these analyses do not completely resolve the uncertainty of the effects that may arise from nonrandom dropouts.

Of the 3 outcome measures, the CGIC failed to demonstrate a significant difference in the efficacy of the 2 treatments. Several factors may have contributed to this. First, the treatment effects may not have been large enough to allow a discrimination from placebo. Second, the CGIC appears to have low sensitivity for measurement of change in dementia over the long term. It asks the clinician to quantify the amount of change in the patient's condition compared with baseline. However, it is not a structured instrument nor is it guided by anchored criteria. Thus, its reliability suffers as the interval between the follow-up visit and the baseline evaluation increases, particularly if relevant information is not systematically elicited at each follow-up visit. . . .

The failure to find differences using the CGIC, however, raised the question of whether the improvements in cognition and social behavior in the EGb group, although statistically significant, were sufficiently large to be "clinically meaningful." In this respect, the . . . analysis of the proportions of patients whose performance improved or worsened reflects more closely how the treatment effects are manifested clinically. In clinical terms, improvement on the ADAS-Cog of 4 points may be equivalent to a 6-month delay in the progression of the disease. In this study, it is noteworthy that 29% of the patients with AD treated with EGb for at least 26 weeks improved by 4 or more points compared with 13% treated with the placebo. These ratios compare favorably with those obtained in a study of an evaluable group of patients with AD receiving a 30-week "high-dose" (160-mg) regimen of tacrine (40% of the tacrine group improved by at least 4 points vs. 25% of the placebo group).

The present trial, however, does not permit conclusions regarding sustained benefits, particularly if drug treatment is subsequently interrupted. In addition, this study tested a single EGb dose. It does not address whether the proportion of treatment responders will increase with higher dosages, as indicated by previous pilot studies, or will remain the same but with an increase of the treatment effect. The latter finding would be more in accordance with the results obtained with 240 mg of EGb in a recent controlled trial in dementia. Additional study testing multiple EGb dosages and applying a design that would distinguish a temporary stemming of the symptoms from a change in the course of the disease would be necessary to explore these important aspects.

. . . [P]ersons with MID as defined by *DSM-III-R* criteria appear to be a heterogeneous group. . . . [T]he results of the AD subgroup have been presented since its criteria have high reliability and it represented the majority of the study sample. However, the present findings should be considered within the limits of our study population. The number of mildly impaired vs. moderately and severely impaired patients may not be representative of the AD population at large. A sizable number of mild cases may have contributed to the fairly modest changes that were observed at end point. For example, the placebo group showed only a 1.5-point worsening on the ADAS-Cog score after an average elapsed time of 35 weeks, compared with 2.0- to 2.5-point changes observed with placebo groups of previous studies. A pervasive learning effect also could be suspected in view of the relatively high percentage of improvers in the placebo group. Nevertheless, considering that the baseline characteristics of the 2 treatment groups are similar and that there is no significant interaction between severity of impairment and treatment, EGb appears to stabilize and, in an additional 20% of cases (vs. placebo), improve the patient's functioning for periods of 6 months to 1 year. Regarding its safety, adverse events associated with EGb were no different from those associated with placebo.

The EGb extract contains multiple compounds that are thought to act synergistically on diverse processes involved in the homeostasis of inflammation and oxidative stress, providing membrane protection and, neurotransmission modulation, which may be the basis for EGb effects at the central nervous system. However, further research is needed to elucidate the precise mechanism of action of EGb, to fully explore the therapeutic potential of this plant extract, and to help better understand the pathogenesis of dementia.

Paul R. Solomon et al.

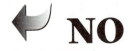

Ginkgo for Memory Enhancement: A Randomized Controlled Trial

Some over-the-counter treatments are marketed as having the ability to improve memory, attention, and related cognitive functions. These claims are generally not supported by well-controlled clinical studies. Ginkoba claims to "enhance mental focus and improve memory and concentration." Several published studies reported beneficial effects of ginkgo on cognition. These studies, however, either report cognitive improvement in only 1 of many memory tests administered or report cognitive enhancement in cognitively impaired clinical populations such as patients with cerebrovascular or Alzheimer disease. In contrast, advertising claims imply that the compound is broadly beneficial to those both with and without clinically significant cognitive impairments. Specific advertising claims cite more than 50 clinical trials that demonstrate benefit centered around concentration and memory. These studies were conducted for periods ranging from 14 days to 2 months. The manufacturer claims benefit with "at least 4 weeks of uninterrupted use."

The purpose of the present study was to evaluate ginkgo in healthy elderly volunteers in a randomized, double-blind, placebo-controlled trial using standardized tests of memory, learning, attention and concentration, and expressive language as well as subjective ratings by participants and family.

Methods

Participants

Following approval by the Williams College institutional review board, participants were recruited from newspaper advertisements that solicited individuals who would participate in a study designed to improve memory. An initial telephone interview was conducted to determine if the participant was likely to meet entry criteria for the study. Those who passed the screen provided informed consent and a medical history including current medications, neurologic or psychiatric illness, and incidence of head trauma, stroke, mental

From Paul R. Solomon, Felicity Adams, Amanda Silver, Jill Zinner, and Richard DeVeaux, "Ginkgo for Memory Enhancement: A Randomized Controlled Trial," *Journal of the American Medical Association,* vol. 288, no. 7 (August 21, 2002), pp. 835–840. Copyright © 2002 by The American Medical Association. Reprinted by permission. References omitted.

illness, mental retardation, or life-threatening illness over the last 5 years. Participants were included in the study if they were community dwelling, older than 60 years, and could provide informed consent. They also needed to have a companion who had contact with them on a regular basis (>4 times per week for ≥1 hour) and was willing to complete a questionnaire. The baseline Mini-Mental State Examination score was required to be greater than 26. All participants reported to be independent in instrumental activities of daily living including shopping, transportation, and managing finances. Participants were excluded if they had a history of psychiatric or neurologic disorder or had a life-threatening illness in the last 5 years. They were also excluded if they had taken antidepressant or other psychoactive medications in the past 60 days. A total of 338 community-dwelling participants were screened over a 26-month period from July 1996 to September 1998, and 230 participants (98 men and 132 women) aged 60 to 82 years were randomized in the study.

Study Design

A 6-week double-blind placebo-controlled study was conducted at a single site. FIGURE 1 summarizes the study participation. Participants were randomly assigned to 1 of 2 conditions: ginkgo (Ginkoba, Boehringer Ingelheim Pharmaceuticals) or placebo control (1:1 ratio). Random assignment of participants to each condition was determined by 1 of the investigators (P.R.S.) using a table of random numbers. Medication was placed in sealed envelopes by a research assistant and provided to the participants by 1 of 3 other investigators (F.A., A.S., J.Z.). Dosages for ginkgo were determined by following the manufacturer's label instructions: 1 tablet (40 mg) 3 times a day, with meals. The placebo group took lactose gelatin capsules of similar appearance and on the same schedule as the ginkgo group. At the beginning of the double-blind period, participants were provided with sealed and dated envelopes, each containing medication for 1 day.

One day prior to taking ginkgo or placebo and again at the end of the 6-week double-blind period (while still taking ginkgo and within 3 days of the end of the study), participants underwent neuropsychological evaluation including tests of learning, memory, attention and concentration, and expressive language. They also completed a questionnaire regarding subjective impressions of their memory. Additionally, at the end of the 6 weeks of treatment, the companion was asked to complete a global questionnaire designed to provide an overall impression of change in memory for the participant. Evaluators (F.A., A.S., J.Z.) were blinded to which randomized treatment the participants received.

Participants were contacted by telephone twice (at the end of weeks 2 and 4) during the 6-week period to evaluate compliance. They were excluded from the study if they missed 6 doses in any 2-week period or did not take 3 consecutive doses. At this time, they were asked to stop taking study medication. As an additional measure of compliance, participants were asked to return all dated envelopes at the end of the study.

Figure 1

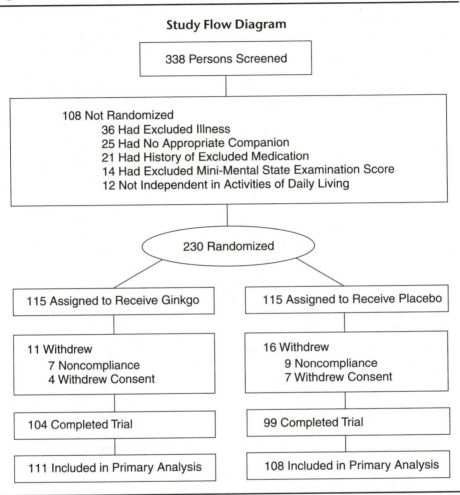

Study Flow Diagram

338 Persons Screened

108 Not Randomized
  36 Had Excluded Illness
  25 Had No Appropriate Companion
  21 Had History of Excluded Medication
  14 Had Excluded Mini-Mental State Examination Score
  12 Not Independent in Activities of Daily Living

230 Randomized

115 Assigned to Receive Ginkgo

115 Assigned to Receive Placebo

11 Withdrew
  7 Noncompliance
  4 Withdrew Consent

16 Withdrew
  9 Noncompliance
  7 Withdrew Consent

104 Completed Trial

99 Completed Trial

111 Included in Primary Analysis

108 Included in Primary Analysis

Outcome Measures

Outcome measures consisted of the following standardized tests of learning, memory, attention and concentration, expressive language, and mental status. Tests of learning and memory included the California Verbal Learning Test (CVLT), in which the participant is asked to learn a 16-item shopping list over 5 trials and then to later recall and subsequently recognize the information; the Logical Memory sub-scale of the Wechsler Memory Scale–Revised (WMS-R), in which the participant is asked to recall paragraphs both immediately after hearing them and then after a 30-minute delay; and the Visual Reproduction sub-scale, in which the participant is asked to draw designs both immediately after seeing them and after a 30-minute delay.

Tests of attention and concentration included the Digit Symbol subscale of the Wechsler Adult Intelligence Scale–Revised (WAIS-R), in which the participant must rapidly copy symbols that are paired with numbers; the Stroop Test, which requires the participant not to be distracted by extraneous aspects of stimuli; the Digit Span (WMS-R), which requires the participant to repeat increasingly longer strings of numbers immediately after hearing them; and Mental Control (WMS-R), in which the participant must recite strings of numbers and letters.

Tests of expressive language included the Controlled Category Fluency test, which requires the participant to name members of a particular category (animals) over a 1-minute period; and the Boston Naming Test, which requires the participant to name pictures of items.

Additionally, the Memory Questionnaire as well as a global evaluation completed by a spouse, relative, or friend with whom the patient had regular contact (at least 4 interactions per week) was completed. The Memory Questionnaire consisted of 27 questions that asked the participant to rate how often certain memory lapses occurred. The participant answered on a 4-point scale with descriptors used as anchors: 1 indicating very often, 2 indicating sometimes, 3 indicating rarely, and 4 indicating not at all, The global evaluation was based on the Caregiver Global Impression of Change rating scale. Informants were asked to indicate the option that best described the change in memory over the preceding 6 weeks. The options included: (1) very much improved, (2) much improved, (3) minimally improved, (4) no change, (5) minimally worse, (6) much worse, or (7) very much worse.

All outcome measures, with the exception of the global evaluation, were administered at both the beginning and end of the study. The global evaluation was administered only at the end of the study. Participants who withdrew from the study, or who were dropped because of noncompliance, were asked to return at the end of the study for evaluation. Adverse events were not specifically monitored in this study. Patients who experienced an adverse event were instructed to discontinue study medication and to contact their primary care physician. . . .

Results

A total of 230 participants were enrolled in the study over a 26-month period, with 203 participants (88%) completing the study (Figure 1). The percentage of participants who completed the study did not differ significantly by treatment group. Of the 27 participants who did not complete the study, 16 (7 ginkgo and 9 placebo) did not comply with the medication dosage regimen and 11 (4 ginkgo and 7 placebo) withdrew consent. All participants were requested to return at the end of week 6 for evaluation.

Modified Intent-to-Treat Analysis

A total of 219 participants (111 ginkgo and 108 placebo) returned at the end of the 6-week period for reevaluation. This included the 203 participants who completed the protocol as well as 13 of 16 participants (6 ginkgo and 7 placebo) who were noncompliant and 3 of the 11 participants (2 ginkgo and 1 placebo) who withdrew consent. The remaining 11 participants (4 ginkgo and 7 placebo) did not return for evaluation and were excluded from the analysis. There were no significant differences between the ginkgo and placebo groups for any of the outcome measures. Neither demographic characteristics nor Mini-Mental State Examination scores varied as a function of treatment condition at baseline.

There were no significant differences between the ginkgo and placebo groups on any of the objective neuropsychological tests. In general, participants performed better during their second evaluation than during their first, but there were no significant test-by-treatment condition interactions as tested by a repeated-measures analysis of variance. . . . Superior performance in all groups at the second testing session was likely due to a practice effect.

When tested by individual *t* tests, measures of attention and concentration, including the Digit Symbol sub-scale of the WAIS-R, the Stroop Test, and the Mental Control and Digit Span (forward and backward) subscales of the WMS-R, showed no significant differences between the ginkgo and placebo groups (FIGURE 2). Similarly, tests of verbal and nonverbal learning and memory, including the Logical Memory (I and II) and Visual Reproduction (I and II) subscales of the WMS-R, and the CVLT (initial acquisition, short and long delay, and recognition), also showed no significant differences between the ginkgo and placebo groups. There were no differences in tests of naming (Boston Naming Test) or verbal fluency (Controlled Category Fluency) between the ginkgo and placebo groups. Finally, self-report on the Memory Questionnaire was scored on a scale of 27 to 108 with higher scores indicating more difficulties. There was no difference in the mean reported scores for participants in the ginkgo and placebo groups. . . .

At the end of the second testing session, participants were asked if they thought they had been taking ginkgo or placebo. Self-report in the ginkgo group indicated that 79 participants (71%) thought they were taking . . . ginkgo, and self-report in the placebo group indicated that 81 participants (75%) thought they were taking ginkgo. . . . Informant response to the global rating indicated no difference between the ginkgo and placebo groups. . . .

Figure 2 shows the 95% confidence intervals (CIs) for differences (treatment group minus control) for performance on each test in the modified intent-to-treat analysis. Each interval contains a zero, indicating that none of the differences are statistically significant. Moreover, 7 of the point estimates are positive (favoring ginkgo) and 7 are negative (favoring placebo).

Evaluable Participant Analysis

A total of 203 participants completed the protocol (fully evaluable population). There were no significant differences between the ginkgo and placebo groups for any outcome measure.

Figure 2

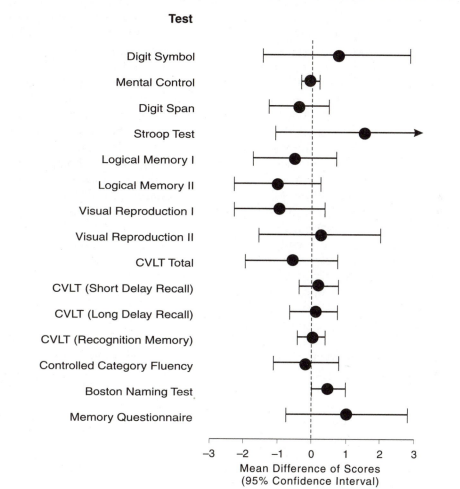

Differences (Treatment Group Minus Control) for Performance on Each Test

CVLT indicates California Verbal Learning Test. Data are based on the modified intent-to-treat analysis with 111 participants in the ginkgo group and 108 participants in the placebo group.

Comment

The results of this 6-week study indicate that ginkgo, marketed over-the-counter as a memory enhancer, did not enhance performance on standard neuropsychological tests of learning, memory, naming and verbal fluency, or attention and concentration. Moreover, there were no differences between ginkgo participants and placebo controls on subjective self-report of memory function or on global rating by spouses, friends, and relatives. These data suggest that when taken following the manufacturer's instructions, this compound provides no measurable benefit in cognitive function to elderly adults with intact cognitive function.

In total, 14 different measures of cognition were evaluated in the present study. Seven of the measures were better in the placebo group, and 7 of the measures were better in the ginkgo group. None of the differences between the means of the 2 groups were statistically significant. The 95% CIs were calculated for each mean difference. Even if one assumes that the true difference between treatments is the upper limit of the 95% CI, it would still be difficult to argue that meaningful benefit was derived from taking ginkgo. For example, the Logical Memory portion of the WMS-R measures the participants' ability to recall 2 paragraphs that they initially heard 30 minutes earlier. There are 25 possible discrete items in each paragraph that the participant could recall. The upper limit of the 95% CI for the mean difference between ginkgo and placebo was 0.20 items (ie, participants in the ginkgo group remembered less than 1 item more than participants in the placebo group). Similarly, on the CVLT, participants learn a 16-item shopping list over 5 trials. A perfect score is 80. The upper limit of the 95% CI for the mean difference between ginkgo and placebo was 1.01 items. It would be difficult to argue that either of these differences are of any clinical significance, even if they are real. The results of the Caregiver Global Impression of Change rating scale further support the failure of ginkgo to provide clinically significant improvement in memory. In general, caregivers did not rate changes in memory over the 6-week trial any differently in participants randomized to ginkgo vs placebo participants. Sixty-six percent of those randomized to placebo and 70% to ginkgo were judged by caregivers as showing no change over 6 weeks. Thirty-three percent of placebo and 28% of ginkgo participants were judged as minimally improved, and 3 participants were judged to be much improved; 2 were in the ginkgo group and 1 was in the placebo group.

Ginkgo has been evaluated in several double-blind studies that have reported beneficial effects, but these effects were not broad or consistent. Wesnes et al conducted a 3-month double-blind, randomized, placebo-controlled study in 54 patients. Patients were evaluated at weeks 4, 8, and 12. Patients receiving Tanakan (ginkgo extract) performed better on only 2 of 8 tests of memory . . . and attention and concentration . . . and in each case at only 1 evaluation point. There was not a consistent effect for any outcome measure. Additionally, neither physicians nor patients could distinguish between placebo and compound on an overall scale. Rai et al compared 12 ginkgo-treated with 15 placebo-treated participants who were classified as having mild to moderate memory impairment in a double-blind study and reported significant differences in favor of the gingko group only on the Kendrick Digit Copying task, but not on tests of learning or memory. Rigney et al evaluated 31 participants and 4 doses of ginkgo in a crossover design. They only reported improvement with 1 dose of ginkgo (120 mg), in only the oldest group of participants (50–59 years), and only in 1 of the multiple tests of memory administered. Other studies that have reported positive effects in favor of ginkgo have also either studied small numbers of participants in uncontrolled studies, have found benefit in one of many cognitive tasks administered, or have found changes in objective tests relative to controls but not in physician ratings in clinical populations. Despite the manufacturer's claims of improved memory in healthy adults, we were unable to identify any well-controlled studies that document this claim.

Recently, ginkgo was reported to be beneficial in a sample of patients with dementia. Mildly to severely demented patients characterized as having either Alzheimer disease or multi-infarct dementia were given either ginkgo (120 mg/d) or placebo for 52 weeks in a randomized double-blind study. The intent-to-treat analysis on 202 patients indicated a 0.1-point decline on the Alzheimer Disease Assessment Scale–Cognitive portion (ADAS-Cog) in the ginkgo group compared with a 1.48-point decline in the placebo group. No subjective differences were reported by either family members or physicians. While provocative, these differences on the ADAS-Cog are significantly smaller than those reported for approved cholinesterase inhibitors in treating patients with Alzheimer disease. Moreover, the failure to find any differences in either physician or family rating raises the issue of whether the small difference on the ADAS-Cog is clinically significant.

Despite the paucity of well-controlled studies, ginkgo continues to be marketed and widely used. Sales in the United States reached $240 million in 1997 and more than 5 million prescriptions are written each year in Germany primarily for dementia, cerebral decline, and peripheral arterial insufficiency.

Our study has limitations. It is certainly possible that higher doses or longer periods of exposure than used in this study are necessary to detect changes; however, we administered the compound following the manufacturer's instructions. The manufacturer's label indicates that ginkgo should be administered at a dose of 120 mg/d and that doses of greater than 120 mg show no additional benefit. This is also the dose suggested by the German Commission E. The daily dose in the present study was 120 mg/d. The label also states that a noticeable benefit should be apparent after 4 weeks of usage. The present study evaluated cognition after a 6-week interval. Moreover, there was no indication of a statistical trend toward significance for any of the compounds on any of the measures. Nevertheless, it is possible that longer exposures could produce beneficial effects.

We did not monitor adverse effects in the present study. Although ginkgo is generally characterized as a benign compound, it is not without adverse effects. Reported adverse effects include bleeding, mild gastrointestinal upset, and headache. None of the participants in the present study discontinued treatment due to adverse effects and none spontaneously reported any adverse effects. This finding is generally consistent with studies that did systematically monitor adverse effects.

The issue of quality control has also been raised as a potential source of variance in studies using over-the-counter compounds. One limitation of the present study is that we did not analyze the content of the ginkgo used in this study. However, the manufacturer claims that ginkgo "is processed under strict guidelines . . . ensured through extensive quality control."

We recognize the possibility that ceiling effects may have contributed to the nonsignificant findings in the present study. However, we selected tests that are normalized for the age group that we studied and, as such, have an appropriate range of scores. For example, in the Logical Memory WMS-R scale (Logical Memory I), the potential range of scores is 0 to 50. The ginkgo participants in the present study scored a mean of 20.49 (SD, 5.08) and the placebo participants scored a mean of 23.61 (SD, 4.65). Each of these is well below the maximum score of 50. In addition, none of the participants obtained a maximum score on this scale or any of the other scales used in this study.

We also recognize that the method of blinding in this study could have resulted in unblinding for some participants. However, the finding that participants taking ginkgo as well as those taking placebo reported in equal proportions taking the active compound ginkgo (71% vs 75%) mitigates this concern.

In summary, this study does not support the manufacturer's claims of the benefits of gingko on learning and memory. Treatment over a 6-week period following the manufacturer's dosing suggestions did not produce objective benefit on any of 14 standard neuropsychological tests, nor were any benefits detected in self-report by the participants or observation by a family member or friend.

POSTSCRIPT

Will Taking Herbal Supplements Enhance Mental Ability?

Herbal supplements cause controversy for reasons of science and politics. Although many people take them and have done so for thousands of years, few have been tested for safety and efficacy. Gingko supplements are promoted as memory enhancers.

One might argue that even small benefits might be useful for conditions like dementia for which there is no effective treatment, but this line of reasoning requires attention to the possibility of adverse effects. Herbal supplements are plant extracts, and plants contain many toxic as well as beneficial substances. Both selections suggest that if gingko produces adverse effects, these effects also are small.

In an article in *Scientific American* (April 2003), scientists reviewed several studies on gingko and cognitive function and concluded that, although "the proof for even a mild benefit is weak," the true test of gingko requires more research. Tests of other herbal supplements have produced equally controversial and inconclusive results (see *Journal of the American Medical Association,* April 10, 2002). Mary Palmer and her colleagues, for example, counted and categorized the number of adverse reactions to supplements reported by 11 poison control centers in the United States. They found hundreds of cases varying in severity but affecting all organ systems and age groups (*The Lancet*, January 11, 2003). More troubling, an investigative report in the *The New York Times* (June 23, 2003) revealed efforts by supplement companies to pressure researchers to alter the results of research studies that did not demonstrate that their products were beneficial.

Herbal supplements also raise political questions. In the United States, the Dietary Supplement Health and Education Act of 1994 removed supplements from effective oversight by the Food and Drug Administration (FDA). In passing this legislation, Congress permitted the makers of herbal supplements to market their products with "structure/function" claims that the products could improve aspects of body structure or function without requiring the makers to prove that the products were safe or effective for those purposes. Under this act, the makers of gingko supplements are permitted to advertise their products as helping to improve memory or thinking. They often cite the study by LeBars et al. as evidence for this benefit, but the regulations do not require them to mention contrary results. As a further result of the legislation, federal agencies do not monitor the contents of herbal supplements and cannot remove potentially harmful products from the market without first filing lawsuits—and winning them—against the manufacturers.

ISSUE 12

Can Functional Foods and Nutraceuticals Benefit Health?

YES: Cyndi Thomson, Abby S. Bloch, and Clare M. Hasler, from "Position of The American Dietetic Association: Functional Foods," *Journal of The American Dietetic Association* (October 1999)

NO: Editors of *Consumer Reports on Health*, from "The New Foods: Functional or Dysfunctional?" *Consumer Reports on Health* (June 1999)

ISSUE SUMMARY

YES: Cyndi Thomson et al., representatives of the American Dietetic Association (ADA), say that fortified, enriched, or enhanced "functional" foods can improve health.

NO: The editors of *Consumer Reports on Health* say that the purpose of functional foods is not to improve health but rather to boost the profits of manufacturers.

The idea that foods might confer specific health benefits has long roots in history, and many world cultures value certain foods—yogurt, garlic, soybeans, and teas, for example—for their therapeutic properties. Scientists have determined the chemical composition of these and other foods and have identified hundreds of compounds that might reduce disease risk. Any food containing a beneficial compound can be considered "functional" in the sense that it provides essential nutrients or confers health benefits, but most experts define functional foods as those that contain healthful substances in addition to those provided by its vitamins, minerals, and other naturally occurring components. Foods *fortified* with vitamins and minerals are considered functional and, therefore, include calcium-supplemented sweetened beverages as well as vitamin- and mineral-supplemented breakfast cereals. Thus, functional foods include a vast array of products with added components: nutrients, phytochemicals, fiber, or other substances designed specifically to lower cholesterol or produce other specific health benefits. Such products are also known by other names: nutraceuticals, designer foods, and techno-foods. No matter what they are called, they do not fit into any standard regulatory category in the United States, meaning that the regulatory environment does nothing to discourage development and sales of such products.

With so much public interest in health, marketing foods as nutritionally enhanced should—and does—increase sales. But do such products really improve the health of people who eat them? Or is their main benefit one of profits to manufacturers? The following selections debate such questions. Cyndi Thomson and her coauthors state the position of the American Dietetic Association (ADA): functional foods are likely to benefit health. To support this position, they cite data from clinical, animal, biochemical, and epidemiologic studies demonstrating the specific roles of nutrients and other food components in health. They also review the ways in which foods provide health benefits that exceed those provided by supplements. Furthermore, they consider fruits and vegetables to be functional foods because consuming such foods is linked to reduced risk of heart disease and certain cancers. The editors of *Consumer Reports on Health*, however, dismisses functional foods as "a triumph of marketing ingenuity." Such foods, the editors argue, have no other purpose than to allow manufacturers to make health claims and, therefore, to increase product sales.

To understand why health claims are a point of contention, it is necessary to review a few basic facts about food regulatory policy. Prior to 1990, the U.S. Food and Drug Administration (FDA) did not permit food manufacturers to place claims about health benefits on the labels of their products. The FDA viewed statements such as "helps lower cholesterol" or "helps prevent heart disease or cancer" as claims similar to those for prescription drugs. If food manufacturers wanted to say that their products conveyed the same benefits as drugs, they would need to follow the rules that applied to drugs. These rules require manufacturers to demonstrate that their products are safe and effective through the use of tests on animals and placebo-controlled clinical trials. Understandably, food manufacturers wanted to avoid such requirements and argued that they were unnecessary.

Food manufacturers were convinced that health claims on package labels would stimulate sales, and they encouraged Congress to mandate such claims as part of the Nutrition Labeling and Education Act of 1990. In 2003, the FDA has allowed 15 claims that health can be improved by eating specific foods or food components, among them calcium (osteoporosis), soy (heart disease and cancer), potassium (high blood pressure and stroke), and folate (neural tube defects). Health claims on product labels are well documented to increase market share.

But doesn't an increased market share suggest that more people will benefit from eating foods that are better for health? The following selections debate that issue. The ADA argues that functional foods offer great potential for improving the health of Americans. The editors of *Consumer Reports on Health* say that most functional foods make no dietary sense, as adding single nutrients or chemicals to foods does not convert them to health foods. As the article explains, "juiced-up junk is still junk."

Cyndi Thomson, Abby S. Bloch,
and Clare M. Hasler

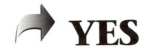 **YES**

Position of The American Dietetic Association: Functional Foods

Position Statement

It is the position of The American Dietetic Association (ADA) that functional foods, including whole foods and fortified, enriched, or enhanced foods, have a potentially beneficial effect on health when consumed as part of a varied diet on a regular basis, at effective levels. The Association supports research to further define the health benefits and risks of individual functional foods and their physiologically active components. . . .

Defining Functional Foods

There is no universally accepted definition of functional foods; however, several organizations have attempted to define this emerging food category. The International Food Information Council (IFIC) defines functional foods as foods that provide health benefits beyond basic nutrition. This definition is similar to that of the International Life Sciences Institute of North America (ILSI), which has defined functional foods as foods that, by virtue of physiologically active food components, provide health benefits beyond basic nutrition. The Institute of Medicine of the National Academy of Sciences limits functional foods to those in which the concentrations of one or more ingredients have been manipulated or modified to enhance their contribution to a healthful diet.

According to these definitions, unmodified whole foods such as fruits and vegetables represent the simplest example of a functional food. For example, broccoli, carrots, or tomatoes would be considered functional foods because they are rich in such physiologically active components as sulforaphane, beta carotene, and lycopene, respectively. Modified foods, including those that have been fortified with nutrients or enhanced with phytochemicals or botanicals, also fall within the realm of functional foods. In addition, food biotechnology will continue to provide new venues for functional food development. . . .

Although the term "functional foods" may not be the ideal descriptor for this emerging food category, recent focus-group research conducted by IFIC

From Cyndi Thomson, Abby S. Bloch, and Clare M. Hasler, "Position of The American Dietetic Association: Functional Foods," *Journal of The American Dietetic Association,* vol. 99, no. 10 (October 1999), pp. 1278–1279, 1282–1284. Copyright © 1999 by The American Dietetic Association. Reprinted by permission of Elsevier. References omitted.

showed that this term was recognized more readily and was also preferred by consumers over other commonly used terms such as "nutraceutical" or "designer foods." Recent broad use and acceptance of the term "functional foods" by media, scientists, and consumers has led ADA to work within this framework rather than introduce a new, more descriptive term, because of concern that new terminology could lead to further confusion among consumers.

As the largest organization of dietetics professionals, ADA, classifies all foods as functional at some physiological level. The term functional food should not be used to imply that there are good foods and bad foods. *All* foods can be incorporated into a healthful eating plan—the key being moderation and variety.

Rationale

Development of functional food products will continue to grow well into the 21st century as consumer demand for these products is heightened. Factors contributing to this reshaping of the food supply include:

- an aging population,
- increased health care costs,
- self-efficacy and autonomy in health care,
- advancing scientific evidence that diet can alter disease prevalence and progression, and
- most importantly, changes in food regulation.

Nutrients and nonnutritive food components have also been associated with the prevention and/or treatment of chronic diseases such as cancer, coronary heart disease, diabetes, hypertension, and osteoporosis. As the data supporting the role of diet in health promotion and disease prevention continue to mount, it is likely that the quantity of enhanced foods will expand substantially. Functional foods are viewed as one option available to Americans seeking cost-effective health care and improved health status, and they will continue to transform the American food supply.

Regulation of Functional Foods

The regulation of functional foods remains confusing. Under the current regulatory environment, functional foods or components can be placed into a number of existing categories, including conventional foods, food additives, dietary supplements, medical foods, or foods for special dietary use. . . . The category used to define a specific functional food or component will depend on how the manufacturer positions and markets the product for intended use as well as its associated label claims.

The most well established and scientifically sound approach to labeling and marketing a functional food is through the use of FDA-approved health claims delineated by law under the Nutrition Labeling and Education Act (NLEA) of 1990. The health claims authorized under NLEA are statements that describe a relationship between a food substance and a disease or other health-related condition (ie, a "risk reduction" relationship). The law mandates that a health claim be authorized in the labeling of FDA-regulated products only if significant scientific agreement among qualified experts exists about the validity of the relationship described in that claim. Under NLEA, companies petition the FDA to consider new health claims through rule-making. . . .

Substantial clinical efficacy and documentation are an important part of a company's petition packet to FDA. For example, 43 human clinical intervention trials were included in the soy health claim petition submitted to FDA. Based on the strong scientific underpinning of the NLEA health claims provisions, ADA supports the use of such preauthorized claims on food products, including functional foods.

A provision in the FDA Modernization Act of 1997 (FDAMA) provided an additional process for manufacturers to use health claims if such claims are based on current, published, authoritative statements from certain federal scientific bodies. These include only those "with official responsibility for public health protection or research relating to human nutrition" such as the National Institutes of Health, the Centers for Disease Control and Prevention and the National Academy of Sciences. . . .

A great boon to the marketplace for functional foods and components occurred with the enactment of the Dietary Supplement Health and Education Act (DSHEA) of 1994. DSHEA exempts dietary supplements from the stringent approval required for food additives. This legislation permits the use of dietary supplement "structure/function" claims without prior FDA authorization. Such statements describe how a food component or ingredient affects the structure and/or function of the body (eg, calcium builds strong bones) without linking it to a specific disease. Because these statements can be made without prior FDA approval, many companies are choosing to market functional foods as dietary supplements, which is a legal loophole permissible as long as the company notifies the FDA 30 days after first marketing the product bearing the claim. The label with the claim must also include the following disclaimer: "This statement has not been evaluated by the Food and Drug Administration. This product is not intended to diagnose, treat, mitigate, cure or prevent any disease." Although manufacturers are required to notify FDA within 30 days of marketing a product, there is currently no requirement for the notification packet to include the scientific basis in support of a structure/function claim. Therefore, the scientific underpinning of such claims is often inaccessible and potentially disputable. There is also little consumer research on the impact of structure/function claims on consumer knowledge and purchasing behaviors. Until such information is known, and until there is full assurance that structure/function claims are based on significant scientific agreement, dietetics professionals and consumers must be cautious about such claims.

One example of a functional food marketed as a dietary supplement has been soups containing St John's Wort or echinacea, which purport to improve mood or immunity, respectively. However, the FDA notified the manufacturer that these soups are not legitimately dietary supplements and must not be sold and labeled as such because the products clearly represent conventional foods.

Initial attempts were also made to market a cholesterol-lowering table spread as a dietary supplement until the FDA informed the manufacturer that the plant stanol esters contained in the product were considered unapproved food additives. Thus, the product's manufacturer was required to demonstrate to the FDA, through sufficient scientific documentation, that these additives are generally recognized as safe (GRAS) before the product could be marketed as a food in the United States.

Several other food products have also used structure/function claims in their marketing approach, which may or may not be supported by scientific evidence. ADA recommends cautious evaluation of the clinical efficacy of individual products before recommending their use to promote a specific health outcome. The proliferation of claims on a variety of products has created an environment of confusion and distrust among health professionals and consumers.

Another route to marketing functional foods that is used by food manufacturers to disseminate information about their products is advertising, which is regulated by the Federal Trade Commission (FTC). The FTC has a more lenient standard for advertising claims about diet-disease relationships than does the FDA for food labeling. Therefore, the potential exists for the advertising medium to permit mention of an association between a food product and prevention of disease. A good example is the advertisement that appeared in magazines in recent months stating that "lycopene (found in tomato products) may help reduce the risk of prostate and cervical cancer." The FDA would refuse such a labeling claim until the scientific evidence was substantial and supported by a sufficient number of controlled, clinical intervention trials that currently do not exist. ADA supports efforts for consistency and a scientific basis for the development of consumer diet-health messages and therefore recommends collaboration among the food industry, health professionals, and government agencies to communicate the health benefits of specific functional foods.

ADA supports the need for all foods and dietary supplements, including functional foods, to be regulated to ensure that the products are safe; that the products have been manufactured using recognized good manufacturing practices; and that all label claims—health, nutrient content, and structure/function—are truthful, not misleading, and are based on significant scientific agreement. Regulating functional foods as such will protect consumers, provide informative and scientifically sound labeling claims that will improve food selections, and potentially advance wellness. This approach will provide the food industry with specific guidelines that, in turn, will direct research and development for future functional foods. Current and future functional foods should be labeled with specific information as to any ingredient (eg, nutrient, phytochemical, zoochemical, or botanical) used to market the product as well as the specific amount available in an average serving. Without disclosing this information, consumers, along with dietetics and other health professionals, will be unable to make an educated assessment as to the appropriate use of the product. Regulating functional foods as described above will ensure that such information is routinely made available. . . .

Scientific Research

The scientific evidence for functional foods and their physiologically active components can be categorized into 4 distinct areas: (a) clinical trials, (b) animal studies, (c) experimental in vitro laboratory studies, and (d) epidemiologic studies. Much of the current evidence for functional foods lacks well-designed clinical trials; however, the foundational evidence provided through the other types of scientific investigation is substantial for several of the functional foods and their health-promoting components. . . .

The strongest scientific evidence of clinical efficacy is for functional foods that are available or have been developed in accordance with the NLEA guidelines for preapproved health claims as discussed previously. For such foods, there is substantial scientific agreement among scientists that a diet-disease relationship exists. Scientific support under NLEA includes all types of research from in vitro to randomized, controlled clinical trials and focuses on the reduction of common chronic diseases in the United States. Basic examples of functional foods that fall into this realm are foods naturally rich in soluble fiber, such as oat bran or psyllium, which have been associated with reduced incidence of coronary heart disease. Another example would be fruits and vegetables and the association between increased consumption and reduced risk for cancer or coronary heart disease. Soy protein is an additional example; however, a final regulation authorizing a health claim related to soy protein intake and reduction of risk for coronary heart disease has yet to be issued by FDA.

Other functional foods may have substantial scientific support, but currently lack an FDA-approved health claim because the food industry has not yet petitioned the FDA. Examples would be garlic and n-3 fatty acids found in fish, which have been shown in clinical trials to reduce serum cholesterol levels in subjects with elevated levels. This group of functional foods might also include new products such as the plant stanol-enriched or sterol-enriched table spreads that have been shown in clinical trials to significantly reduce serum cholesterol levels in subjects with mild to moderate hyperlipidemia.

A third category of functional foods are those that have been fortified to enhance the level of a specific nutrient or food component that has been associated with the prevention or treatment of a disease or other clinical condition. Many of these products bear authorized health claims for product marketing. This category would include products such as calcium-fortified orange juice, pasta, or rice marketed to maintain good bone health and reduce osteoporosis risk, as well as fiber-supplemented snack bars or folate-enriched cereals. Many other functional foods in this category may lack sufficient evidence to warrant an authorized health claim at this time. This would include, for example, beverages with added vitamin E for reduced heart disease risk and salad dressings with n-3 fatty acids to reduce the inflammatory response of rheumatoid disease.

A fourth category of functional foods includes whole foods that have been associated with reduced risk of disease. For these whole foods, in vitro, in vivo, or epidemiologic research is available to support the health benefits of these whole foods; however, no health claim exists, partially because of the limited or improperly designed clinical trial data or lack of scientific agreement as to the strength of the evidence. This category includes:

- tomato products rich in lycopene, a carotenoid, whose consumption is associated with reduced cancer rates in epidemiologic studies;
- eggs with n-3 fatty acids, which may potentially reduce cholesterol levels;
- black and green tea, which are rich in polyphenols, has been associated experimentally and in human studies with cancer prevention and control;
- nondigestible oligosaccharides (prebiotics), especially fructans, which may potentially provide health benefits for cardiovascular disease, type 2 diabetes, and intestinal infectious diseases;
- fermented dairy products (probiotics), which have been shown to improve gastrointestinal health; and
- dairy products and red meat with conjugated linoleic acid, which may alter cancer carcinogenesis.

For each of these, an association with reduced disease risk has been observed but has not reached scientific consensus.

Finally, there exists a growing selection of functional food components marketed under the umbrella of dietary supplements. For the majority of these products, the evidence for their structure/function claims is currently limited, incomplete, or unsubstantiated. Examples include antioxidant-enriched beverages or candies, chewing gum with phosphatidylserine, and snack bars with chromium. This category also includes a large number of herbal-enriched products that make a variety of structure/function claims. Examples include cereal fortified with ginkgo biloba, which is marketed as reducing symptoms of dementia, or juices with echinacea, which are marketed for boosting the immune system. Both claims do have support in controlled clinical trials. Other evidence for botanical-enriched products have shown conflicting results in clinical trials such as the use of echinacea to reduce cold and flu symptoms or kava to reduce anxiety. Still other structure/function claims have no clear therapeutic efficacy, such as the use of goldenseal for immune enhancement or ginseng for energy or enhanced physical performance. Others, such as ma huang, may be harmful. Historically, evidence for the clinical efficacy of select botanicals was limited primarily because of poor research design (eg, inconsistency in dosage form or amount, small sample size, and frequently the lack of a placebo control, in part resulting from insufficient funding for research in this area). Yet many of these botanicals are being introduced into our food supply—sometimes irresponsibly—in the form of functional foods. ADA must call on industry to fund additional research in this emerging area.

Evaluation of the efficacy of individual functional foods must be completed using a scientifically valid risk-benefit model that clearly assesses all physiological effects, both positive and negative. Review of the in vitro, animal, epidemiologic, and clinical data is essential before functional foods are marketed to consumers for their health-promoting qualities.

The Value of a Varied Diet

The weight of scientific evidence indicates that the optimal approach for achieving a health benefit from the intake of nutrients and other physiologically active constituents is through the consumption of a varied diet that is rich in plant foods. In reality, each vegetable contains numerous different nutrients and phytochemicals—a biological circumstance that is not currently replicated in pill form. In addition, the assumption that a combination of plant constituents that are naturally occurring is maintained at equivalent levels of biological activity when extracted, dried, and compacted into pill form is likely unfounded.

Pharmaceutical companies have isolated many food components into supplement form, including allyly sulfides, genistein, anthocyanin (bilberry extract), and glycyrrhizin (licorice) to name only a few. In the United States, tens of billions of dollars are spent annually on dietary supplements. The rapid growth in functional foods might be considered the food industry's response to growing sales of dietary supplements. Supplements can provide nutrients and other physiologically active components in a potentially unbalanced and concentrated form that may be far different from the form used in research studies. Nutrients and other bioactive food components that occur naturally in foods act synergistically with other dietary elements such as fiber to promote health. . . .

Levels of Intake

Safe levels of intake must be considered when evaluating functional foods in the context of a healthy diet. For the majority of research studies, the optimal levels of nutrients and other physiologically active components in functional foods have yet to be determined. Animal research has provided some indication of desired intake; however, these data are difficult to extrapolate to human dietary requirements. . . .

Many functional foods or food components will require continued in vivo and in vitro research, as well as pharmacokinetic studies, before specific levels for clinical trial investigations can be determined. . . .

Current dietary measurement tools are limited in data collection related to herb, spice, condiment, and/or flavoring intake, despite the fact that several physiologically active components have been identified in these foods. The adequacy of intake of nutrients and other physiologically active dietary components found in functional foods must include evaluation of these foods (eg, herbs, spices) and the interactions among the various nutrients and bioactive food components in the diet.

Dietary constituents appear to act synergistically to improve absorption of nutrients or physiologically active dietary components. One example is lycopene in tomatoes and the enhancement of its absorption when consumed along with fat. The specific intake levels recommended to reduce the risk of disease in a healthy population can be altered in the presence of a disease such as cancer or cardiovascular disease. Therefore, dietary advice regarding approximate levels of intake for functional foods and their components will need to be evaluated based on currently available scientific information in the context of the specific populations or individual variance. . . .

Summary

Never before has the focus on the health benefits of food been so strong. The philosophy that food can be health promoting beyond its traditional nutritional value is gaining acceptance among scientists and health professionals. Dietetics professionals are uniquely qualified and positioned to translate scientific evidence into practical dietary applications for consumers and to provide the food industry, policy makers, and the media with valuable insight and expertise for future research, product development, regulation, and communication regarding functional foods. Increasing the availability of health-promoting foods in the US diet will help to ensure a healthier population. Dietetics professionals must be leaders in this evolving area of food and nutrition.

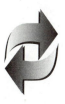

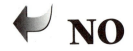
The New Foods: Functional or Dysfunctional?

As you wander through your local food store, you may wonder whether you've stumbled into a drugstore by mistake. The soup aisle features Hain's *Kitchen Prescription Chicken Broth and Noodles with Echinacea* to "support your immune system" and *Chunky Tomato with St. John's Wort* to "give your mood a natural lift." The snack section has Robert's American Gourmet *Kava Kava Corn Chips* to "promote relaxation," and *Ginkgo Biloba Rings,* a potato-corn snack, to "increase memory and alertness." You see sodas, juices, drinks, gum, candy, frozen desserts—all spiked with supposedly health-enhancing herbs. Even products from mainstream food-manufacturing giants like Kellogg, Procter & Gamble, and Tropicana are taking on a decidedly pharmaceutical cast these days, with specially added nutrients and special health claims against heart disease or osteoporosis, the brittle-bone disease.

Welcome to the weird new world of "nutraceuticals," or "functional foods," the hottest new terms in food marketing. Americans have been eating *fortified* foods since 1924, when manufacturers started adding iodine to salt to prevent the nutritional deficiency that causes goiters. But functional foods represent a new concept in several ways—and a triumph of marketing ingenuity. The various added ingredients are generally intended to treat or prevent either symptoms or diseases, not deficiency; many of them aren't normally found in foods at all; and most of them are added primarily to let the manufacturer make enticing health claims.

Such products are flooding the market due largely to relaxed and fuzzy rules governing what's allowed in foods and what their manufacturers can say about them. First, the Food and Drug Administration began to approve specific disease-fighting claims. Then Congress allowed the manufacturers to make "structure and function" claims—"helps maintain healthy cholesterol levels," for example—without FDA approval, provided they don't actually mention a specific disease. But while that rule applies to all supplement manufacturers, *food* companies can make such unapproved claims only if the proposed benefit stems from the food's "nutritive value." Not even the FDA—let alone your average food manufacturer—knows exactly what that phrase means.

Some companies try to sidestep the morass and legitimize an unapproved claim by marketing their food as a dietary supplement. Others simply ignore the rules, in hopes that the overloaded FDA won't challenge them.

But even foods that bear FDA-approved health claims aren't necessarily healthful. And foods that carry unapproved claims—or that contain impressive-sounding special ingredients—may be nutritionally worthless, or worse.

Capitalizing on Claims

The FDA opened the functional-food floodgates in 1993, when it ruled that products high in calcium, such as milk and yogurt, could sport labels claiming protection against osteoporosis. Seizing the opportunity, several manufacturers promptly started *adding* calcium—about 350 milligrams, a bit more than the amount in a glass of milk—to items that are not naturally rich in the mineral, such as *Tropicana Pure Premium* orange juice, Procter & Gamble's *Sunny Delight* orange beverage and Kellogg's *Eggo Homestyle* frozen waffles. For a while, you could even buy *Pringle's Potato Chips* with extra calcium.

Most Americans, particularly women, don't get the recommended amounts of calcium: 1,200 milligrams a day for post-menopausal women if they take bone-bolstering drugs, and 1,500 milligrams if they don't; 1,000 milligrams for other adults up to age 50, then 1,200 milligrams from age 50 to 65 and 1,500 after 65. The best way to meet those recommendations is by eating a variety of healthful, calcium-rich foods, such as low-fat dairy products, dark-green leafy vegetables, beans, tofu prepared with calcium salts—and, yes, even calcium-fortified orange juice. Those foods, including OJ, are rich not only in calcium but also in numerous other nutrients, and they've all been linked to a variety of benefits beyond strong bones, such as reduced risk of coronary disease and cancer.

In contrast, calcium-fortified waffles (mainly refined flour) and orange drink (mainly sugar and water), have little to offer except calcium. If you can't get enough calcium from your diet, you'd be better off eating unrefined foods like whole-wheat products, or drinking 100 percent fruit juices, and taking a modest calcium supplement than consuming the nutritionally weak waffles or drink.

A Slick Ensemble

Kellogg's *Ensemble* product line, the first offering from the company's new functional-foods division, takes the nutraceuticals idea one step further: Unlike calcium, the psyllium husks that are added to these foods aren't found in the ordinary diet at all.

Kellogg laid the groundwork for introducing its new product line by convincing the FDA that the soluble fiber found in psyllium husks, like the soluble fiber in oats, reduces the blood-cholesterol level and thus should reduce the risk of developing coronary disease. After the FDA approved that health claim in February of last year, Kellogg quickly released its psyllium-fortified line, including frozen pasta entrees, dry pasta, breads, breakfast cereals, snacks, and desserts—

many in packages emblazoned with a claim about cholesterol, heart disease, or heart health. All the products are sold at premium prices: For example, a 20-ounce loaf of *Ensemble Split-Top Sandwich Bread* costs $2.29, nearly twice as much as most other white breads, and slightly more than many whole-wheat breads.

It's true that the various *Ensemble* products are good sources of soluble fiber. So they're better than the same foods without the added fiber. But that's damningly faint praise. Like the calcium-containing waffles and orange drink, almost none of the *Ensemble* products offers much except the added ingredient: Nearly all the products are made from refined flour, several of them pack too much fat or salt to qualify for the health claim, and several are loaded with sugar. The three breakfast cereals are made from oat flour, another good source of soluble fiber, but even the cereals are moderately high in sugar.

Instead of stocking up on those products, you can get all the fiber you need—and a host of other important nutrients as well—by eating the recommended 5 to 9 daily servings of produce and 6 to 11 servings of whole grains. Among many other things, those foods supply lots of *in*soluble fiber, which helps prevent constipation and possibly colon cancer as well.

Margarine Medicine?

Two brand-new margarines contain added ingredients that, like soluble fiber, help reduce cholesterol levels. But those ingredients are even more obscure than psyllium, and the FDA hasn't yet allowed any health claim.

Regular margarine contains little saturated fat but lots of trans fat, which makes the spread roughly as bad for your cholesterol levels as butter (which is loaded with saturated fat). Several margarines, including Lipton's *Take Control* and Johnson & Johnson's *Benecol,* are specially formulated to minimize or eliminate the trans fat. But *Take Control* also contains concentrated plant compounds called sterols, which help keep the cholesterol that the body produces or ingests from getting into the bloodstream, where it can contribute to clogged arteries. *Benecol* contains a similar-acting sterol derivative. Clinical trials have shown that consuming three pats of *Benecol* spread a day instead of other low-trans margarines can reduce the blood-cholesterol level by an average of 10 to 14 percent. *Take Control* may have a similar though slightly smaller benefit.

But for both margarines, the studies tested only modest amounts and lasted no longer than a year. Further, they still contain as much *total* fat and as many calories as the other margarines. So don't regard their potential benefits as license to indulge your fat tooth. These products, which cost several times more than regular spreads and some low-trans spreads, may be worth trying only if you have an elevated cholesterol level and don't mind the uncertainty about safety if you plan to use them for a long time.

Johnson & Johnson initially hoped to sell *Benecol* as a dietary supplement, but the FDA rejected that proposal. Whether the company will now try to peg a health claim on *Benecol's* "nutritive value"—and how the FDA might react—remains to be seen.

Off the Deep End

While the world of herbs is largely uncharted territory, there are at least trends toward standardized doses of the pills and extracts and toward warnings about risks. But the addition of herbs to *foods* is a step backward into the darkest jungle. Such products may be worthless or even harmful, for any of these reasons:

The herb may not work   Journey's *Tropical Herb Ginseng Soda* highlights its "Brazilian Suma ginseng." But the variety of ginseng thought to offer possible benefits is Asian Panax; Brazilian Suma isn't even real ginseng. And the herb added to Hain's *Chunky Tomato with St. John's Wort* consists of stems, while the active ingredient (which may indeed ease mild depression) appears to come mainly from the leaves and flowers.

The amount is absurdly small   A serving of that Hain's soup contains 98 milligrams of St. John's wort *stems.* The apparently effective dose of the leaves and flowers, on the other hand, is 20 to 30 times higher—and it's supposed to be taken three times a day for at least a month. *Peace Cereal Vanilla Almond Crisp,* described as "an herbal brain power cereal," contains some 2 milligrams of ginkgo-leaf extract, while the possibly effective dose is 120 to 240 milligrams—and any benefit from the herb is probably limited to people who have cognitive problems such as those in early-stage Alzheimer's disease.

The herb may sometimes be unsafe   If certain products do contain any significant doses, the herb might cause harm in some cases. For example, if Robert's American Gourmet *Kava Kava Corn Chips* actually contain much kava kava, pigging out on them theoretically might relax your muscles enough to precipitate a fall or an accident—particularly if you're drinking alcohol or taking another muscle-relaxing drug. SoBe's *Energy* drink contains yohimbe at what the maker calls "supplement" levels. If that's true, the herb may pose certain risks, especially for people who have diabetes or heart, liver, or kidney disease or who take antidepressants known as MAO inhibitors. And if the echinacea added to several functional foods constitutes a substantial dose, it might harm people who have autoimmune disorders such as rheumatoid arthritis. While many herbal *supplements* carry that warning, it's not on any of the echinacea-fortified *foods* that we've seen.

Juiced-up junk is still junk   The main ingredient in such products as Blue Sky's *Ginseng Creme Soda,* RJ Corr's *Ginseng Rush Natural Soda,* and Ben & Jerry's new *Tropic of Mango Frozen Smoothie* with echinacea—apart from an uncertain amount of an herb with uncertain benefits—is sugar.

Summing Up

Most "functional foods" function mainly to boost manufacturers' profits, not to improve your health. Apart from calcium-fortified orange juice and possibly the *Ensemble* breakfast cereals and the two margarines for people with a high blood-cholesterol level, none of the functional foods makes good dietary sense. Adding a single healthful ingredient, like calcium or psyllium, does not turn a nutritional nonentity into a desirable food—particularly since you can get the same or equivalent ingredients from foods loaded with additional nutrients, often at a lower price. Dumping *herbs* into foods is even more dubious, since the herb or the dose may be ineffective or unsafe.

FOODS IN THE MEDICINE CABINET?

"The first medical food recommended by doctors for the dietary management of vascular disease." That's the claim on *HeartBar,* a $1.95 snack bar that debuted in January. *HeartBars* contain the amino acid L-arginine which, the company says, relieves angina, or heart-related chest pain, by dilating the coronary arteries.

If *HeartBar* were a drug, the Food and Drug Administration would require reams of evidence from the maker, Cooke Pharma, documenting its safety and effectiveness. If it were a dietary supplement or just a food, the FDA could prohibit claims about a specific disease (though the agency might allow more general claims—see story). But Cooke has sidestepped those restraints by selling the bars as a "medical food," an obscure regulatory category for foods that treat diseases with clear nutritional requirements, such as malnutrition or intractable diarrhea.

The labels must state that such foods should be eaten only under a doctor's supervision. But they can be sold without a prescription (usually in drugstores), and manufacturers can make specific claims without FDA approval. In recent years, a few companies hoping to take advantage of that loophole have developed products for common diseases with less-definite nutritional links. And the FDA has started to reconsider how it deals with such foods. Here's the lowdown on the most common medical foods:

HeartBar   A growing body of evidence—mostly from animal research—does suggest that L-arginine can help relax the arteries. And a few clinical trials in humans have shown that it can relieve angina in at least some patients. But other trials have found no benefit. And there's no long-term evidence on L-arginine's safety or effectiveness. The bottom line: A serious problem like angina should be managed only with proven medications, not with a *possibly* helpful snack bar.

NiteBite and Choice dm   These chocolate-flavored snack bars are loaded with starch; that carbohydrate is meant to prevent the hypoglycemia, or low blood-sugar level, that afflicts some diabetic individuals, usually when they sleep or work out. But any carbohydrate-rich snack eaten shortly before bedtime or exercise can help prevent hypoglycemia. And sometimes the best way to avoid the problem is not by eating a snack but by adjusting the dosage or type of antidiabetic medication you take. Your doctor may suggest a safer, more effective option than downing starch bars (which cost $1.20 apiece).

Cardia When this salt alternative hit the shelves two years ago it was marketed as a medical food, complete with a claim that it helps control hypertension. The manufacturer has now dropped that claim, in order to drop the accompanying warning about medical supervision. But the claim never amounted to much in the first place.

Some research does suggest that *Cardia*—which basically contains half the sodium of regular salt, plus potassium and magnesium—can reduce blood pressure in hypertensive people. But that effect is typically modest. Further, people who have kidney disease or take either an ACE inhibitor or a "potassium-sparing" diuretic should indeed check with a doctor first, since the potassium in *Cardia* theoretically may cause excessive potassium buildup. As for people with normal blood pressure, it's not clear whether they benefit even from salt restriction—and there's no evidence they'd benefit from *Cardia.*

POSTSCRIPT

Can Functional Foods and Nutraceuticals Benefit Health?

Astroll through any American supermarket today immediately illustrates the basis of the arguments in these selections. Food manufacturers say that health claims help to inform consumers about the nutritional value of food products. Thus, nutrient-fortified cereals, fruit drinks, and candies are abundant, along with fiber-supplemented candy bars, soy-supplemented "dairy" drinks, and margarines (fats) containing substances designed to lower cholesterol. The labels of many such products inform the public about the content of added vitamins and minerals or the ability of the food to help reduce the risk of heart disease, cancer, osteoporosis, or other chronic diseases. Orange juices well known to be sources of vitamin C now display statements about their ability to help people reduce high blood pressure (because of their natural potassium content). The FDA and the analogous agency that regulates advertising, the Federal Trade Commission (FTC), have documented impressive gains in sales advantage when products display or advertise health claims.

But do these products really improve health? Such a connection is difficult to demonstrate, and not only for the usual scientific reasons. People who typically choose to buy nutritionally enhanced products are among the best educated and wealthiest segments of the population. They typically eat more healthful foods (fruits and vegetables, for example) than the general population; they also tend to be more physically active and to avoid excessive intake of alcohol. This "tracking" of health behaviors makes research on the benefits of functional foods especially difficult. It also explains why both selections recommend further research, emphasize that dietary patterns are more important than intake of single nutrients, and agree on the need for appropriate regulation of functional foods.

Clare M. Hasler, one of the authors of the ADA paper, later reviewed the current status of functional foods in the *Journal of Nutrition* (December 2002). She concludes that studies provide very strong evidence for the health benefits of fortified margarines, soy foods, and whole oat products, and strong evidence for the benefits of fatty fish with omega-3 fatty acids. Because the evidence is weaker for other food components, she thinks more research is needed to establish the benefits of most functional foods. Consumers, she says, must realize that functional foods are not "magic bullets" and that they cannot compensate for poor health habits. Such concerns explain why the ADA qualifies its position on functional foods, stating that such foods are beneficial "when consumed as part of a varied diet on a regular basis, at effective levels." The editors of *Consumer Reports on Health* are likely to agree with this qualification.

Elizabeth Sloan, an editor of *Food Technology,* wrote in that journal in April 2002 that the worldwide market for functional foods was close to $50 billion, an increase of $20 billion just since 1995. The rapid growth in this market is alone sufficient to explain the interest of food manufacturers in developing such products. She predicted that manufacturers will be producing increasing numbers of fortified foods, as well as functional foods developed and marketed to reduce disease risks, enhance sports performance, improve children's health, and manage body weight. Such trends reinforce the point made by the authors of both selections: much remains to be learned about the health effects of functional foods, and more research needs to be done to address their scientific, medical, and social implications. Such research is emerging rapidly, as indicated by a comprehensive review of recent studies and international perspectives on development of functional foods (*British Journal of Nutrition* supplement, November 2002).

On the Internet . . .

Food Security Institute

The Food Security Institute at Brandeis University provides a frequently up-dated guide to studies on hunger and food security, demands for food and wel-fare assistance, and the effects of food insecurity on health.

http://www.centeronhunger.org/FSI/fsiguide.html

The International Baby Food Action Network

The International Baby Food Action Network Web site promotes breastfeeding and monitors the actions of international companies that promote formula feeding and the use of commercial baby food.

http://www.ibfan.org/english/gateenglish.html

Organic Farming Research Foundation

The Organic Farming Research Foundation supports studies demonstrating the health, nutritional, and environmental benefits of organic agricultural prac-tices.

http://www.ofrf.org

Food Safety Information: Irradiation

This Web site concerning food safety information contains links to United States government agencies and their answers to basic questions about food irradiation. The site also provides details about the current regulatory status of irradiation.

http://www.foodsafety.gov/~fsg/irradiat.html

The International Consultative Group on Food Irradiation

The International Consultative Group on Food Irradiation site provides infor-mation about methods and regulation of food irradiation in countries through-out the world.

http://www.iaea.or.at/icgfi/

PART 5

Nutrition and Food Policy

*A*dvice about almost any aspect of nutrition and health has implications for federal policy and for the economic interests of food companies. The United States government is heavily involved in food and nutrition policies that affect matters as diverse as dietary guidance, farm production, food assistance, food safety regulation, monitoring of the food supply and dietary intake, and food labeling and advertising. Because food is such big business, food companies are sensitive to almost any action taken by the government that might affect profits, and the economic implications of federal regulatory policies underlie many of the debates in this field. In this part, debates about issues that might affect the cost of federal expenditures for food assistance or the profitability of industries that sell infant formulas or foods that are irradiated or genetically modified, as opposed to conventionally grown, are examined. Because industries affected by federal regulations often attempt to influence governments to protect their interests, the debates enter the realm of politics and require political as well as scientific resolution.

- Does Widespread Hunger Exist in America?

- Should Mothers Infected With the AIDS Virus Breastfeed Their Infants?

- Is Organically Grown Food Better Than Conventionally Grown Food?

- Will Irradiation Improve the Safety of the Food Supply?

- Does the World Need Genetically Modified Foods?

ISSUE 13

Does Widespread Hunger Exist in America?

YES: Mark Nord, Margaret Andrews, and Steven Carlson, from "Measuring Food Security in the United States: Household Food Security in the United States, 2001," *Food Assistance and Nutrition Research Report Number 29*, A Report of the Food and Rural Economics Division, Economic Research Service, United States Department of Agriculture (October 2002)

NO: Robert E. Rector, from "The Myth of Widespread American Poverty," *The Heritage Foundation,* http://www.heritage.org/Research/ PoliticalPhilosophy/BG1221.cfm (September 18, 1998)

ISSUE SUMMARY

YES: Mark Nord et al., U.S. Department of Agriculture (USDA) economists, estimate that 11.5 million U.S. households do not have enough food to meet basic needs; of these, 3.5 million households sometimes go hungry for lack of resources to buy food.

NO: Robert E. Rector, policy analyst for the Heritage Foundation, a Washington, D.C.–based think tank, finds little evidence of hunger among the poor; on the contrary, he argues that their principal nutrition problems are overweight and obesity.

The U.S. food supply is so abundant that it provides an average of 3,900 kilocalories (kcal) per day for every man, woman, and child in the country, nearly twice the average need. Income, however, is distributed unequally, and it is possible that some people might not have enough resources to obtain adequate food every day. In the 1960s the discovery of malnutrition in rural areas of the deep South shocked the nation and led President Lyndon Johnson to declare a "War on Poverty." Congress enacted legislation creating welfare and food assistance programs such as food stamps and WIC (Special Supplemental Nutrition Program for Women, Infants, and Children). As a result of these programs, the prevalence of malnutrition declined. In the early 1980s, however, reductions in federal expenditures and rising inflation widened the income gap, and advocates for the poor began to conduct surveys to document the lack of *food security* (defined as assurance of regular access to adequate food) and consequent *hunger* (the physiological effect of involuntary food insufficiency). Subsequently, advocates in hundreds of communities throughout the United States conducted hunger surveys; these surveys invariably found large numbers of people to have unreliable access to food, even among recipients of federal food and income assistance. Also invariably, critics argued that the methods used to define food security and count the hungry lacked validity. In response, university and government researchers refined the methods and developed statistically validated survey questions that could be used to assess food insecurity and hunger in communities.

Since 1995 the U.S. Department of Agriculture (USDA) has used precisely such questions to probe the extent of food insecurity in the U.S. population. The Census Bureau includes food security questions as part of a supplement to its monthly survey of 50,000 households (adults and children sharing the same dwelling). In 2001, on the basis of the answers to such questions, USDA economists concluded that 89 percent of U.S. households were food secure, but 11 percent—representing 11.5 million households with 20.9 million adults and 12.7 million children—were not. They also concluded that two-thirds of these households were marginally food insecure. The household members managed to meet dietary needs by relying on a few basic foods. The USDA defined the remaining one-third, meaning 6.1 million adults and 3 million children, as food insecure and said that among the children from households defined as food insecure, 467,000 were hungry some of the time. The USDA economists noted that the most food-insecure segments of the population were inner-city households with children headed by a single woman, especially if she was black or hispanic.

Robert E. Rector charges that the methods used by the USDA to obtain such data are too flawed and misleading to draw such conclusions. Hunger may exist in the United States, he says, but not to any appreciable extent. The poor eat just as well as the middle class, and their nutrient intakes greatly exceed requirements. Poor children are taller and heavier on average than they were in the 1950s. Indeed, he argues that overconsumption of food—not underconsumption—is the principal diet-related health problem of the poor. Even if hunger does exist, says Rector, its cause is not poverty. Instead, inappropriate welfare policies have so increased dependency on federal programs that families no longer take care of themselves.

The following selections address clashing issues of science and values. How valid is the method used by the USDA to evaluate the extent of food insecurity and hunger? What factors might influence the way people respond to such questions? How do economic and social factors interact in influencing food security and obesity among the poor? How might personal, social, or political values influence opinions on this issue?

In the following selections, Mark Nord et al. report that millions of Americans experience food insecurity and hunger as a result of inadequate income. In contrast, Rector says that hunger is minimal in America and occurs mainly as a result of a welfare-induced erosion of family values.

Mark Nord, Margaret Andrews,
and Steven Carlson

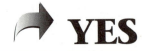 **YES**

Measuring Food Security in the United States: Household Food Security in the United States, 2001

Introduction

Since 1995, the U.S. Department of Agriculture (USDA) has collected information annually on food spending, food access and adequacy, and sources of food assistance for the U.S. population. The information is collected in yearly food security surveys, conducted as a supplement to the nationally representative Current Population Survey (CPS). A major impetus for this data collection is to provide information about the prevalence of food insecurity and hunger in U.S. households. USDA reports in the series *Measuring Food Security in the United States* have summarized the findings of this research for each year from 1995 to 2000. . . .

This report updates the national statistics on food security, using data collected in the December 2001 food security survey. The report also updates the statistical series initiated in last year's report on household food spending, how food-insecure households use Federal and community food assistance, and the numbers of households using community food pantries and emergency kitchens. These statistics provide additional insight into the nature of food insecurity and how low-income households meet their food needs. . . .

Household Food Security

Food security—access by all people at all times to enough food for an active, healthy life—is one of several conditions necessary for a population to be healthy and well nourished. This section provides information on food security, food insecurity, and hunger in U.S. households based on the December 2001 food security survey—the seventh annual survey in the Nation's food security monitoring system.

From Mark Nord, Margaret Andrews, and Steven Carlson, "Measuring Food Security in the United States: Household Food Security in the United States, 2001," *Food Assistance and Nutrition Research Report Number 29,* A Report of the Food and Rural Economics Division, Economic Research Service, United States Department of Agriculture (October 2002). References and some notes omitted.

Methods

The results presented in . . . this report are based on data collected in the Current Population Survey (CPS) food security surveys for the years 1995–2001. The statistics . . . are based on a measure of food security calculated from responses to a series of questions about conditions and behaviors known to characterize households having difficulty meeting basic food needs. Each question asks whether the condition or behavior occurred during the previous 12 months and specifies a lack of money or other resources to obtain food as the reason for the condition or behavior [see Box]. Voluntary fasting or dieting to lose weight is thereby excluded from the measure. . . . Full-question wordings are presented in Bickel et al., 2000, and are available from the ERS Food Security Briefing Room at http://www.ers.usda.gov/briefing/foodsecurity/

EXAMPLES OF QUESTIONS FROM THE CPS FOOD SECURITY SURVEY

"We worried whether our food would run out before we got money to buy more." Was that often, sometimes, or never true for you in the last 12 months?

"The food that we bought just didn't last and we didn't have money to get more." Was that often, sometimes, or never true for you in the last 12 months?

In the last 12 months did you or other adults in the household ever cut the size of your meals or skip meals because there wasn't enough money for food?

In the last 12 months were you ever hungry, but didn't eat, because you couldn't afford enough food?

(For households with children) In the last 12 months did any of the children ever not eat for a whole day because there wasn't enough money for food?

Interviewed households are classified into one of three categories—food secure, food insecure without hunger, food insecure with hunger—based on the number of food-insecure conditions and behaviors the household reported. Households classified as food insecure with hunger that include children are further classified as to whether both children and adults were hungry or only adults. The presence of hunger among children in food-insecure households is measured by a subset of the food security questions that ask specifically about the conditions and experiences of children (Nord and Bickel, 2002). Appropriate weighting factors are then applied to the surveyed households to obtain nationally representative prevalence estimates.

Prevalence of Food Insecurity and Hunger—National Conditions and Trends

Eighty-nine percent of U.S. households were food secure throughout the entire year 2001. "Food secure" means that all household members had access at all times to enough food for an active, healthy life. The remaining 11.5 million U.S. households (10.7 percent of all households) were food insecure at some time during the year. That is, they were uncertain of having, or unable to acquire, enough food to meet basic needs for all household members because they had insufficient money and other resources for food. About two-thirds of food-insecure households avoided hunger, in many cases by relying on a few basic foods and reducing variety in their diets. But 3.5 million households (3.3 percent of all U.S. households) were food insecure to the extent that one or more household members were hungry, at least some time during the year, because they couldn't afford enough food. In most households, children were protected from substantial reductions in food intake and ensuing hunger. However, in some 211,000 households (0.6 percent of households with children) food insecurity was sufficiently severe that one or more children in each household were also hungry on one or more days during the year because the household lacked money for enough food. In some households with more than one child, not all the children experienced hunger. In particular, younger children are often protected from hunger even when older children are not.

When interpreting food security statistics, it is important to keep in mind that households are classified as food insecure, or food insecure with hunger if they experienced the condition at any time during the previous 12 months. The rates of food insecurity and hunger on any given day are far below the annual rates. For example, the prevalence of hunger on a typical day is estimated to be about 13 to 18 percent of the annual rate, or 0.4 to 0.6 percent of households (460,000 to 630,000 households) on a typical day in 2001.

How Often Were People Hungry in Households With Hunger?

When poverty-linked hunger occurs in the United States, it is, in most cases, occasional or episodic, not chronic. The food security scale on which the statistics in this report are based is designed to register these occasional or episodic occurrences. Most of the questions ask whether a condition, experience, or behavior occurred at any time in the past 12 months. Three of the questions ask how many months a specific condition or behavior occurred, but households can be classified as food insecure or hungry based on a single, severe episode during the year. It is important to keep this aspect of the scale in mind when interpreting food security and hunger statistics. ERS analysis of CPS Food Security Supplement data has found that:

- About one-third of the hunger measured by the standard 12-month measure is rare or occasional, occurring in only 1 or 2 months of the year. Two-thirds is recurring, experienced in 3 or more months of the year.

- For about one-fifth of households classified as food insecure and one-fourth of those classified as hungry, occurrence of the condition was frequent or chronic. That is, it occurred often, or in almost every month.
- The monthly prevalence of resource-constrained hunger in the United States is about 70 percent of the annual prevalence, and the daily prevalence of hunger is 13 to 18 percent of the annual prevalence. . . .

The prevalence of food insecurity and hunger increased somewhat from 1999 to 2001 after having declined from 1995 to 1999 (fig. 1). The year-to-year deviations from a consistent downward trend from 1995 to 2000 included a substantial 2-year cycle that is believed to result from a seasonal influence on food security prevalence rates (Cohen et al., 2002b). The CPS food security surveys over this period were conducted in April in odd-numbered years and August or September in even-numbered years. Measured prevalence of food insecurity was higher in the August/September collections, suggesting a seasonal response effect. In 2001, the survey was conducted in early December. Data collection is planned for December in future years, which will avoid further problems of seasonality effects in interpreting annual changes.

Figure 1

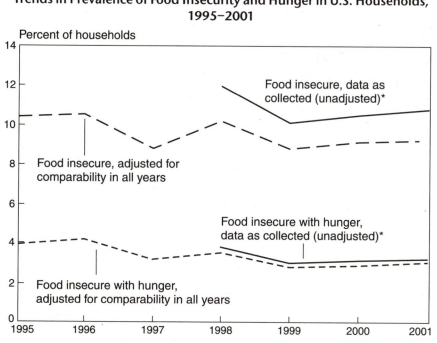

Trends in Prevalence of Food Insecurity and Hunger in U.S. Households, 1995–2001

*Data as collected in 1995–97 are not directly comparable with data collected in 1998–2001.
Source: Calculated by ERS based on Current Population Survey Food Security Supplement data.

A smaller food security survey was also conducted in April 2001 to provide information to bridge the new December series to the previous years' statistics, since seasonal effects of conducting the survey in December were unknown. Comparison of food security statistics from the April 2001 survey with those from April 1999 and December 2001 suggests that seasonal effects in early December were similar to those in April. At the national level, the measured prevalence of food insecurity was slightly higher and the prevalence of hunger was slightly lower in the December 2001 survey than in the April 2001 survey, but the differences were not statistically significant. From April 1999 to April 2001, prevalences of both food insecurity and hunger increased, and these increases were statistically significant.[1] Thus, the April 2001 survey confirms that the observed increases in food insecurity and hunger from April 1999 to December 2001 represented genuine changes from 1999 to 2001 and were not artifacts of the month in which surveys were conducted. Throughout this section, therefore, statistics from the December 2001 survey are compared with those from April 1999.

The prevalence of food insecurity rose from 10.1 percent in 1999 to 10.7 percent in 2001 and the prevalence of food insecurity with hunger rose from 3.0 percent to 3.3 percent (table 1). The number of food-insecure households increased from 10.5 million in 1999 to 11.5 million in 2001, an increase of 9.4 percent, and the number of households that were food insecure with hunger rose from 3.1 million to 3.5 million during the 2-year period, an increase of 12.9 percent. (During this period, the total number of households in the Nation grew by 3.0 percent.) The prevalence of food insecurity with hunger among children was unchanged from 1999 to 2001.

Prevalence of Food Insecurity and Hunger—Conditions and Trends, by Selected Household Characteristics

The prevalence of food insecurity and hunger varied considerably among household types. Rates of food insecurity were well below the national average of 10.7 percent for households with more than one adult and no children (6.0 percent) and for households with elderly persons (5.5 percent).[2] Rates of food insecurity substantially higher than the national average were registered by the following groups:

- households with incomes below the official poverty line (36.5 percent),[3]
- households with children, headed by a single woman (31.9 percent),
- Black households (21.3 percent), and
- Hispanic households (21.8 percent).

Overall, households with children reported food insecurity at more than double the rate for households without children (16.1 vs. 7.7 percent). Among households with children, those with married-couple families showed the lowest rate of food insecurity (10.7 percent).

The prevalence of food insecurity for households located in central cities (13.9 percent) and nonmetropolitan areas (11.5 percent) substantially exceeded

Table 1

Prevalence of Food Security, Food Insecurity, and Hunger by Year

| Unit | Total[1] | Food secure | | Food insecure | | | | | |
| | | | | All | | Without hunger | | With hunger | |
	1,000	1,000	Percent	1,000	Percent	1,000	Percent	1,000	Percent
Households									
1998	103,309	91,121	88.2	12,188	11.8	8,353	8.1	3,835	3.7
1999	104,684	94,154	89.9	10,529	10.1	7,420	7.1	3,109	3.0
2000	106,043	94,942	89.5	11,101	10.5	7,786	7.3	3,315	3.1
2001	107,824	96,303	89.3	11,521	10.7	8,010	7.4	3,511	3.3
All individuals (by food security status of household)[2]									
1998	268,366	232,219	86.5	36,147	13.5	26,290	9.8	9,857	3.7
1999	270,318	239,304	88.5	31,015	11.5	23,237	8.6	7,779	2.9
2000	273,685	240,454	87.9	33,231	12.1	24,708	9.0	8,523	3.1
2001	276,661	243,019	87.8	33,642	12.2	24,628	8.9	9,014	3.3
Adults (by food security status of household)[2]									
1998	197,084	174,964	88.8	22,120	11.2	15,632	7.9	6,488	3.3
1999	198,900	179,960	90.5	18,941	9.5	13,869	7.0	5,072	2.5
2000	201,922	181,586	89.9	20,336	10.1	14,763	7.3	5,573	2.8
2001	204,340	183,398	89.8	20,942	10.2	14,879	7.3	6,063	3.0

| | Total[1] | Food secure | | Food insecure | | | | | |
| | | | | All | | Without hunger among children | | With hunger among children | |
	1,000	1,000	Percent	1,000	Percent	1,000	Percent	1,000	Percent
Households with children									
1998	38,036	31,335	82.4	6,701	17.6	6,370	16.7	331	.9
1999	37,884	32,290	85.2	5,594	14.8	5,375	14.2	219	.6
2000	38,113	31,942	83.8	6,171	16.2	5,916	15.5	255	.7
2001	38,330	32,141	83.9	6,189	16.1	5,978	15.6	211	.6
Children (by food security status of household)[2]									
1998	71,282	57,255	80.3	14,027	19.7	13,311	18.7	716	1.0
1999	71,418	59,344	83.1	12,074	16.9	11,563	16.2	511	.7
2000	71,763	58,867	82.0	12,896	18.0	12,334	17.2	562	.8
2001	72,321	59,620	82.4	12,701	17.6	12,234	16.9	467	.6

[1]Totals exclude households whose food security status is unknown because they did not give a valid response to any of the questions in the food security scale. In 2001, these represented 353,000 households (0.3 percent of all households).

[2]The food security survey measures food security status at the household level. Not all individuals residing in food-insecure households are appropriately characterized as food insecure. Similarly, not all individuals in households classified as food insecure with hunger nor all children in households classified as food insecure with hunger among children were subject to reductions in food intake or experienced resource-constrained hunger.

Sources: Calculated by ERS using data from the August 1998, April 1999, September 2000, and December 2001 Current Population Survey Food Security Supplements.

the rate for households in suburbs and other metropolitan areas outside central cities (8.3 percent). Regionally, the prevalence of food insecurity was higher in the South and West (12.3 and 11.9 percent, respectively) than in the Northeast and Midwest (8.2 and 9.0 percent).

The prevalence of hunger in various types of households followed a pattern similar to that observed for food insecurity. Hunger rates were lowest for married couples with children (2.1 percent), multiple-adult households with no children (2.1 percent), and households with elderly persons (1.5 percent). Hunger rates were higher than the 3.3 percent national average among families headed by single women (8.7 percent), Black and Hispanic households (6.2 and 5.4 percent, respectively), and households below the poverty line (12.9 percent). Geographically, hunger was more common in central-city households (4.8 percent) and in those in the South and West (3.6 and 3.7 percent, respectively).

Households showing the lowest rates of hunger among children were married-couple families, single male-headed households, and households with higher incomes. Children living with a single mother were more affected by resource-constrained hunger, as were Black and Hispanic children.

The increases in food insecurity and hunger from 1999 to 2001 appear to have affected most regions and types of households. The prevalence of food insecurity increased for all regions except the Northeast, and for all types of households except single fathers with children, individuals living alone, households with elderly, and households with incomes below 130 percent of the poverty line. Few of the changes were statistically significant, but except as noted, the observed rates of food insecurity increased for all groups analyzed. Changes in the prevalence of food insecurity with hunger were less consistent across household types, with small, statistically insignificant changes for most groups.

Food Insecurity and Hunger in Low-Income Households

Food insecurity and hunger, as reported here, are by definition conditions that result from insufficient household resources. In 2001, food insecurity was six times as prevalent, and hunger seven times as prevalent, in households with annual income below 185 percent of the poverty line as in households with income above that range. However, many factors that might affect a household's food security (such as job loss, divorce, or other unexpected events) are not captured by an annual income measure. Some households experienced episodes of food insecurity, or even hunger, even though their annual income was well above the poverty line (Gundersen and Gruber, 2001). On the other hand, many low-income households (including almost two-thirds of those with income below the official poverty line) were food secure.

. . . Almost one-third of . . . low-income households [with annual incomes below 130 percent of the poverty line] were food insecure, and in 10.9 percent, household members experienced hunger at times during the year. Low-income households with children were more affected by food insecurity than households without children (41.4 percent vs. 24.8 percent), although the prevalence of hunger differed only slightly between the two categories. Low-income single mothers with children were especially vulnerable to both food insecurity and hunger; 45.5 percent of these households were food insecure, including 13.2 percent in which one or more persons, usually the mother, experienced hunger at times during the year because of lack of money or other resources for food.

Number of Persons by Household Food Security Status and Household Type

The food security survey is designed to measure food security status at the household level. While it is informative to examine the number of persons residing in food-insecure households, these estimates should not be used to characterize the number of individuals affected by food insecurity and hunger; not all persons in food-insecure households are food insecure. Similarly, people who live in households classified as food insecure with hunger, especially young children, are not all subject to reductions in food intake and do not all experience hunger.

In 2001, 33.6 million people lived in food-insecure households, up from 31.0 million in 1999 (table 1). They constituted 12.2 percent of the U.S. population and included 20.9 million adults and 12.7 million children. Of these individuals, 6.1 million adults and 3 million children lived in households where someone experienced hunger during the year. The number of children living in households classified as food insecure with hunger among children was 467,000 (0.6 percent of the children in the Nation; table 1). . . .

Prevalence of Food Insecurity and Hunger by State, 1999–2001

Prevalence rates of food insecurity and hunger varied considerably from State to State. Data for 3 years, 1999–2001, were combined to provide more reliable statistics at the State level. Measured prevalence rates of food insecurity during this 3-year period ranged from 6.5 percent in New Hampshire to 14.6 percent in New Mexico; measured prevalence rates of hunger ranged from 1.5 percent in Virginia to 5.8 percent in Oregon.

Notes

1. Prevalence rates of food insecurity were 10.1 percent in April 1999, 10.6 percent in April 2001, and 10.7 percent in December 2001; corresponding rates of food insecurity with hunger were 3.0, 3.4, and 3.3 percent.
2. "Elderly" in this report refers to persons age 65 and older.
3. The Federal poverty line was $17,960 for a family of four in 2001.

Robert E. Rector 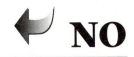 **NO**

The Myth of Widespread American Poverty

In the last week of September, the U.S. Census Bureau will issue its annual report on the number of Americans who are "living in poverty."

Census Bureau poverty reports vary little from year to year. For the past decade, the Census Bureau has declared that between 31.5 million and 39 million persons were living in poverty each year. Last year, for example, the Census Bureau declared there were 36.5 million poor Americans—nearly 14 percent of the U.S. population. But a close look at the actual material living standards of persons defined as "poor" by the Census Bureau demonstrates that the Bureau's official poverty report is misleading. For most Americans, the word "poverty" means destitution, an inability to provide a family with nutritious food, adequate clothing, and reasonable shelter. But only a small number of the 36.5 million persons classified as "poor" by the Census Bureau fit such a description.

In fact, numerous government reports indicate that most "poor" Americans today are better housed, better fed, and own more personal property than average Americans throughout most of this century. Today, inflation-adjusted expenditures per person among the lowest-income one-fifth (or quintile) of households equal those of the average American household in the early 1970s.

The following facts about persons defined as "poor" by the Census Bureau are taken from various government reports:

- In 1995, 41 percent of all "poor" households owned their own homes.
- The average home owned by a person classified as "poor" has three bedrooms, one-and-a-half baths, a garage, and a porch or patio.
- Over three-quarters of a million "poor" persons own homes worth over $150,000; and nearly 200,000 "poor" persons own homes worth over $300,000.
- Only 7.5 percent of "poor" households are overcrowded. Nearly 60 percent have two or more rooms per person.
- The average "poor" American has one-third more living space than the average Japanese does and four times as much living space as the average Russian.

- Seventy percent of "poor" households own a car; 27 percent own two or more cars.
- Ninety-seven percent have a color television. Nearly half own two or more televisions.
- Nearly three-quarters have a VCR; more than one in five has two VCRs.
- Two-thirds of "poor" households have air conditioning. By contrast, 30 years ago, only 36 percent of the entire U.S. population enjoyed air conditioning.
- Sixty-four percent of the "poor" own microwave ovens, half have a stereo system, and over a quarter have an automatic dishwasher.
- As a group, the "poor" are far from being chronically hungry and malnourished. In fact, poor persons are more likely to be overweight than are middle-class persons. Nearly half of poor adult women are overweight.
- Despite frequent charges of widespread hunger in the United States, 84 percent of the "poor" report their families have "enough" food to eat; 13 percent state they "sometimes" do not have enough to eat, and 3 percent say they "often" do not have enough to eat.
- The average consumption of protein, vitamins, and minerals is virtually the same for poor and middle-class children, and in most cases is well above recommended norms.
- Poor children actually consume more meat than do higher-income children and have average protein intakes that are 100 percent above recommended levels.
- Most poor children today are in fact super-nourished, growing up to be, on average, one inch taller and ten pounds heavier that the GIs who stormed the beaches of Normandy in World War II.

Why the Census Data Are Badly Flawed

The Census Bureau counts as poor any household with cash income that is less than the official poverty threshold—which, in 1997, was $16,404 for a family of four. But the Census Bureau dramatically undercounts the incomes of these less affluent Americans. Other government surveys consistently show that spending by low-income households greatly exceeds the income the Census Bureau claims they have.

Why does this happen? Careful examination reveals that the annual Census poverty report dramatically exaggerates poverty and misrepresents the living conditions of lower-income Americans. The inaccuracy of the report is the result of three errors:

1. The Census Bureau deems that a family is "poor" if its annual cash income falls below certain specified "income thresholds." These thresholds were set in the early 1960s and have been raised upward in each subsequent year to adjust for inflation. For example, the poverty threshold for a family of four was roughly $3,100 in 1963 and reached

$16,404 in 1997. This official poverty measurement served initially as a public relations instrument in President Lyndon Johnson's larger "War on Poverty." Therefore, the initial income thresholds were set artificially high in order to enlarge the apparent numbers of the poor and build public support for Johnson's welfare policies. Although families with incomes below the thresholds will face many financial difficulties, they are not necessarily poor in the sense of lacking adequate food, shelter, and clothing.

2. In determining whether a family is poor, the Census Bureau considers only current income and ignores all assets accumulated in prior years. Thus, a businessman who suffers temporary business losses resulting in a negative net income for the year will be labeled as "poor" even if he has a million dollars sitting in the bank.

3. The most critical error by far is that the Census radically undercounts the true economic resources or annual income received by the American public. This may be seen by comparing Census income figures with the U.S. Department of Commerce's National Income and Product Accounts (NIPA), which provide the figures measuring the gross national product (GNP). In 1996, NIPA figures show that aggregate "personal income" of Americans was $6.8 trillion. By contrast, aggregate personal income according to the Census Bureau's official definition of income was only $4.8 trillion. In other words, the Census missed $2 trillion in annual income, or roughly $20,000 for each U.S. household. The missing $2 trillion of personal income exceeds the entire economies of most of the world's nations. Much of the missing income belongs to the middle class and the rich; but low-income families receive a large slice as well. . . .

Food Shortage and Hunger

There are frequent charges of widespread hunger and malnutrition in the United States. Reliable survey data show that while hunger definitely exists in the United States, it is relatively restricted in scope and frequency. For example, the Third National Health and Nutrition Examination Survey conducted by the U.S. Department of Health and Human Services in 1988–1989 found that 96 percent of U.S. households reported they had "enough food to eat." Some 3 percent reported that they "sometimes" did not have enough food, and around a half percent said they "often" did not have enough food. Among the poor, 84 percent reported having enough food, while 13.2 percent reported shortages "sometimes," and 2.7 percent "often." [See Figure 1]

Poverty and Food Quality

It is widely believed that lack of financial resources forces poor people to eat low-quality diets that are deficient in nutriments and high in fat. However, survey data show that nutriment density (amount of vitamins, minerals, and protein per 1,000 calories of food) does not vary by income class. Nor do the poor

Figure 1

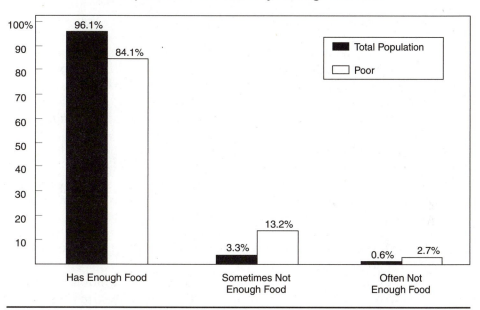

Self-Reported Food Sufficiency Among Americans

Source: Department of Health and Human Services, *Third National Health and Nutrition Examination Survey, 1988–91;* cited in the USDA Third Report on Nutrition Monitoring in the United States, Vol. 2, p. VA95.

Table 1

Fat Intake and Poverty

	Low: Fat Intake At or Below 30% of Calories		Medium: Fat Intake Between 30% and 40% of Calories		High: Fat Intake Greater than 40% of Calories	
	Male	Female	Male	Female	Male	Female
Adults with Income Below 131% of Poverty Level	21.7%	25.9%	50.9%	53.0%	27.4%	21.0%
Adults with Income Above 350% of Poverty Level	22.3%	23.6%	52.0%	53.0%	25.7%	23.0%

Source: USDA Continuing Survey of Food Intakes by Individuals 1989–91, cited in *Third Report on Nutrition Monitoring,* Vol. 2, p. VA 167.

consume higher-fat diets than the middle class. Table 1 shows the percentage of calories derived from fat for low-income and high-income adult men and women; there is little variation by income level. The percentage with high fat intake (as a share of total calories) is virtually the same for low-income and upper-middle-income persons.

Poverty and Nutrition

The U.S. Department of Agriculture periodically surveys the food and nutriment consumption of American households. These surveys provide little evidence of widespread under-nutrition among the poor; in fact, they show that the average nutriment consumption among the poor closely resembles that of the upper middle class. Example: Children in families with incomes below the poverty level actually consume more meat than do children in families with incomes at 350 percent of poverty or higher (roughly $57,000 for a family of four in today's dollars).

. . . The intake of nutriments is very similar for poor and middle-class children, and is generally well above the recommended daily level. For example, the consumption of protein (a relatively expensive nutriment) among poor children is, on average, between 150 and 267 percent of the RDA.

When shortfalls of specific vitamins and minerals appear (for example, among teenage girls), they tend to be very similar for the poor and the middle class. For example, while poor teenage girls, on average, tend to under-consume Vitamin E, Vitamin B-6, calcium, phosphorus, magnesium, iron, and zinc, a virtually identical under-consumption of these same nutriments appears among upper-middle-class teenage girls.

Overall, examination of the average nutriment consumption of Americans reveals that age and gender play a far greater role in determining nutritional patterns than does income. The average nutriment intakes of adult women in the upper middle class (above 350 percent of poverty) more closely resemble the intakes of poor women than they do those of upper-middle-class men, children, or teens. The nutriment consumption of upper-middle-income preschoolers, as a group, is virtually identical to that of poor preschoolers, but not to the consumption of adults or older children in the upper middle class. This same pattern holds for adult males, teens, and most other age and gender groups.

It is important to note that the nutriment intake . . . represent[s] only the average nutriment intakes for poor children in various age categories . . . [and] do[es] not necessarily rule out the possibility that there could be pockets of under-nutrition within each age group of poor children even while the average consumption of the group remains high. The data do, however, refute any claim of widespread under-nutrition and hunger among poor children in general.

Increase in Children's Size

During this century, improvements in nutrition and health have led to increases in the rate of growth and ultimate height and weight of American children. Poor children have been affected by this trend. Poor boys today at ages 18 and 19 are actually taller and heavier than similar aged boys in the general U.S. population in the late 1950s. Poor boys living today are one inch taller and some ten pounds heavier than GIs of similar age during World War II, and nearly two inches taller and 20 pounds heavier than American doughboys back in World War I.

This does not mean, of course, that all poor children have now reached optimal levels of health and nutrition. In particular, poor children remain more likely to be born at low birth weight than are children of higher income groups. Low birth weight, in turn, contributes to a slightly disproportionate number of poor children being short for their age, particularly in the preschool years. However, the general trend among poor children has been one of marked improvements in health and nutrition, leading to rapid growth and large stature.

Poverty and Obesity

The principal nutrition-related health problem among the poor, as with the general U.S. population, stems from over-consumption, not the under-consumption, of food. While overweight and obesity are prevalent problems throughout the United States, they are found most frequently among poor adults. . . . [N]early half of poor adult women are overweight, compared with a third of women who are not poor.

Recently, health experts have expressed concern over the growing problem of obesity among children. Poor children have not been immune to this problem, and some studies actually have found obesity to be more prevalent among poor children than among middle-class children. For example, a recent pediatric study examined height and weight of school children aged 5 to 12 in inner-city Harlem. The children in the study were black or Hispanic, and nearly all were from low-income households. As a whole, these economically disadvantaged inner-city children were found to be above average in height and weight, compared with government norms. A large sub-group was markedly obese: The study noted that "more than a quarter of central Harlem children could be considered obese; of whom nearly 14% would be super obese." The authors noted the contrast between these inner-city children and the image of the lean black child that emerged from studies in the late 1960s.

Dr. Sue Kimm of the University of Pittsburgh used data from the Growth and Health Study (NGHS) of the National Heart, Lung, and Blood Institute to examine the relationship between obesity and socioeconomic status, based on a sample of nine- and ten-year-old girls drawn from Ohio, California, and the District of Columbia in 1987. The study found 19 percent of white girls and 31 percent of black girls were overweight. White girls from low-income families (below $10,000) were two to three times more likely to be overweight than were middle- and upper-income girls. The prevalence of obesity among blacks did not vary according to family income.

Conclusion

If poverty is defined as generally lacking adequate nutritious food for one's family, suitable clothing, and a reasonably warm, dry apartment in which to live, or lacking a car to get to work when one is needed, then there are few poor persons remaining in the United States. Real material hardship does occur in America, but it is limited in both extent and severity. The bulk of the "poor" live in material conditions that would have been judged comfortable or well-off just a few generations ago.

The old maxim that "the rich get richer and the poor get poorer" is simply untrue. Material conditions of lower-income Americans have improved dramatically over time. In fact, living conditions in the nation as a whole have improved so much that American society can no longer clearly remember what it meant to be poor or even middle class in earlier generations.

But higher material living standards should not be regarded as a victory for the War on Poverty. Living conditions were improving dramatically and poverty was dropping sharply long before the War on Poverty began. The principal effect of the War on Poverty has been not to raise incomes, but to displace self-sufficiency with dependence. A second consequence of welfare has been the destruction of families. When the War on Poverty began, 7.7 percent of children were born out of wedlock. Today, the figure is 32 percent. Using the Census Bureau's own standards, a child born to a never-married mother is 700 percent more likely to live in poverty than is a child born to a husband and wife whose marriage remains intact.

The Census poverty report has been tightly linked to the War on Poverty since its inception. The implicit message of the poverty report is that government should throw more and more welfare benefits at low-income communities in an effort to artificially raise family incomes above the official poverty thresholds. Such welfare policies have been disastrous.

Despite spending $7 trillion, the War on Poverty—by eroding the work ethic and marriage—has failed. By undermining families' capacity for self-support, the War on Poverty expanded the clientele of needy persons. Government became caught in a trap: The more aid that it gave, the more persons in apparent need of its aid emerged. With the Welfare Reform Act of 1996, the federal government finally began to break away from this failed entitlement mentality. But the Census Bureau report continues to embody the old, failed philosophy of unending free handouts.

The Census poverty report also has had a distorting effect on the national dialogue by focusing attention exclusively on income and material living standards while ignoring values and behavior. The report is rooted in the belief that "poverty" causes social problems such as crime, drug use, school failure, illegitimacy, and dependence. This belief, although common, is false. Clearly, there were far more truly poor persons in earlier generations than there are today. (In fact, nearly all adults alive today had parents or grandparents who grew up "poor" in the sense of having incomes below the current Census thresholds, adjusted for inflation.) If it were true that "poverty" causes social and behavioral problems, then earlier generations should have been awash in drugs, crime, and promiscuity. But this was not the case. Most social problems have expanded as incomes have increased.

In reality, it is the norms and values within a family, rather than its income, that are critical to a child's well-being and prospects for success in future life. Ironically, conventional welfare, with its misplaced emphasis on artificially boosting income, has a strongly damaging effect on the very values that are critical to a child's success. By ignoring values and undermining the norms of work, self-control, and marital stability, the War on Poverty has harmed those whom it intended to help.

Overall, the Census poverty report is deeply flawed as a measurement tool and misleading as a policy indicator. The report not only exaggerates poverty, but, even more tragically, encourages policymakers to focus on the symptom of income shortage while ignoring behavioral problems, which are the root causes of the lack of income. As such, the report serves both society and the poor badly.

POSTSCRIPT

Does Widespread Hunger Exist in America?

Since the days of the War on Poverty, advocates for the poor have maintained that federal welfare policies fail to provide an adequate safety net for the most vulnerable segments of the population. For years, they conducted small, local hunger surveys to demonstrate the need for more food and income assistance. The Heritage Foundation and other such groups argued that the survey results were too flawed to constitute a basis for expanding the welfare system. They argued that rather than aiding the poor, welfare causes poverty by increasing dependency and undermining self-reliance. In response to such criticisms, university and government researchers improved the reliability of their survey methods and developed questions that correlated highly with other measures of food insecurity. On the basis of answers to these questions, the USDA has produced estimates of the extent of food insecurity in the U.S. population since 1995. The agency finds food insecurity and hunger not only to exist in America but also to have increased slightly in the past few years. Supporting this finding is the possibility that the USDA is underestimating the extent of food insecurity because its surveys do not include the homeless. Furthermore, the Brandeis University Center on Hunger and Poverty (http://www.centeronhunger.org/index.shtml) has performed its own analyses and confirmed the USDA's results in August 2002. Although the USDA economists do not offer policy recommendations, their work has obvious implications for federal policies and programs. The United States is a wealthy country, with resources that are more than adequate to feed everyone in the population. If people do not have enough food for lack of personal resources, shouldn't the government expand welfare and food assistance benefits to make sure that no adult or child goes hungry?

Opposing this view are conservative policy analysts like Rector who view welfare and food assistance not as a solution to problems of poverty but as their *cause*. As evidence, Rector cites studies finding that the nutrient intake of the poor is no different from that of wealthier Americans and that their rates of overweight and obesity are higher than among the general population. Indeed, researchers have shown that people who report not getting enough food to eat are more likely to be obese (Townsend et al., *Journal of Nutrition*, June 2001). However, recent evidence contradicts the first contention. New York University professor Beth Dixon and her colleagues, for example, reporting in the *Journal of Nutrition* (April 2001), found that adults in food-insufficient families consumed less of several key vitamins and minerals than their food-sufficient counterparts. They found the intake of some nutrients to be so far below standard as to constitute a health risk. Similarly, a study published in the *American*

Journal of Public Health (May 2001) reported that food-insufficient children display higher rates of iron deficiency than children living in food-sufficient households.

On the other hand, much evidence supports Rector's contention that rates of overweight and obesity are higher among the poor. Researchers examining this "unexpected and paradoxical association" conclude that food insecurity is a significant *predictor* of overweight, particularly among recipients of federal food stamps (*Journal of Nutrition,* June 2001). Although food stamps permit recipients to purchase food at lower cost, the benefits typically run out after about three weeks. According to these researchers, inadequate resources to purchase food leads to cycles of food surplus and inadequacy. Recipients overeat when they receive food stamps but go hungry when the benefits run out. If this as yet unproven supposition is correct, it argues for increasing food stamp benefits. Opponents of this view, however, are likely to argue that doing so would only increase dependency and, therefore, be counterproductive.

Rector agrees that hunger exists, but he views the magnitude of the problem as minimal. Whether nearly half a million children reported as hungry is a large or small problem depends on point of view. Advocates for the poor find such figures shameful in so rich a country. Conservatives tend to minimize their significance. Because this argument depends on values rather than science, efforts to improve the methods used to define hunger and food security are unlikely to resolve debates about the significance of the numbers of the hungry and food insecure. Questions of values require political rather than scientific resolution.

ISSUE 14

Should Mothers Infected With the AIDS Virus Breastfeed Their Infants?

YES: Jean Humphrey and Peter Iliff, from "Is Breast Not Best? Feeding Babies Born to HIV-Positive Mothers: Bringing Balance to a Complex Issue," *Nutrition Reviews* (April 2001)

NO: Dorothy Mbori-Ngacha et al., from "Morbidity and Mortality in Breastfed and Formula-Fed Infants of HIV-1–Infected Women: A Randomized Clinical Trial," *Journal of the American Medical Association* (November 21, 2001)

ISSUE SUMMARY

YES: Johns Hopkins public health researcher Jean Humphrey and her Zimbabwe-based colleague Peter Iliff argue that the mortality risks of formula feeding are so high that infants of mothers infected with Human Immunodeficiency Virus (HIV), the virus that causes Acquired Immunodeficiency Syndrome (AIDS), have a better chance of survival if they are breastfed.

NO: Pediatrician Dorothy Mbori-Ngacha and her research colleagues argue that formula feeding is a safe alternative to breastfeeding and ensures longer survival of infants of HIV-infected mothers.

$\mathbf{B}$reast milk is a perfect food for human infants, and nearly all mothers are fully capable of breastfeeding. Despite these undeniable facts, many mothers choose to feed their infants substitutes for breast milk—commercial formulas. Formulas contain cow's milk or soy proteins with added sugars, vitamins, and minerals. They reproduce most of the nutritional characteristics of breast milk but lack immune substances that protect against microbial infections. Furthermore, most formulas must be diluted to appropriate concentrations; this requires adequate supplies of clean, uncontaminated water. Clean water is often unavailable in developing areas. Formulas are an excellent medium for growth of bacteria and must be stored under refrigeration to avoid microbial contaminants that might cause infants to develop diarrhea. Diarrheal diseases deplete infants of fluids and essential nutrients and are a principal cause of infant mortality. One additional problem is that breast milk substitutes must be purchased. Their appropriate use requires income, education, a clean water supply, and refrigeration. Because such conditions are not always available in Africa and other developing areas, the use of commercial infant formulas has long been associated with diarrhea-induced malnutrition, stunted growth, and deaths of children and adults in such areas. As a result, breastfeeding advocates have long opposed efforts of formula manufacturers to market their products in developing countries.

In recent years, advocacy of breastfeeding has been complicated by issues related to the transmission of the Human Immunodeficiency Virus (HIV) from infected mothers to their infants. This virus causes the Acquired Immunodeficiency Syndrome (AIDS). In some areas of Africa, nearly 50 percent of all pregnant women are infected with HIV and can transmit it to up to half of their children. Because appropriate use of breast milk substitutes can prevent nearly 50 percent of such infections, commercial infant formulas might seem to be the solution to the problem of HIV transmission. But are they?

Jean Humphrey and Peter Iliff argue that the mortality risk associated with the use of infant formulas is so great that it offsets the benefits of preventing mother-to-child transmission of HIV. Even when mothers are educated and have access to clean water, use of infant formulas still carries a substantial risk. Instead, they say, efforts to make breastfeeding safer are a better alternative for ensuring the health and survival of African infants born to HIV-infected women.

Dorothy Mbori-Ngacha and her colleagues, however, have evaluated the infant mortality risks associated with formula feeding by low-income mothers infected with HIV. They found little difference in rates of diarrhea and mortality among breastfed and formula-fed infants during the first two years of life. At age two, however, formula-fed infants were much more likely to remain uninfected with HIV. Furthermore, infants infected with HIV during the first two months of life were more likely to die than those infected after the age of two months, suggesting that early transmission of HIV through breastfeeding is particularly harmful. In addition, the mothers of formula-fed infants were more likely to be alive after two years. On the basis of these findings, the researchers conclude that formula feeding is not only a safe alternative to breastfeeding but also is better for the health of mothers as well as their children.

In reading the following selections, it is worth noting how the approaches of the investigators differ. The study by Humphrey and Iliff is an analysis of the body of research published on this question through April 2001. The single study by Mbori-Ngacha et al. appeared later that year. Would Humphrey and Iliff be likely to change their opinion on the basis of the more recent study? Why might HIV-infected mothers live longer if their infants are fed formula rather than breast milk? The policy implications of this argument are also of interest. How might positions on this question affect public health advice for pregnant women in general as opposed to advice for an individual pregnant woman? How might the interests of formula manufacturers enter into this debate?

In the following selections, public health researchers Humphrey and Iliff argue that breastfeeding remains best for infants of HIV-infected mothers, but Mbori-Ngacha et al. maintain that formula feeding is preferable.

Jean Humphrey and Peter Iliff 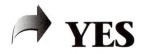 **YES**

Is Breast Not Best? Feeding Babies Born to HIV-Positive Mothers: Bringing Balance to a Complex Issue

Introduction

Surely one of the most poignant tragedies of the HIV pandemic is this: whereas breastfeeding prevents an estimated 6 million infant deaths each year throughout the world, it also results in 200,000–300,000 infant HIV infections. (An estimated 620,000 children became infected with HIV in 1999 and of these, ⅓–½ are estimated to have been infected during breastfeeding.) Furthermore, the first 6 months of life, when breastfeeding is most critical to preventing infant deaths and *not* breastfeeding is associated with a two- to tenfold higher risk of infant death in many developing countries, is the same period when the majority of breastfeeding-associated HIV transmission probably occurs.

This [selection] will review the paradigm shift regarding infant feeding in the context of the HIV epidemic from 1985—when the first case of breastfeeding-associated transmission was reported—up to and focusing on the first published randomized breastfeeding versus formula feeding trial from Kenya in 2000, which confirmed that mother-to-child transmission (MTCT) of HIV during breastfeeding can be substantial. We will then examine the delicate balance between the life-saving benefits and the HIV infection risks of breastfeeding for babies born to HIV-positive women in Africa. The factors that are likely to determine the net balance of these opposing risks for an individual baby will be explored. Finally, we will estimate the number of HIV-positive African women for whom the Kenyan study results are likely to be applicable.

Chronology of the Breastfeeding Transmission of HIV Problem

The first case of MTCT of HIV during breastfeeding was reported in 1985. This report, based on a breastfeeding mother who had been infected with HIV soon after delivery by way of an infected blood transfusion, established that it is

From Jean Humphrey and Peter Iliff, "Is Breast Not Best? Feeding Babies Born to HIV-Positive Mothers: Bringing Balance to a Complex Issue," *Nutrition Reviews,* vol. 59, no. 4 (April 2001). Copyright © 2001 by The International Life Sciences Institute. Reprinted by permission. References omitted.

biologically possible for HIV to be transmitted from mother to baby via breast-feeding. This was quickly confirmed by other case reports mostly of breastfeeding mothers who were at low risk for HIV infection and who were presumed HIV-negative until they received an infected blood transfusion soon after delivery. Many authors suggested that breastfeeding shortly after maternal seroconversion may represent a special high-risk situation; this is because the viral load in milk probably parallels the peak viremia associated with primary infection. It was therefore thought that this risk should *not* be extrapolated to lactating women with previously established HIV infection, who, globally, made up the vast majority of HIV-positive breastfeeding women. Because these cases demonstrated a theoretical risk for previously infected women, however, the U.S. Centers for Disease Control and Prevention immediately recommended that known HIV-positive women avoid breastfeeding. Other industrialized countries soon followed suit.

From the late 1980s to the mid-1990s, data steadily accumulated from studies comparing infection rates of babies born to HIV-positive mothers who had self-selected breastfeeding or formula feeding. Though two studies reported similar rates of MTCT for breastfed and formula-fed infants, the majority observed excess rates of infection ranging from 12% to 46% among the breastfed compared with the formula-fed babies. Six of these studies were included in a meta-analysis published in 1992 that estimated the average excess risk of MTCT attributable to breastfeeding by women with established HIV infection to be 14%. Among women seroconverting [blood tests changing from no HIV to HIV positive] during lactation, the estimated risk was twice that, namely 29%. These figures became the most frequently cited estimates on this issue for the remainder of the decade.

In 1987 and 1992, the World Health Organization published consensus statements recommending that, "where the primary causes of infant deaths are infectious diseases and malnutrition . . . breastfeeding should remain the standard advice to pregnant women, including those known to be HIV infected." The recommendation continued, however, that, "where infectious diseases are not the primary causes of death during infancy, pregnant women known to be infected with HIV should be advised not to breastfeed but to use a safe feeding alternative for their babies."

Though this policy was meant to recommend the feeding option that would result in the greatest probability of HIV infection–free survival for babies in each environment based on evidence available at that time, it was often viewed by developing country authorities as a "double standard" and the issue became highly emotive and polarized. One breastfeeding expert wrote in *The New England Journal of Medicine* in 1992, "The role of breastfeeding in the transmission of HIV-1 remains doubtful and at worst minuscule," whereas in the same year an HIV expert pointed out that, " . . . nine cases that strongly suggest transmission of HIV-1 through breastfeeding have been described . . . careful, large-scale, prospective cohort studies . . . are of the utmost priority."

Between 1994 and 1997, four carefully analyzed prospective cohort studies were published. All estimated the excess risk of HIV transmission attributable to breastfeeding as ranging from a minimum of 4% to a maximum of 22%, depending on how infants were classified. This stronger evidence led to a major shift in policy of the relevant United Nations organizations (WHO, UNICEF, and UNAIDS), who jointly published revised recommendations in 1997 and 1998. These recommendations acknowledged that more than one-third of all pediatric HIV infections were acquired during breastfeeding and that if (but only if) babies of HIV-positive mothers could be ensured uninterrupted access to nutritionally adequate, safely prepared breast milk substitutes, they would be at less risk of illness and death. The reports recommended that women have access to testing and counseling and "be empowered to make fully informed decisions about infant feeding."

Over the past couple of years, formula feeding has become the standard for babies of HIV-positive women in some intermediate-economy countries (Thailand, Brazil, and some parts of South Africa). This is not the case in the rest of sub-Saharan Africa, however, which is home to more than 10.6 million HIV-infected women of reproductive age (two-thirds of the global total). These women experience a gross national product of $US375 (roughly equivalent to the cost of a 6-month supply of infant formula), an infant mortality rate of 100/1000 live births, and 45% do not have access to safe water. Most of these women have not had access to HIV testing, let alone information or resources enabling them to make and implement "fully informed decisions about infant feeding."

The Role of "Exclusive" Breastfeeding, Breast Pathology, and Other Practices

In 1999, a seemingly paradoxical study was published from Durban, South Africa. HIV-positive women who chose to breastfeed were counseled to do so exclusively—giving nothing at all except breast milk for up to 6 months, at which point they were counseled to wean rapidly. Transmission rates at 3 months of age among infants who received exclusively breast milk, exclusively formula, and mixed feedings were 14.6%, 18.8%, and 24.1%, respectively. The rates for exclusively breastfed and exclusively formula-fed infants were not statistically different, but the difference between exclusive breastfeeding and mixed feeding was large (a 48% reduction in risk of transmission after adjustment for potential confounders) and significant. . . . At 6 months, the cumulative probabilities of HIV infection were nearly identical between babies who were exclusively breastfed for at least 3 months and babies who were exclusively replacement-fed (19.4% in both groups); the rate among babies who received mixed feedings was 26.1%. The authors suggested that feeding non–breast milk foods may impair gut integrity by way of infection, allergy, or trauma. When the baby is also fed HIV-containing breast milk, the damage to the gut may facilitate viral absorption. Thus, "mixed feeding" may represent the riskiest feeding mode for babies of HIV-positive mothers.

Criticism of this study has included the possibility of reverse causality: perhaps HIV-associated illness of the mother, baby, or both was an impetus to begin mixed feeding. The authors addressed this by comparing morbidity rates among children who continued exclusive breastfeeding with those of children who received mixed feedings and found no differences in reported diarrhea, lower respiratory tract infections, or candida infection (personal communication, Anna Coutsoudis, October 2000).

In 1999, Semba and colleagues in Malawi showed that high sodium content in breast milk, first suggested to be an indicator of subclinical mastitis by Ball and colleagues, was associated with higher viral loads in breast milk and increased rates of HIV transmission from mother to child. This corroborated an earlier case report of a breastfed infant who became infected soon after his HIV-positive mother developed a breast abscess. These findings suggested that breast pathology may be an important risk factor for breastfeeding-associated HIV transmission. A more recent study among HIV-negative Bangladeshi women showed that sodium content of breast milk can be reduced by practicing good lactation management, which minimizes engorgement, mastitis, and nipple disease. This intervention has not yet been formally evaluated among HIV-positive lactating women. Semba's work was also the first to document that high viral load of breast milk is associated with higher transmission rates. Because we know that unprotected sex can reinfect HIV-positive women and increase plasma viral load, it makes sense that practicing safe sex during the breastfeeding period may limit milk viral concentrations, and thereby reduce breastfeeding-associated transmission. All of these studies indicated that we could no longer think only about "ever" versus "never" breastfed babies when considering the risk of postnatal MTCT transmission of HIV. Weaning patterns, breast pathology . . . and positioning during breastfeeding, and maternal sexual practices may all influence this risk.

Nairobi Randomized Trial of Feeding Method

The cohort studies followed women who self-selected their infant feeding method. Though care was taken to control for baseline differences in all studies, and the consistency between them strengthened their conclusions, several writers suggested over the years that only a randomized controlled trial of breastfeeding versus formula feeding would provide an unbiased estimate of the risk of transmission through breastfeeding. In 1992, Dr. Ruth Nduati and colleagues in Nairobi, Kenya started such a trial. It was completed in 1998 and the long-awaited results were published in March 2000. A total of 16,529 pregnant women were screened for HIV and 2315 (14%) were identified as HIV-positive. Of these, 425 (18% of the HIV-positive women identified) returned for their test results and agreed to join the trial. The two major reasons for women declining to join were unwillingness to be randomized to formula feeding and plans to leave Nairobi after delivery.

The authors did an impressive job of successfully meeting the many ethical challenges of such a study. One of the ways they did this was by setting stringent criteria that would limit the risk of infant illness owing to not breastfeeding among those randomized to formula feeding. For example, only women with access to municipal water were enrolled. The study population was therefore "highly selected," of ethical necessity. All women received extensive counseling by a study physician on MTCT and the relative risks and benefits of breastfeeding and formula feeding. Participants were described as being of lower socioeconomic status, but were relatively well educated (mean 8 years schooling). They were enrolled and randomly allocated to formula feeding or breastfeeding at approximately 32 weeks gestation.

Women in the formula feeding arm were instructed in safe formula preparation, and in a subsequent visit were asked to demonstrate their skills. Key tasks included use of boiled water in mixing formula and feeding by cup rather than by bottle. Free dried milk commercial infant formula was provided for the first 6 months of life. The authors reported no special feeding instructions for the mothers in the breastfeeding group. Home visits were conducted at 2 weeks postpartum and then as needed. Mother-baby pairs were followed up monthly for the first year and quarterly for the second year, and given free clinical care. HIV was diagnosed in infants by DNA–polymerase chain reaction on blood taken at birth, 6 weeks, 14 weeks, and every 3 months thereafter until 24 months of age. Intention to treat analyses were carried out to calculate MTCT rates, timing of transmission, mortality rates, and infection-free survival rates using a sophisticated method for estimating joint distribution of death and HIV-1 infection.

The key findings of this study were:

1. At 24 months, 36.7% of breastfed compared with 20.5% of formula-fed infants were HIV-infected, representing a 16.2% excess risk of transmission in the breastfeeding arm. Most of this excess transmission occurred early. Sixty-three percent, 75%, and 87% of the overall difference had already occurred at 6 weeks, 6 months, and 12 months, respectively. Thus, this study confirmed the findings of many observational studies: breastfeeding can nearly double the risk of MTCT and early breastfeeding carries the greatest risk.

2. Mortality at 24 months was high in both groups: 244/1000 and 200/1000 in the breastfeeding group and formula feeding group, respectively. In the first 6 weeks of life, mortality among all children was four times greater among the formula-fed children compared with the breastfed children. . . . The point estimates for cumulative mortality continued to be higher in the formula-fed group compared with the breastfed group (though not statistically different) until 12 months of age, when mortality among the breastfed babies began to exceed that of the formula-fed babies (differences were again not statistically significant). A recent analysis showed that among children who were HIV-negative, those in the formula group were six times more likely to die in the first 6 months of life compared with those in the breastfeeding group (5% of the formula-fed babies versus 0.8% of the breastfed babies died). Thus, this study also confirmed decades of work demonstrating that *not* breastfeeding is associated with substantial risk of death, especially for the youngest babies.

3. HIV-free survival was greater at 24 months in the formula-fed group compared with the breastfed group (70% versus 58%). This calculation shows that, *in this study population* the balance of risks favored those in the formula group.

4. Compliance with the formula arm of intervention (defined as complete avoidance of breast milk) was 70%. Compliance with the breastfeeding intervention (defined as any use of breast milk) was 96%.

Under the conditions of this study, therefore, formula feeding nearly halved MTCT of HIV and increased HIV infection–free survival by 12%. These benefits are substantial and immediately beg these questions: Will formula feeding, or more generally, replacement feeding, result in a better outcome for *all* HIV-positive women in developing countries (more than 80% of whom live in sub-Saharan Africa)? . . .

For How Many Women Are the Nairobi Results Valid?

As a first step in estimating the number of HIV-positive African women to whom the Nairobi results might be relevant, we estimated the number who are likely have a similarly low R [R: Relative risk of death attributable to *not* breastfeeding] based on access to safe water and literacy. Of the nearly 13 million HIV-positive women of reproductive age living in sub-Saharan Africa, 55% (7.2 million) have access to safe water and nearly the same number (7.1 million) are literate. They are no doubt mostly the same women. Therefore, replacement feeding might be favorable for roughly 7 million babies if factors to minimize R are put in place (as they were carefully implemented in the Nairobi study) and if women accept and comply with these interventions.

The first assumption requires huge resources and ingenuity. The second assumption is more difficult to estimate: what proportion of these 7 million women will be willing to learn their HIV status, disclose it to others, prepare and feed the replacement feeding safely, limit rural travel so they can attend frequent medical care and access replacement feedings, and have husbands and other close family members who will support them in this process? In the Nairobi study, 18% of the identified HIV-positive women agreed to know their HIV results, stay in Nairobi where they could access formula supplies, counseling, and clinical follow up, and said they would be willing to formula-feed if they were randomized to that arm of the study.

Why was this proportion so low? The proportion of antenatal women willing to be tested and told their HIV status varies greatly across African settings, but is frequently low. Frequent travel between rural and urban homes and being away from an urban setting for prolonged periods (e.g., planting or harvesting times) is the norm for most African populations. Finally, breastfeeding is universal in most of Africa; *not* breastfeeding may label a woman as being HIV-positive, as having an evil spirit, or as being sexually promiscuous and unfaithful to her husband. Thus, it is not surprising that only 18% of the screened HIV-positive women in Nairobi agreed to comply with these conditions. Applying the 18% acceptance rate to the 7 million women with adequate education and safe water implies that replacement feeding will increase HIV infection−free survival for 1.3 million babies (approximately 10% of all babies born to the 13 million HIV-positive African women). . . .

It is critical to understand that this discussion is not just a description of how hard it is to put these programs in place—the answer to that would be to work harder. This is an estimate of how many of these mothers will not be able to comply with the conditions that will make replacement feeding favorable; it is an estimate of the number of babies whose chance of HIV infection−free survival would be better if they were breastfed, even though their mothers are relatively educated and have access to safe water.

Compliance With "Exclusive" Feeding: A Core Issue

The findings from South Africa suggest that mixed feeding is twice as risky as either exclusive replacement feeding or exclusive breastfeeding. If these findings are confirmed, and in situations where minimum maternal education, access to safe water, uninterrupted supply of replacement feeding, and accessible clinical care are in place, counseling sessions with an individual HIV-positive mother should focus on helping her decide with which mode—exclusive replacement feeding or exclusive breastfeeding—she is most likely to comply. Both of these "exclusive" feeding modes have proved difficult to implement. Of the "highly selected" women in the Nairobi study that were randomized to the formula feeding arm, received intensive counseling to avoid breastfeeding, and initially agreed to comply with the study protocol, 30% admitted to partially breastfeeding. Given all the social constraints *not* to replacement feed in Africa, the pressure to breastfeed, even occasionally or for a short time, can be intense for some women. In our work in Zimbabwe, some women have told us that they formula-feed in private, but breastfeed in public. Anecdotal reports from some of the MTCT pilot projects offering antiretroviral drugs and free infant formula suggest that many women accept the formula, but then also breastfeed.

On the other hand, exclusive breastfeeding is also not the norm in most of the world, including Africa. In 1999, 38.6% of Zimbabwean infants ages 0−3 months and 7.2% of those ages 4−6 months were exclusively breastfed. In Kwazulu Natal, nearly half of the mothers in a longitudinal study of infant feeding had supplemented breast milk within 48 hours of delivery, mostly because of perceived "insufficient breast milk." However, programs to promote exclusive breastfeeding have been moderately successful. In a peri-urban community in Mexico, ante- and postnatal visiting by peer counselors increased exclusive breastfeeding at 3 months from 12% to 67%. . . . In Bangladesh, home-based counseling by peer counselors (local mothers who had received 10 days training) increased the prevalence of exclusive breastfeeding at 5 months from 6% to 70%.

It is perhaps more than a coincidence that the compliance figures for exclusive formula feeding in Nairobi and exclusive breastfeeding in Mexico and

Bangladesh are remarkably similar (≈70%). Mixed feeding is a hard practice to break. It may be, however, that acceptance of exclusive breastfeeding by African communities will not involve the quantum cultural jump required for exclusive formula feeding. Work is underway in several settings to better understand if this is so.

Through most of this [selection] we have considered the risk benefit balance for the 55% (≈7 million) of all HIV-positive African women who are literate and have access to safe water, assuming these to be the absolute minimal conditions before replacement feeding could provide benefit. We have shown that for these women, the risk-benefit ratio is very tightly balanced, such that it will vary from one woman to the next, even within the same community. For the remaining 45% (≈5.8 million) of HIV-positive women in sub-Saharan Africa who do not have safe water and/or minimal maternal education, it will be the rare woman who will meet the criteria necessary for formula feeding to save lives. This is not to say that these unusual individual women should not be provided with all the information, support, and resources the community, both local and international, can provide. At a public health level, however, inputs to reduce T [T: Risk of transmission attributable to breastfeeding] will probably be more effective in increasing HIV infection−free survival of these women's babies. . . .

Conclusion

It is clear that:

Babies of HIV-positive mothers who are breastfed are substantially more likely to be infected with HIV than those who are replacement-fed.

Even among highly selected African mothers who are relatively well educated, have access to safe water, have access to free, frequent, and careful clinical care, and have access to free medications for illness and free commercial infant formula, the mortality risk associated with replacement feeding is substantial.

The balance of risk versus benefit is finely placed for mothers in sub-Saharan Africa, the area of the world where the HIV epidemic is currently most fierce. As health policy makers and clinicians, we must first clearly acknowledge that none of the available feeding modes for babies of African HIV-positive women are great—none are devoid of risk. With humility we must help each HIV-positive woman to decide which of the available, albeit imperfect options holds the greatest chance of her baby staying HIV-negative and alive. Very importantly, we must then intensively support her as she implements her choice.

It is probable that:

Intense input to support exclusive replacement feeding at community, health service, and individual levels could make it significantly safer for more babies born to HIV-positive African women.

Intense input at the same levels to support "safer breastfeeding" practices could make breastfeeding significantly safer for babies born to HIV-positive African women.

In the short term, efforts to make breastfeeding safer will benefit many more African babies than efforts to make replacement feeding safer.

Countries, ministries of health, clinics, individual health workers, and most importantly, individual mothers will have to decide where the balance of benefit lies. The complexities of the issues are such that the time of simplistic poster messages ("Breast is best" or "Formula for ALL babies of HIV-positive mothers") is past. Finally, these difficult decisions will have to be reviewed repeatedly as new data are reported.

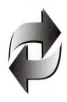

Morbidity and Mortality in Breastfed and Formula-Fed Infants of HIV-1–Infected Women: A Randomized Clinical Trial

We conducted a randomized clinical trial of breastfeeding and formula feeding in Nairobi, Kenya, and previously reported that the estimated risk of breast milk transmission of human immunodeficiency virus type 1 (HIV-1) was 16%. Forty-four percent of all HIV-1 infections among those in the breastfeeding arm were attributable to breastfeeding. This result, in conjunction with results from clinical trials of short-course antiretrovirals that have reported approximately 40% to 50% reductions in perinatal transmission rates, suggest that it may be possible to reduce substantially mother-to-child transmission of HIV-1 in the developing world with interventions of moderate cost.

In resource-poor settings where the most prevalent causes of infant morbidity and mortality are infectious, there is the possibility that breast milk avoidance would be accompanied by an increase in mortality that might offset any gains achieved by decreasing HIV-1 transmission. To enable the formulation of safe infant-feeding policies for HIV-1–infected women in resource-poor settings, it is important to have accurate estimates of the risks associated with the use of artificial feeds by infants of HIV-1–seropositive mothers in developing countries.

The risk of mortality associated with the use of artificial feeding has been reported in a number of observational studies from developing countries. In a recent meta-analysis, the increased mortality risk due to infectious diseases among nonbreastfeeders was substantial, particularly among very young infants. . . . Observational studies have reported substantially increased diarrhea risk in artificially fed infants, with highest risk being noted in the first 2 to 3 months of life. The protective role of breastfeeding with regards to other infectious diseases in developing countries has not been studied as extensively. However, there are some data that suggest that formula fed infants are at increased risk of pneumonia compared with breastfed infants.

From D. Mbori-Ngacha, R. Nduati, G. John, M. Reilly, B. Richardson, A. Mwatha, J. Ndinya-Achola, J. Bwayo, and J. Kreiss, "Morbidity and Mortality in Breastfed and Formula-Fed Infants of HIV-1–Infected Women: A Randomized Clinical Trial," *Journal of the American Medical Association,* vol. 286, no. 19 (November 21, 2001), pp. 2413–2420. Copyright © 2001 by The American Medical Association. Reprinted by permission. References omitted.

One of the major mechanisms of the protection conferred through breast-feeding is by the passive transfer of antibodies, immune-competent cells, and cytokines [chemicals involved in growth regulation]. For mothers with HIV-1-related immunocompromise, it is unknown whether breastfeeding would confer the same magnitude of protection. No study to date has definitively evaluated the degree of protection that breast milk affords infants of HIV-1-infected mothers.

Our randomized clinical trial of breastfed and formula fed infants of HIV-1-seropositive women in Nairobi, Kenya, was conducted with the primary goal of determining the frequency of breast milk transmission of HIV-1. This unique trial also provided an opportunity to compare morbidity and mortality in children according to randomized feeding modality. We previously reported that 2-year mortality rates among children in the formula feeding and breast-feeding arms were similar. In this companion article, we provide additional data regarding mortality as well as analyses of diarrhea, pneumonia, other childhood morbidities, and nutritional status.

Methods

Study Population and Procedures

. . . In brief, HIV-1-seropositive women were recruited from antenatal clinics in Nairobi and randomly assigned to breastfeed or to use formula to feed their infants. Mother/infant pairs were followed-up for 2 years after delivery.

At each visit, information was obtained about feeding status, current and interim morbidity, and history of hospitalization. A physical examination was conducted, including measurement of weight and recumbent length. Ill children received outpatient care from the study clinicians. In the event of diarrhea, mothers were advised to initiate the use of oral rehydration solutions before bringing the child to the research clinic. Children requiring hospital admission were managed by Kenyatta National Hospital staff and pertinent clinical information was abstracted from the hospital records. Verbal autopsies were conducted to assign a possible cause of death for all children who died outside of Kenyatta National Hospital.

Clinical Definitions

Current morbidity was determined by study clinicians using standard diagnostic criteria. Interim infant morbidities were based on maternal history. Diarrhea was defined as the passage of 3 or more loose or watery stools during a 24-hour period for at least 2 days. Chronic diarrhea was defined by diarrhea lasting for more than 1 month. Dehydration was defined as the presence of 1 or more of the following clinical signs and symptoms: abnormal thirst, dry oral mucosa, reduced skin turgor, sunken eyes, or decreased urine output. . . . Weight for height was used to evaluate nutritional status. . . .

Results

Characteristics of the Study Population

. . . Of 425 women enrolled in the study between 1992 and 1998, 213 were randomly assigned to the formula feeding arm and 212 to the breastfeeding arm. The women in each group had similar enrollment characteristics.

Four hundred twenty infants were born to the 408 women who were in follow-up at the time of delivery. After excluding stillbirths and second born twins, there were 204 infants in the formula feeding arm and 197 in the breastfeeding arm. The infants in the 2 groups were comparable at birth with regards to anthropometric measurements, gestational age, sex, and morbidity. . . . Follow-up information on infant morbidity and mortality during the first 2 years of life was available for 186 infants in the formula feeding and 185 in the breastfeeding arm, while HIV-1 infection status information was available for 162 infants in the formula feeding and 171 in the breastfeeding arms.

A total of 4733 infant follow-up visits were made in the first 2 years of life, including 2579 in the formula feeding and 2154 in the breastfeeding arms. Infants in the breastfeeding arm attended significantly fewer scheduled visits to the clinic (median 9, range 1–19) than infants in the formula feeding arm (median 12, range 1–19, . . .). Infants in the breastfeeding arm also tended to have fewer nonscheduled visits (median, 2 vs 3 . . .). The median of the average intervisit interval for infants in the 2 arms was identical (36 days). The median durations of follow-up were 1.7 and 1.3 years in the formula feeding and breastfeeding arms, respectively, yielding total follow-up times of 257 and 228 person-years.

Compliance with randomized feeding modality was significantly higher in the breastfeeding arm than the formula feeding arm of the study (96% vs 70%, . . .). The median duration of breastfeeding among infants randomized to breastfeed was 17 months, and the median age of introduction of supplemental feeds was 3.8 months.

Ninety-two infants acquired HIV-1 infection during the study, 31 in the formula feeding arm and 61 in the breastfeeding arm. The cumulative proportion of HIV-1 infection at 2 years of follow-up was 21% in the formula feeding arm and 37% in the breastfeeding arm of the study. . . .

Mortality

Of the 401 live-born infants in the study, 84 infants died during the course of follow-up, 39 in the formula feeding arm and 45 in the breastfeeding arm.

. . . Mortality rates in the formula feeding and breastfeeding arms did not significantly differ either at 12 months (15.4% vs 16.7%, . . .) or at 2 years (20.0% vs 24.4%. . . .). There was a trend for increased mortality in the formula arm at 6 weeks (3.9% vs 1.0% . . .), but 38% of these deaths were due to complications of delivery and could not be attributable to formula exposure (TABLE 1). Among infants who remained HIV-1 uninfected throughout follow-up, the 2-year cumulative mortality rate was 10.0% in the formula feeding arm and 8.1% in the

Table 1

Potential Contributing Causes of Death by Randomization Arm*

Variables	Deaths Between 0 and 6 mo			Deaths Between 6 and 24 mo			All Deaths		
	Formula Feeding, No. (%) (n = 21)	Breastfeeding, No. (%) (n = 18)	P Value	Formula Feeding, No. (%) (n = 14)	Breastfeeding, No. (%) (n = 26)	P Value	Formula Feeding, No. (%) (n = 35)	Breastfeeding, No. (%) (n = 43)	P Value
Pneumonia	11 (52)**	16 (94)**	.01	5 (36)	9 (35)	.99	16 (46)	25 (58)	.27
Diarrhea	8 (38)	2 (12)	.14	8 (57)	12 (46)	.51	16 (46)	14 (33)	.24
Failure to thrive	7 (33)	5 (29)	.80	6 (43)	14 (54)	.51	13 (37)	19 (44)	.53
Sepsis	6 (29)	1 (6)	.10	1 (7)	0 (0)	.35	9 (20)	1 (2)	.02
Meningitis	2 (10)	2 (12)	.99	1 (7)	3 (12)	.99	3 (9)	5 (12)	.72
Malaria	1 (5)	0 (0)	.99	0 (0)	3 (12)	.54	1 (3)	3 (7)	.62
Measles	0 (0)	0 (0)	...	2 (14)	0 (0)	.12	2 (6)	0 (0)	.20
Tuberculosis	1 (5)	1 (6)	.99	0 (0)	1 (4)	.99	1 (3)	2 (5)	.99
Encephalopathy	0 (0)	0 (0)	...	0 (0)	2 (8)	.53	0 (0)	2 (5)	.50
Cerebral abscess	0 (0)	0 (0)	...	0 (0)	1 (4)	.99	0 (0)	1 (2)	.99
Neonatal noninfectious†	4 (19)	0 (0)	.11	0 (0)	0 (0)	...	4 (11)	0 (0)	.04
Road traffic accident	0 (0)	0 (0)	...	0 (0)	1 (4)	.99	0 (0)	1 (2)	.99

*More than one potential contributing cause of death was present for many children. Ellipsis indicates not applicable.

†Birth asphyxia (n = 2), cord improperly tied (n = 1), prematurity (n = 1).

[**Significantly higher number of infants who were breast-fed died from pneumonia compared with formula-fed infants.]

breastfeeding arm. . . . Among infants who became HIV-1 infected during the course of the study, the 2-year cumulative mortality rates were 40.2% in the formula arm and 46.0% in the breastfeeding arm. . . . [T]here was no significant difference in mortality in the formula and breastfeeding arms. . . . However, HIV-1 infection was associated with a 9.0-fold increased mortality risk. . . .

Two-year mortality rates were much higher for children infected during the first 2 months of life than for children infected after 2 months of age (63.2% vs 8.8%, . . .).

In a separate analysis we found that women who were randomly assigned to the breastfed group had an approximate 3-fold higher mortality rate over 2 years than women in the formula arm, and that maternal death was associated with increased risk of subsequent infant death. We analyzed the infant mortality data controlling for maternal vital status. The relative effect of formula feeding compared with breast-feeding remained unchanged. . . .

One hundred thirty-eight infants died or became HIV-1 infected during the course of follow-up, including 58 in the formula arm and 80 in the breast-feeding arm. The percentage of infants who were dead or infected at 24 months was significantly lower in the formula arm (30% vs 42% . . .). Formula feeding conferred a 28% protective effect from an adverse outcome (HIV-1 infection or death).

Precise information about causes of death was not available because of limited availability of diagnostic tests in health care facilities and reliance on verbal autopsies for children who died at home. For the 78 deaths for which potential contributing causes of death were known, information was obtained by review of hospital records for 41 (53%) and by verbal autopsy for 37 (47%). Pneumonia was the most common cause (53%). Other major contributing causes of death included diarrhea (39%), sepsis (10%), and failure to thrive (41%). Over the 2-year period, children in the 2 groups were comparable for causes of death, except for a higher frequency of sepsis in the formula group . . . as well as a higher frequency of neonatal noninfectious deaths (. . ., Table 1). In a stratified analysis, there were no significant differences in cause of death between the 2 groups for HIV-1−uninfected children. Among HIV-1−infected children, those in the formula arm were more likely to die from sepsis than those in the breastfed group (33% vs 0% . . .). During the first 6 months of life, pneumonia was a more common cause of death in the breastfeeding arm than in the formula arm. . . .

Diarrheal Morbidity

The incidence of diarrhea (defined by history of diarrhea since the last visit) during the 2 years of follow-up was almost identical in infants randomized to receive formula and to breastfeed (155 vs 149 per 100 person-years, respectively. . . . The incidence of diarrhea increased with age and peaked at 9 to 12 months. When analyzed by 3-month quarter, there were no significant differences in diarrheal incidence between the 2 trial groups for any quarter.

Among infants with diarrhea, the severity of diarrhea was similar in the 2 groups. Twelve percent of episodes of diarrhea were associated with bloody stools and 36% with more than 5 stools per day. Forty-five percent of episodes prompted the mother to administer oral rehydration solution and 8% of children with diarrhea at the time of a clinic visit presented with dehydration. Chronic diarrhea was reported by 10% of the study subjects. All of these characteristics were similar in the 2 groups, . . . as was the incidence of these measures of the severity of diarrhea over the 2-year period. Investigating the severity of diarrhea by 3-month quarter, the incidence of dehydration . . . and current diarrhea (at the time of a visit) . . . were significantly higher in the formula group in the first 3 months of life while the incidence of diarrhea with more than 5 stools per day was significantly lower in the formula feeding group between ages 18 and 21 months. . . .

After stratifying by HIV-1 infection status, there was no significant difference in incidence of diarrhea between formula and breastfeeding arms in either HIV-1 infected (241 vs 247 per 100 person-years) or uninfected infants (150 vs 140 per 100 person-years). This was true for the 2-year follow-up period as well as when analyzed by 3 month quarter. Likewise there were no significant differences for any of the measures of severity of diarrhea over the 2-year follow-up period.

Pneumonia

The incidence of pneumonia during the first 2 years of life in infants randomized to the formula and breastfeeding groups was identical (62 per 100 person-years . . .) (TABLE 2). Pneumonia occurred with similar frequency in the 2 groups during every quarter of follow-up. There was no difference in pneumonia incidence over the 2-year period between the 2 groups after stratifying by HIV-1 infection status, either overall or for any quarter. Among HIV-1–infected children, the incidence of pneumonia was 188 per 100 person years among formula fed and 150 per 100 person-years among breastfed. . . . Among HIV-1–uninfected children, the comparable figures were 50 vs 45. . . .

Other Morbidities

The overall incidence of various infant morbidities for the 2 randomization arms is presented in Table 2. There were no significant differences between the study arms for the incidence of any of the infant morbidities over the 2-year follow-up period although there was a trend for lower incidence of otitis media and higher incidence of conjunctivitis in the formula arm. We also compared morbidity incidence between the 2 groups during each quarter of follow-up. There were no significant differences between the 2 groups for any of the morbidities for any quarter of life.

When stratifying by HIV-1 infection status, there was a higher incidence of sepsis in the formula arm compared with the breastfeeding arm among HIV-1–infected infants. . . . No other significant differences were found between the 2 groups. Comparing morbidity incidence between the 2 groups during each quarter of follow-up, the only significant difference was an increased

Table 2

Incidence of Other Morbidities by Randomization Arm

Incidence per 100 Person-Years (No. of Cases)*

Variables	Formula-Feeding (257 Person-Years)	Breastfeeding (228 Person-Years)	Hazards Ratio (95% Confidence Interval)*	P Value
Hospitalization since last visit	18 (47)	20 (46)	0.9 (0.6–1.5)	.71
Fever since last visit	265 (680)	255 (582)	0.9 (0.8–1.1)	.32
Vomiting since last visit	89 (228)	82 (188)	1.0 (0.8–1.3)	.84
Fever on examination	41 (104)	35 (81)	1.0 (0.7–1.5)	.83
Pneumonia	62 (159)	62 (142)	0.9 (0.7–1.3)	.74
Measles	4 (10)	3 (7)	1.1 (0.4–3.1)	.81
Malaria	81 (207)	71 (162)	1.0 (0.8–1.3)	.80
Thrush	43 (110)	45 (102)	0.9 (0.6–1.4)	.78
Otitis media	32 (83)	43 (98)	0.6 (0.4–1.0)	.06
Upper respiratory tract infection	343 (881)	322 (736)	1.0 (0.9–1.1)	.79
Conjunctivitis	30 (77)	22 (50)	1.4 (1.0–2.1)	.09
Sepsis	7 (18)	5 (12)	1.4 (0.6–3.0)	.54

*Hazards ratios are from Anderson-Gill proportional hazards model with robust variance estimate and controlling for number of visits.

risk of reported hospitalization between 9 and 12 months in those infected with HIV-1 in the formula arm. . . .

Nutritional Status

. . . There was a trend for the breastfeeding arm to have better nutritional status overall . . . and significantly better nutritional status in the first 6 months of life. . . . After adjusting for HIV-1 infection status, children in the breastfeeding arm had significantly better nutritional status than those in the formula arm over the 2-year period, . . . particularly during the first 6 months. . . . Malnutrition . . . occurred at some time in 27 (15%) of 183 children in the formula fed and 17 (9%) of 181 children in the breastfeeding arm. . . . The proportion of children with malnutrition was relatively low in the first year of life, but increased with age (2% during the first year of life and 15% during the second year). The proportion of children with malnutrition did not differ significantly by randomization group overall or during any quarter of follow-up. Among HIV-1–infected children, 29% in the formula arm and 14% in the breast-feeding arm had malnutrition at some time during follow-up. . . . Among HIV-1–uninfected children, malnutrition occurred in 11% of those in the formula arm and 7% in the breastfeeding arm. . . .

Comment

In this randomized clinical trial, we found no significant difference in 2-year mortality rates between infants randomly assigned to be formula fed or to be breastfed. Because HIV-1 infections occurred with higher frequency in the breastfeeding arm, we considered the possibility that excess formula-associated deaths might be masked by excess HIV-1–related deaths in the breastfeeding arm. However, even when we performed analyses that adjusted for or stratified by HIV-1 infection status, there was no significant difference in 2-year mortality rates between the 2 trial arms. The major causes of death in the study were infections, and there was no difference in cause-specific infection mortality between the 2 study arms except for an increased frequency of sepsis as a contributing cause of death in the formula arm. Thus, in this study population, formula feeding and breastfeeding were associated with similar mortality risks during the first 2 years of life.

At first glance, our results may seem paradoxical. Breastfeeding was associated with higher rates of HIV-1 transmission; HIV-1 infection in infants was associated with higher mortality; formula resulted in no increased mortality. One might have predicted that we would have seen significantly higher mortality risk in the breastfeeding arm. However, our trial terminated with only 2 years of follow-up, by which time many deaths had occurred among infants infected in utero, peripartum, or through early breastfeeding, but relatively few among infants with later acquisition of HIV-1 through breast milk. Of children infected after 2 months of age, only 9% had died by 2 years but most of the remaining children would be expected to die sometime during childhood. At study end, there were 19 HIV-1 infected children who were alive at their last visit in the formula arm and 35 in the breastfeeding arm. The 2 years of follow-up was sufficient to capture any potential adverse consequences of formula feeding but not all of the adverse consequences of breastfeeding with respect to HIV-1 related mortality. Because of this, HIV-1–free survival (the percentage of children who remained alive and HIV-1 uninfected) best captures the combined risks of feeding modality and HIV-1 infection. In this trial, HIV-1–free survival at 2 years was significantly higher in the formula arm.

The mortality risk among the children in this study was high, largely because of infant HIV-1 infection which was associated with a 9.0-fold increased risk of dying during the first 2 years of life. Among children who remained HIV-1 uninfected, the 12 month infant mortality rate (7.0%; 95% CI, 3.9%-10.0%) was not significantly different than the infant mortality rate of 4.1% reported for Nairobi or 7.4% reported for Kenya as a whole although it is higher than what might have been predicted given the level of medical care available in the research context. This suggests that infants of HIV-1–infected mothers may have a somewhat elevated mortality risk, even if they themselves escape HIV-1 infection.

There have been concerns that the use of formula by women infected with HIV-1 in resource-poor settings would result in increases in diarrheal morbidity and mortality. We found no significant difference in diarrheal incidence in the 2 study groups of the trial over the 2 year follow-up period. This was true for the group of infants as a whole and after stratifying by HIV-1 infection status. We did find an increased incidence of current diarrhea (at the time of a visit) and dehydration in the formula feeding arm during the first 3 months of life. This coincides with the period during which most breastfed infants were fed exclusively by breast milk (the median age of introduction of supplemental feeds was 3.8 months) and were thus at low risk of exposure to diarrheal pathogens from food sources. Our results are consistent with previously published observational studies in which breast milk has been most protective against diarrheal disease in the first 3 months of life, a finding that underscores the necessity of careful follow-up of formula fed infants during early infancy.

In the cohort overall, we did not observe increased risk of any major childhood morbidities, including pneumonia, sepsis, malaria, or otitis media, associated with formula feeding. Among HIV-1–infected formula feeders, there was an increased risk of sepsis during the 2 years of follow-up and an increased risk of hospitalization toward the end of the first year of age. Although our study suggests that formula feeding by HIV-1–infected mothers does not increase the risk of most childhood morbidities, there may be some increased risk among HIV-1–infected infants.

Infants in the breastfeeding arm had better nutritional status than those in the formula feeding arm, particularly during the first 6 months of life, consistent with observational studies. We observed a fairly high prevalence of malnutrition during the second year of life, consistent with patterns of malnutrition seen in sub-Saharan Africa, due in part to repeated infections and introduction of poor weaning diets. However, there was no difference in the prevalence of malnutrition in the 2 study groups. Thus, with adequate supplies of formula and nutrition counseling, the mothers in this trial were able to administer formula feeds without seriously compromising the nutritional status of their infants. However, the better growth in breastfed infants, particularly during the first 6 months, highlights the importance of nutritional counseling for mothers of formula feeding infants.

The major strength of our study was its randomized clinical trial design. Choice of infant feeding modality may be influenced by factors that affect infant health outcomes and not all observational studies have controlled for important confounding factors such as educational level, socioeconomic status, and low birth weight. Nor have most studies addressed the possibility of reverse causality, eg, that changes in infant feeding modality (and in particular a switch from breast milk to formula) may be influenced by childhood illnesses. Our randomized clinical trial design allows us to present data regarding morbidity and mortality associated with formula that are not potentially confounded.

There are several limitations of our trial that warrant discussion. First, compliance with feeding modality in the formula feeding arm was imperfect, and 30% of such infants had some exposure to breast milk. . . . [T]his could potentially result in underestimates of risk associated with formula feeding. However, when we repeated our mortality analyses using true feeding modality rather than randomization group, we found similar results. Two-year mortality was 18.8% among true formula feeders and 22.0% among true breastfeeders. . . .

Among HIV-1−uninfected children, the 2-year mortality was 8.7% among true formula feeders and 7.3% among true breastfeeders. . . . Second, we relied on maternal histories to capture childhood illnesses that occurred between clinic visits, so our estimates of morbidity may be underestimates. In addition, our study was not designed to determine causes of death and these data are imprecise because of limited availability of diagnostic testing and reliance on verbal autopsies. Finally, the number of visits to the clinic was lower for breastfeeding than formula feeding children. Although this would not affect our mortality rates, it could influence our estimates of the incidence of diarrheal disease and other morbidities. We corrected for this in our analyses by adjusting all relative risks for the various infant morbidities of interest by the number of clinic visits made.

Our estimates of morbidity and mortality risk are not generalizable to all women in developing countries. Our results represent the best-case scenario. All women participating in the trial had access to potable water, extensive health education regarding safe preparation of formula, a reliable supply of formula, and access to medical care for their infants. The magnitude of risks associated with formula feeding will vary in different settings depending on differences in these important variables. Because of these differences, we would advocate context-specific counseling for HIV-1−infected expectant mothers so that each woman can select the feeding method that maximizes benefits and minimizes risks given her individual situation, as is recommended by the World Health Organization. In addition, our trial was conducted among HIV-1−infected mothers and the results may not be generalizable to uninfected women. It is possible that the breast milk of HIV-1−infected women lacks factors that confer protection from death, diarrheal disease, and pneumonia.

We previously reported that the use of formula could prevent 44% of HIV-1 infections in infants of HIV-1−seropositive mothers. Our current results demonstrate that in a developing country setting, it is possible for this gain to be realized without increased morbidity or mortality during the first 2 years of life. In our trial, formula-fed infants clearly had a better outcome than breastfed infants because they were more likely to be alive and HIV-1 uninfected at the age of 2 years. Formula feeding conferred a 28% protective effect from an adverse outcome (HIV-1 infection or death). In addition, mothers who used formula were more likely to be alive 2 years after delivery than mothers who breastfed. Thus, formula provided advantages for both mother and child. Our current analyses show that the use of formula to prevent HIV-1 transmission can be a safe and viable option even in resource poor settings, if maternal education, clean water, a supply of formula, and access to health care are available.

POSTSCRIPT

Should Mothers Infected With the AIDS Virus Breastfeed Their Infants?

Public health nutrition issues often require grappling with difficult dilemmas of science and values, but surely none can be as painful to resolve as this one. Should HIV-infected women, who do not have adequate income or education or access to clean water, breastfeed their infants and risk transmitting the virus, or should they feed formula to their infants and risk transmitting malnutrition and death from diarrheal diseases?

In the *British Medical Journal* (June 17, 2000), Michael Latham and Elizabeth Preble, of Cornell University argue that researchers have exaggerated the risks of breastfeeding and that much can be done to support the health of breastfeeding mothers infected with HIV. They note that many breastfeeding mothers use formulas occasionally and that exclusive breastfeeding paradoxically reduces HIV transmission from mothers to infants, perhaps by helping the infant's digestive system to remain intact and functional. Most African women, say Latham and Preble, cannot afford to buy commercial formulas. Even if the formula is free, the women have no means to keep it sterile. Instead of promoting infant formulas, they say, public health officials should be supporting better diets for women of childbearing ages and teaching new mothers how to use breastfeeding in ways that reduce HIV transmission. To further complicate this question, South African researchers put forth a new argument in an accompanying commentary on the *British Medical Journal* paper. They say the feeding question may be unresolved but that this debate really does not matter. Instead, the best method for preventing HIV transmission is to use antiviral drugs. The breastfeeding versus formula-feeding argument, they say, detracts from more important public policies like obtaining adequate drug therapy for infected mothers.

It must be noted that breastfeeding costs nothing, requires no purchases, and is of no benefit to any industry. Neither of the studies offered here—both funded by government grants—discusses the historic role of the formula and drug industries in framing the terms of this debate or in attempting to influence public policy decisions about preventing HIV transmission. For an individual woman, the decision about whether to breast- or bottle-feed necessarily depends on her particular circumstances. For governments, the choice of whether to promote one or the other method cannot help but be influenced by corporations interested in increasing sales of formulas or drugs.

ISSUE 15

Is Organically Grown Food Better Than Conventionally Grown Food?

YES: John P. Reganold et al., from "Sustainability of Three Apple Production Systems," *Nature* (April 19, 2001)

NO: Dennis Avery, from "The Fallacy of the Organic Utopia," in Julian Morris and Roger Bate, eds., *Fearing Food: Risk, Health, and Environment* (Butterworth-Heinemann, 1999)

ISSUE SUMMARY

YES: Agricultural researcher John P. Reganold and colleagues say that organic farming methods produce apples that are sweeter, less tart, more profitable, more energy efficient, and more environmentally and economically sustainable than those grown by conventional farming methods.

NO: Agricultural economist Dennis Avery counters that as a global food production system, organic farming would be an environmental disaster, an imminent danger to wildlife, and a hazard to public health.

Conventional, large-scale methods for growing commercial plant crops routinely use fertilizers and insecticides, herbicides, and other toxic pesticides. These add nutrients to soil or kill weeds and insect pests. Use of these chemicals increases crop productivity in the short term—but at a price. Massive farming promotes "monoculture," the use of just one kind of crop, and reduces biodiversity. It also depletes the soil of nutrients and harms the environment. Fertilizers leak into streams and encourage the growth of algae that clog streams. Pesticides are toxic to workers; they also get into water supplies, enter the food chain, and become incorporated into human tissues. These problems make conventional agriculture potentially unsustainable and unhealthful, and they stimulate interest in organic farming as a meaningful alternative. Organic methods avoid use of synthetic fertilizers and pesticides. Instead, they replace depleted soil nutrients with composted plant matter, use biological methods to control pests, and systematically rotate and diversify crops and livestock. At first glance, organic methods might seem healthier for people and for the environment but perhaps more expensive and less productive. Although all such assumptions could be tested experimentally, few investigators have conducted well-controlled comparative studies of the effects of organic versus conventional farming methods.

In one such test, John P. Reganold and his colleagues grew Golden Delicious apples in Washington State using three methods of cultivation. An *organic* method used compost as fertilizer; bark mulch, cultivation, or mowing to control weeds; organically certified biological controls of insect pests; and hand picking to thin the fruit. In contrast, a *conventional* method used synthetic soil fertilizers, herbicides, insecticides, and chemical fruit thinners. An *integrated* method used some features of both methods: compost and synthetic fertilizers, bark mulch, and herbicides to control weeds and conventional methods to control weeds and thin fruit. The researchers evaluated the quality of the soil and apples grown under these conditions from 1994 to 1999, measured yields, and evaluated costs. Apple yields under all three conditions were similar, but the organic system resulted in the best soil quality, the least damage to the environment, the best tasting and sweetest apples, and the most profits. On this basis, the researchers urge policymakers to find ways to support farmers who would like to produce food under environmentally and economically sustainable conditions.

In sharp contrast, Dennis Avery argues that organic farming methods produce measurably lower yields, thereby requiring greater amounts of land to grow equivalent amounts of food. More land, however, is either unavailable or of such poor quality that attempting to cultivate such land would cause massive erosion. He raises particular objections to the use of biological controls such as the insecticidal toxins produced by *Bacillus thuringiensis* (*Bt*) bacteria. These toxins, he says, are more likely than chemical pesticides to kill wild insects and other forms of life. Overall, Avery argues that organic farming methods are so unreliable that using them would reduce food yields, cause prices to rise and food reserves to fall, and would threaten the food security of the world's most vulnerable populations. He views conventional farming as the only sensible means to prevent starvation among the world's rapidly expanding population. Finally, he adds that world supplies of plant matter available for composting are too limited to support widespread organic farming; chemical pesticides are demonstrably safe for human health; and organic foods provide no advantage in safety, nutritional quality, productivity, or environmental impact.

What are we to make of such divergent views? Clearly, both of these selections deal with matters of science and values. What are the scientific issues? What values do they express? What economic or social matters are affected by the outcome of this debate? How is the interpretation of this argument likely to be affected by the point of view of the reader?

In the following selections, Reganold et al. argue that organic farming methods are superior to conventional methods in several important respects, while Avery argues precisely the opposite.

John P. Reganold et al.

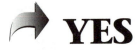
YES

Sustainability of Three Apple Production Systems

Escalating production costs, heavy reliance on non-renewable resources, reduced biodiversity, water contamination, chemical residues in food, soil degradation and health risks to farm workers handling pesticides all bring into question the sustainability of conventional farming systems. It has been claimed, however, that organic farming systems are less efficient, pose greater health risks and produce half the yields of conventional farming systems. Nevertheless, organic farming became one of the fastest growing segments of US and European agriculture during the 1990s. Integrated farming, using a combination of organic and conventional techniques, has been successfully adopted on a wide scale in Europe. Here we report the sustainability of organic, conventional and integrated apple production systems in Washington State from 1994 to 1999. All three systems gave similar apple yields. The organic and integrated systems had higher soil quality and potentially lower negative environmental impact than the conventional system. When compared with the conventional and integrated systems, the organic system produced sweeter and less tart apples, higher profitability and greater energy efficiency. Our data indicate that the organic system ranked first in environmental and economic sustainability, the integrated system second and the conventional system last.

Organic management practices combine traditional conservation-minded farming methods with modern farming technologies but exclude such conventional inputs as synthetic pesticides and fertilizers, instead putting the emphasis on building up the soil with compost additions and animal and green manures, controlling pests naturally, rotating crops and diversifying crops and livestock. Organic farming systems in the US range from strict closed-cycle systems that go beyond organic certification guidelines by limiting, as much as possible, external inputs to more standard systems that simply follow organic certification guidelines. Integrated farming systems reduce the use of chemicals by integrating organic and conventional production methods.

Just because a system is organic or integrated does not ensure its sustainability; nor does sustainability, an inherently complex concept, readily lend itself to quantification. To be sustainable, a farm must produce adequate yields of high quality, be profitable, protect the environment, conserve resources and be socially responsible in the long term. But under conventional economic systems, market and social forces can change the viability of a production system independent of its environmental sustainability. It has been proposed that ecological and economic systems should be linked so that ecosystem services are accounted for in commercial markets, thereby making sustainable land management a prerequisite for economic sustainability.

A crucial step in developing such ecological–economic links is to assess the effects of agricultural systems on specific, measurable properties that are important indicators of sustainability. We measured the effects of an organic, a conventional and an integrated apple production system on the sustainability indicators of soil quality, horticultural performance, orchard profitability, environmental quality and energy efficiency. Perennial food crops such as apples may prove to be more sustainable to produce over the long term than annual crops, and they currently comprise a significant portion of the world's agricultural production. For example, globally, nearly 5.6 million hectares of apples were harvested in 2000 (ref. 17). In the USA alone, apples and other high-value perennial food crops constituted 16% of the total value of food crops in 1998 (ref. 18).

We measured soil quality by analysing physical, chemical and biological soil properties and incorporating the data into a soil quality index. Soil quality is the capacity of a soil to sustain biological productivity, maintain environmental quality and promote plant and animal health. We evaluated soil quality in terms of four soil functions: accommodating water entry; accommodating water movement and availability; resisting surface structure degradation; and supporting fruit quality and productivity. Soil quality ratings in 1998 and 1999 for the organic and integrated systems were significantly higher than those for the conventional system, largely owing to the addition of compost and mulch in 1994 and 1995. Organic matter has a profound impact on soil quality, enhancing soil structure and fertility and increasing water infiltration and storage. Because of poorer ability to accommodate water entry and to resist surface structure degradation, the conventional system (no organic amendments added) scored lowest overall in soil quality.

We assessed horticultural performance by measuring fruit yields, size and grade; tree growth; leaf and fruit mineral contents; fruit maturity; and consumer taste preference. There were no observable differences in pests, disease or physiological disorders among plots during each growing season. Differences in annual fruit yields were inconsistent among the three systems (Fig. 1). Cumulative yields were similar for all three systems. In 1995–1997, fruit size was similar across systems, except in 1996 when apples were larger in the integrated system. In 1998 and 1999, the organic system produced smaller fruit. In 1995–1997, all marketed fruit produced from the three systems was sold for processing because it was downgraded primarily owing to skin russetting, a physiological skin disorder that reduces the fruit's visual appeal but not its taste or other attributes. (Although russetted Golden Delicious apples are not sold as fresh fruit in the US marketplace, Italy domestically markets a fully russetted Golden Delicious apple, and in the world market fully russetted Bosc pears are preferred to non-russetted ones.) The low landscape position of the experimental site in the orchard resulted in early season cool, humid conditions that contributed to the unusually high level of russetting. Fruit damage due to other physiological disorders, pests and diseases were minimal and equal for each of the three systems. In 1998 and 1999, marketable fruit not graded as Washington Extra Fancy or Fancy was sold for processing.

Tree growth was similar in all three systems. Although there were some differences in leaf nutrient contents among the three systems, analyses indicated satisfactory levels of nutrients. Fruit tissue nutrient analyses indicated some inconsistent differences.

Mechanical analysis of fruit firmness at harvest and after storage in 1998 and 1999 showed that organic fruit was firmer (a positive consumer attribute for apples) than or as firm as conventional and integrated fruit. Ratios of soluble solids (sugar) content to acidity (tartness), an indication of sweetness, were most often highest in organic fruit. These data were confirmed in taste tests by untrained sensory panels that found the organic apples to be sweeter after six months of storage than conventional apples and less tart at harvest and after six months storage than conventional and integrated apples. The same taste tests, however, could not discern any difference in firmness among apples in the three systems at harvest or after storage. Taste tests also indicated that the integrated apples had a better flavour after six months storage but found no differences among organic, conventional and integrated apples in texture or overall acceptance.

Enterprise budgets were generated each year to calculate net returns from total costs and gross receipts. Receipts for the integrated system were estimated

Figure 1

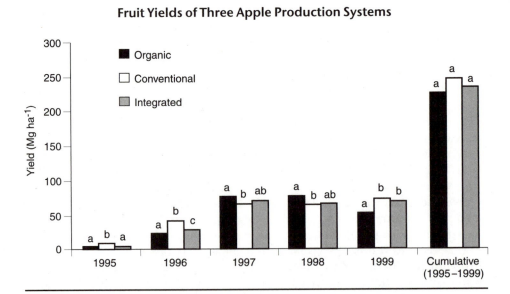

Differences between values in a year followed by different letters are significant at the 0.05 level (least significant difference).

using prices for conventionally produced fruit, as unlike organic fruit there was no price premium for integrated fruit. Receipts for the organic system were estimated using prices for conventionally produced fruit in the first three years (1994–1996), the number of years necessary to convert from conventional to certified organic. The price premium to the grower for each grade of organic fruit in the next three years (1997–1999) averaged 50% above conventional prices.

The three systems did not show a net annual profit until 1999 under measured fruit quality conditions (with skin russetting). When we adjusted the economic analysis by eliminating the effects of russetting but maintained the estimated crop loss of 15% due to other factors and the measured size, grade and firmness of fresh fruit in this study, the organic system was more profitable than the conventional and integrated systems in 1997 and 1998. Higher production costs for the organic system in 1995 and 1997 (under measured and non-russetted fruit quality conditions) were largely due to differences in weed control practices, fruit thinning and compost applications. Production costs in 1999, however, were significantly lower for the organic system than for the other two systems due to reduced carryover interest costs resulting from faster repayment of the original investment.

The breakeven point, when cumulative net returns equal cumulative costs, can vary depending on several factors, such as fruit prices, input costs, yields and fruit quality. The breakeven point in this study is projected to occur nine years after planting (in 2002) for the organic system under measured fruit quality conditions. The conventional and integrated systems would break even 15 and 17 years after planting, respectively, under measured conditions. Under non-russetted fruit quality conditions, the breakeven point would occur six, eight and nine years after planting for the organic, conventional and integrated systems respectively. Assuming similar non-russetted fruit quality conditions, estimated breakeven points for conventional apple orchards in central Washington range from 8 to 11 years from planting.

Without price premiums for organic fruit, the conventional system would break even first, the integrated second and the organic third under measured or non-russetted fruit quality conditions. For breakeven points of the organic and integrated systems to occur in the same year as the conventional system, price premiums of 12% for the organic system and 2% for the integrated system would be necessary under measured fruit quality conditions. Under non-russetted fruit quality conditions, premiums of 14% for the organic system and 6% for the integrated system would be necessary to match the breakeven point of the conventional system.

We assessed the environmental impact of the three production systems by using a rating index employed by scientists and growers to determine the potential adverse impact of pesticides and fruit thinners, including naturally occurring certified organic products. The higher the rating, the greater the negative impact. As only 35% of conventional Washington apple growers use pheromone-mating disruption (PMD), an environmentally benign biological control used in our conventional treatment, we also included a conventional system in which synthetic pesticides were used in place of PMD. The total environmental impact rating of our conventional system was 6.2 times that of the organic system, whereas the integrated system rating was 4.7 times greater and the non-PMD conventional system rating was 7.7 times greater (Fig. 2).

Energy accounting was divided into inputs (labour, fuel, fertilizers and so on), output (yield) and output/input ratios (energy efficiency). Cumulative energy inputs and output for the six-year study period were lower for the organic system than for the conventional and integrated systems. The output/input ratio for the organic system during the six-year study period, however, was 7% greater than that for the conventional system and 5% greater than that for the integrated system, making the organic system the most energy efficient.

Our results show that organic and integrated apple production systems in Washington State are not only better for soil and the environment than their conventional counterpart but have comparable yields and, for the organic system, higher profits and greater energy efficiency. Although crop yield and quality are important products of a farming system, the benefits of better soil and environmental quality provided by the organic and integrated production systems are equally valuable and usually overlooked in the marketplace. Such external benefits come at a financial cost to growers. Currently, growers of more sustainable systems may be unable to maintain profitable enterprises without economic incentives, such as price premiums or subsidies for organic and integrated products, that value these external benefits. Equally important, upon

Figure 2

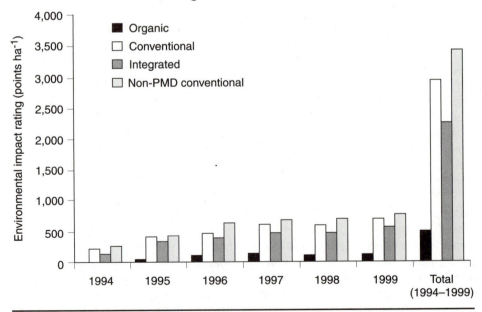

Environmental Impact Ratings of Four Apple Production Systems: Organic, Conventional, Integrated and Non-PMD Conventional

Higher ratings indicate greater potential for negative environmental impact. . . .

incorporation of external costs into economic assessments of farming systems, we may find that many currently profitable farming systems are uneconomical and therefore unsustainable. The challenge facing policymakers is to incorporate the value of ecosystem processes into the traditional marketplace, thereby supporting food producers in their attempts to employ both economically and environmentally sustainable practices.

METHODS

Study Area

In May 1994, we planted four replicate plots for each of the three apple production systems with 'Golden Delicious' apples (*Malus* × *domestica* Borkh.). . . . The experiment was part of a 20-ha commercial apple orchard in the Yakima Valley, Washington. . . .

Farming Systems

In cooperation with the farmers, professional consultants and extension agents, we chose appropriate management practices for the three systems. The organic system included compost and foliar sprays. In the first three years (1994–1996), bark mulch and landscape fabric controlled weeds; thereafter, cultivation and mowing were used for weed control. Organically certified biological controls, including applications of *Bacillus thuringiensis* and PMD to control codling moth (*Cydia pomonella* L.), were used for pest management. Fruit thinning was by hand. The conventional system included synthetic soil fertilizers and foliar sprays, pesticides, chemical fruit thinners and PMD. The integrated system used both compost and synthetic fertilizers and controlled weeds with both bark mulch and herbicides. Pest management and fruit thinning were similar to those of the conventional system. The three systems had similar total soil nitrogen inputs. Pests, diseases and physiological disorders were monitored throughout each growing season by the farmers and professional consultants, who recommended organic, conventional or integrated treatments for their control.

Soil Analyses

All soil samples were taken from the inner two rows of each experimental plot to minimize edge effects, excluding the first 20 trees from each end of these sample rows. Samples were collected midway between trees within tree rows. In 1998 and 1999, soil analyses included bulk density, water content, total nitrogen, nitrate-nitrogen, extractable phosphorus, cation-exchange capacity, pH, electrical conductivity, organic carbon content, aggregate stability, microbial biomass carbon and nitrogen, and earthworm populations. Details of analytical procedures are described elsewhere.

Horticultural Performance

All components of horticultural performance were measured from trees, leaves and fruit sampled in the middle two rows of each plot, excluding the first 20 trees from each end of these sample rows. We recorded yields and size (average mass) of fruit at harvest in 1995–1999. The proportions of fruit suitable only for processing (due to small size or defects) and fruit suitable for fresh market and divided by grade were also recorded. Grading of fresh fruit was based on Washington State's apple industry standards. We used trunk cross-sectional area to estimate unit tree growth. We analysed leaf mineral contents . . . in 1994–1999 from pooled samples of mid-shoot leaves taken randomly from each plot in midsummer. We analysed fruit flesh mineral contents . . . in 1995 and 1997–1999 from pooled samples of uniformly sized fruits taken three weeks before harvest. Mineral analyses were carried out according to standard methods. We assessed fruit maturity parameters, including flesh firmness, soluble solids and acidity, according to standard procedures at harvest and after three and six months of controlled atmosphere storage in 1998 and 1999. Untrained sensory panels were used to determine preferences for overall acceptance, texture, flavour, firmness, sweetness and tartness of 1999 fruit from each production system and storage treatment.

Economic Analyses

We calculated gross receipts using farmgate prices paid by packing houses to farmers for apples sold at harvest or after storage. Prices for the specific size, grade and firmness of 'Golden Delicious' organic and conventional apples from our study were based on prices from *Washington Growers Clearing House Bulletins* and fruit packing houses in Washington State. Total costs included non-harvest variable costs (fertilizers, pesticides, fuel, labour and water), harvest variable costs (picking, grading, packing and storage) and fixed costs (machinery, interest and taxes). Projected returns for 2000 and beyond were estimated from average fruit sizes (1998–1999) and yields (1997–1999) for each treatment, assuming a 15% cullage rate for all three treatments and a 50% price premium for organic fruit.

Environmental Impact Assessment

We determined environmental impact ratings for each farming system using an index developed by Stemilt Growers, Inc. of Wenatchee, Washington, as part of their 'Responsible Choice' program. Similar to Cornell University's Environmental Impact Quotient but updated to include fruit thinners and certified organic products, the index takes into account chemical efficacy, potential worker and consumer exposure, leaching potential, soil sorption index, chemical half-life and the effects of chemicals on beneficial organisms, all based on toxicological studies and chemical characteristics of each product. The active ingredient of each pesticide and the dose and frequency of application were used to calculate the environmental impact ratings.

Energy Use

Energy use for each production system was calculated from energy data specific to agricultural production.

NO ↰

Dennis Avery

The Fallacy of the Organic Utopia

Introduction

Organic farming has been put forward as one of the major pillars of a new, more-sustainable human society that would be 'kinder to the earth.' Unfortunately, organic farming cannot deliver on that promise. In fact, organic farming is an imminent danger to the world's wildlife and a hazard to the health of its own consumers.

Organic farming today supplies less than 1 per cent of food for affluent countries and a declining proportion of the food in the Third World. This is good. A thoughtful world would not allow organic farming to be more than a niche source of fruits and vegetables for chemophobes who might otherwise endanger their health by refusing to eat fresh produce.

However, as a global food production system, organic farming would be an environmental disaster:

- Organic farming would force us to plough up an additional 5 to 10 million square miles of wildlands to make up for its lower yields and the global shortage of organic nitrogen. We would trade wildlands for huge tracts of clover and alfalfa.
- Expanding agriculture onto poorer-quality land would inflict severe losses on wildlife species. The world is already farming most of its good-quality land. A major expansion would clear large tracts of poorer-quality land, which typically have more biodiversity (Huston 1993). For example, there are more wildlife species in a few square miles of tropical rain forest than in the whole of North America.
- Organic farming uses biological controls instead of modern pesticides. Unfortunately, biological controls are far more likely to wipe out wild species than farm chemicals. Pesticides have not caused a single known species extinction in 50 years of broad use. Farm pesticides are applied only on fields, with very limited spillover into wildlands where most of the wild species live. Bio-controls move out on their own into the ecosystem. We already know that introduced species are one of the major

threats to the world's wild species. One bio-control insect released by the US government (the European flowerhead weevil) now threatens to eradicate two of America's native thistle species and the pictured-wing fly that depends on one of them.

- Global organic farming would incur staggering levels of soil erosion as millions more square miles of more-fragile land would have to be farmed to provide food. Equally unfortunate, organic farmers refuse to use the only truly sustainable tillage systems available to most of the world (conservation tillage and no-till farming) because those systems depend on chemical weed killers.

Worldwide organic-only farming would also be dangerous to public health:

- The world's food supply would become far more erratic and uncertain under organic farming. Low organic yields would force the use of far more marginal land, prone to drought, pests and early frosts. The fields would be far more susceptible to periodic plagues of pests because biological pest controls are the weakest and most erratic in the farmers' defence arsenal.
- Food costs would be prohibitively high for the poor in the low-production years. The world would also have to store more food reserves—unprotected by storage pesticides—and thus suffer much higher losses to cereal beetles, weevils, moulds and other threats to stored food.
- Eating five fruits and vegetables per day is humanity's strongest weapon against cancer; it cuts total cancer risk in half, no matter how the produce was grown. Only about one-tenth of First World consumers eat enough produce for full protection, even though the stores are full of cheap and attractive fruits and vegetables. Organic produce is often twice as expensive and typically less attractive due to pest damage. How many consumers would eat enough fruits and vegetables if the stores had only organic suppliers?

Saving Room for Wildlife With High-Yield Farming

High-yield farming gained fame as a way to feed the world's expanding human population and lower food costs for the poor—but today its biggest advantage is that it feeds more people from less land.

The crop yield increases achieved since World War II have saved at least 15 million square miles of wildlife habitat from being ploughed for low-yield crops. We are feeding more than twice as many people today and feeding them better diets—on the same amount of cropland used in 1950. Africa is the exception to this happy state of affairs, because Africa is not yet using high-yield farming.

Additional land has been saved by modern meat production, with its highly bred genetics, effective veterinary medicines, scientifically balanced feed rations and confinement housing systems. (Without 'hog hotels' the world might need more than a million square miles of land in 2050 just to house its breeding hogs outdoors. The US would need all the cropland in the State of Pennsylvania just to raise its chickens on free range.)

Modern food processing also saves wildlands because it allows us to grow crops where the yields are highest (often two or three times as high). Processing prevents post-harvest losses as we transport the food wherever the people choose to live.

Why We Will Have to Triple Farm Output by 2050

The human population is rapidly stabilising. Births per woman in the Third World have plummeted from 6.5 in 1960 to 3.1 today. As stability is 2.1 births per woman, poor countries have come three-fourths of the way to stability in one generation. First World families average 1.7 births per woman reflecting an inverse population growth curve. Affluence, urbanisation and food security have encouraged this decline in birth rates.

These human population trends project to a peak of 8.5 to 9 billion humans, reached about the year 2035. That peak will be followed by a slow, modest decline in human numbers. However, the price of population stability is that we will have to feed virtually all these people high-quality diets, including lots of meat, milk, fruit, vegetables and provide the cotton and natural fibre wardrobes that affluent people will demand for themselves and their children.

There is no vegetarian trend in the world and it is probably too late to count on vegetarianism to save the wildlands. 'Vegetarian conservation' would require at least 50 per cent of the world population to become vegan, foregoing all livestock products. The First World average is currently less than 0.5 per cent vegan.

Instead of becoming vegetarians, the world is in the midst of the biggest surge in meat and milk demand ever seen. China's meat consumption has doubled in the past seven years. India has doubled its milk consumption since 1980. Indonesia is clearing tropical forest to grow chicken feed and cattle pasture.

In addition to feeding the people, the world will have to feed its pets. The US has 113 million cats and dogs living amongst its 270 million people. Pet stores in Hong Kong and Shanghai are now beginning to get beyond the traditional caged birds and crickets, selling a few kittens and the occasional small puppy. With a one-child population policy how many companion pets will an affluent Chinese population of 1.3 billion have in 2050? And woe unto whoever stands between a pet-owner and that animal's preferred diet.

All told, experts predict that the world must be prepared to produce three times as much food from its farms in 2050 as today. Hopefully, we will be able to harness enough selective breeding, chemistry, engineering and biotechnology to again triple the yields on the land we are already farming.

It is impossible to believe that we can triple the yields on organic farms or that humans will voluntarily give up high-protein diets.

Organic Yields Are Too Low

A British farm manager who handles 50,000 acres of organic and mainstream crops summed up the objective data from a dozen First World countries. He said, 'I'm lucky to get half as much yield from my organic acres.'

The *American Journal of Alternative Agriculture* recently published a best-case organic yield achievement. The Rodale Institute, a famous organic research centre, acquired a field near its headquarters and shifted it from chemically supported farming to organic production. The field has good soils and lies in a well-watered region. Rodale spent eight years building up the organic content of the field's soils, adding manure imported from nearby feedlots and testing the most productive crop rotations. Then, under ideal conditions, the newly organic field produced yields that were only 21 per cent below those of neighbouring mainstream farms—using 40 per cent more labour.

Researchers at Texas A&M concluded that US field crop production would drop by 24–57 per cent without pesticide protection. They concluded fruit and vegetable yields would drop by 50 to 100 per cent without pesticides and that many production areas would have to quit producing altogether.

The Shortage of Organic Plant Nutrients

Despite the substantial penalty of low yields, organic farming's biggest environmental shortcoming is the global shortage of 'natural' nitrogen fertiliser. Experts at the US Department of Agriculture have calculated that the available animal manure and sustainable biomass resources in America provide only about one-third of the plant nutrients needed to support current US food production. And, most of the world has far less pasture and manure per capita than the US. Globally, we may have less than 20 per cent of the organic plant nutrients needed to sustain current food output—let alone tripling farm output for the 21st century.

Organic proponents talk of millions of tons of compostable materials, such as urban sewage sludge, being 'wasted.' But the nitrogen in all of America's sewage sludge equals only about 2 per cent of the nitrogen being applied through commercial fertilisers. Nor could we ignore the problems of heavy metals and live pathogens in the sewage sludge.

There are indeed 'millions of tons' of compost materials, such as tree chippings and grass clippings, that could be gathered. However, a recent New Jersey recycling report suggests it would cost perhaps $100 per ton just to gather the wastes—with additional costs for hauling and distributing them on farmland.

Moreover, the 'millions of tons' of compost must be compared to the 2 billion tons of manure, corncobs and other farm waste already being spread annually on American farms. They make compost look like just an expensive way to add 1 or 2 per cent to the American agricultural biomass.

The only realistic way for the world to get millions of additional tons of organic nitrogen is to plough millions of square miles of forest to expand the world's green manure crops. Growing six million square miles of clover and alfalfa would take a land area equal to all of Europe and half the US away from wildlife.

The Safety of Modern Pesticides

It is a continuing mystery how organic believers can be so casual about the pathogens in manure and sewage sludge—which cause thousands of First World deaths per year—and so incredibly fearful of pesticide residues which have never caused a documented consumer death.

The World Health Organisation estimates that pesticides cause about 200,000 human deaths per year. However, more than 90 per cent of these deaths are suicides. For example, pesticides are a relatively cheap and painless aid to suicide in India, while chewing the leaves of a local tree produces an agonising death. Another 7 per cent of the pesticide deaths are accidental household poisonings: children getting into rat poison, or an adult drinking something from an unlabelled bottle. The remaining few percentage points of the 200,000 deaths are farm workers who apply products carelessly, or return to a field too soon after the spraying of one of the harsher pesticides, such as methyl parathion.

The US National Research Council has published *Carcinogens and Anti-Carcinogens in the Human Diet,* a conclusive 417-page report which says pesticide residues are no significant health risk to consumers. By implication, this report also says the much-weaker traces of pesticides found in drinking water are even less of a threat. The report was careful to emphasise that consumers should not let any fear of pesticides interfere with eating lots of fruits and vegetables.

The National Cancer Institute of Canada's Panel on Pesticides and Cancer came to the same conclusion in 1997: 'The Panel concluded that it was not aware of any definitive evidence to suggest that synthetic pesticides contribute significantly to overall cancer mortality. The Panel also concluded that it did not believe that any increased intake of pesticide residues associated with increased intake of fruits and vegetables poses any increased risk of cancer.'

In other words, we are still looking for the first victim of pesticide residues, 50 years after we began using them broadly and after billions of dollars in medical research spent trying to find such a victim.

> All substances are poisons. There is none which is not a poison. The right dose differentiates a poison from a remedy (Paracelsus 1492–1541). . . .

No Nutritional Advantage From Organic Foods

For decades, organic believers have claimed organic foods had higher nutritional value. This defied logic, since virtually all crop plants need exactly the same menu of plant nutrients. Without them, the plants will not grow. With them, the plants will produce their normal grains and fruits, with their normal nutritional content.

Tufts University in Massachusetts hosted an international conference in 1997 on 'Agricultural Production and Nutrition.' For the most part, the following studies were done by alternative agriculturists trying to demonstrate that their products are more nourishing. Researchers from dozens of countries reported they could find no nutritional differences between organic and chemically-supported foods.

- Colorado State compared the vitamin contents of carrots and broccoli and found no differences between conventional and organic produce. Colorado State also grew potatoes under four different systems, analysed nine minerals and seven vitamins—and found no clear differences.
- A Lithuanian study compared three farming systems on carrots, potatoes and cabbage. 'Traditional chemical analyses of nutritional value did not show strong, consistent effects . . . on produce quality.'
- A Norwegian study found *conventional* carrots had more beta-carotene and more carotinoids (both important anti-oxidants). The organic carrots had more aluminium.
- An American study found more soluble iron in conventional spinach, but modestly more available iron in the organically grown spinach.

The varieties of vegetables grown seem to make a bigger difference in nutritional levels than the farming system and even the impact of the varieties was not large.

Modern Farming Is the Most Sustainable

People are rightly concerned about the sustainability of agriculture. Nothing is more important to the long-term sustainability of human society. It is clear, however, that modern high-yield farming is the most sustainable practised by humanity in the 10,000 years since we left the forests and created fields.

Soil Erosion

Soil erosion has always been a major problem. We have only to visit the Mediterranean Basin to realise that early farming systems allowed too much soil degradation and erosion. Primitive plough-based farming systems went straight up and down the hillsides. Ploughing also allowed water to run off the surface, taking too much soil with it and released carbon and reduced organic matter in the soils, making them even more vulnerable to wind and water.

Asia's wet rice culture was one of the few early farming systems that was truly sustainable, in large part because of the laborious land terracing that prevented erosion.

High-yield farming, which really only got started in the 1930s, has delivered major victories in the war against erosion. Tripling the yields on the best-quality land almost automatically cut erosion per ton of food by two-thirds. It allows us to avoid farming steep hillsides and fragile soils, so can cut erosion per ton by *more* than two thirds. High-yield conservationists of that era also developed some important weapons against erosion, including contour ploughing, strip cropping and cover crops.

Conservation Tillage

However, it was not until modern chemistry collided with the oil-price crisis of the 1970s that modern farming gained its biggest weapon against erosion—conservation tillage. Chemists of that era were beginning to develop chemical weed killers at the same time farmers were looking for ways to cut fuel costs after oil prices quadrupled. The result was that farmers put away their deep mouldboard ploughs, began using shallow disc-ploughs and relied on herbicides to control weeds. The conservation tillage revolution was born.

Conservation tillage chops crop residues into the top few inches of the soil, creating billions of tiny dams to prevent erosion. Or, in no-till farming, it uses cover crops to protect the soil all year round, using a herbicide to kill the cover crop just before the new seeds are planted through the killed sod.

Conservation tillage cuts water run-off from the field by up to 90 per cent, traps more of the rainfall for the crop and cuts erosion per acre by another 65 to 90 per cent. Subsoil populations of earthworms and soil microbes thrive with year-round supplies of decomposing vegetation and the freedom from being ploughed.

Conservation tillage is now being used on hundreds of millions of acres of land in North America, South America, Australia and Asia. It has even been tested successfully in Africa, where too few farmers can yet afford herbicides.

Paul Johnson, President Clinton's former Administrator of the Natural Resources Conservation Service in the US Department of Agriculture, said that conservation tillage was allowing farmers, for the first time, to build topsoil even as they produced some of the highest crop yields in the history of the world.

Ironically, organic farmers refuse to use conservation tillage, even though it emulates their own long-cherished emphasis on maintaining soil tilth and encouraging subsoil biota. Organic farmers continue to use 'bare-earth' farming systems featuring mouldboard ploughs, steel cultivator shanks and tractor-drawn rotary hoes. This means leaving themselves far more vulnerable to erosion. It also leaves them vulnerable to wet springs, when mechanical cultivators can't get into the fields and weeds can overwhelm the organic crops. The same year, the next-door farmer who used a pre-emergence herbicide, is producing high yields.

Pesticide Sustainability

Critics say pesticides aren't 'sustainable' because pests keep developing resistance. That's true of modern antibiotics as well—but we keep investing in the research to develop new antibiotics, instead of accepting death from pneumonia. In the same way, we must increase our research efforts and develop still more pest control strategies. Crop and livestock pests multiply so rapidly that we've never beaten them with any static defence. Moreover, modern monoculture fields create an ideal environment for pests to attack (but they also produce the highest yields per acre).

Biological pest controls offer much promise but to date they have been the weakest and most erratic of the farmers' pest weapons. They are often slow to build up in the fields, allowing the pests to get a head start on crop destruction. They can often be thrown off stride by unfavourable weather. As mentioned earlier, they also present potential threats to the local eco-systems and thus must be used with great care.

Integrated pest management tries to combine all our weapons against pests: crop rotation, biological pest controls, baited traps, crop timing and many other techniques besides pesticides. This helps minimise pesticide use and costs and helps maintain the effectiveness of a given pesticide for a longer period. However, even IPM ultimately depends on the synthetic chemicals as the last line of defence against crop loss.

Hopefully our next generations of pesticides will be even safer than the ones used now. However, Roundup and atrazine, key herbicides used in conservation tillage, are among the safest chemicals ever tested.

Glyphosate, the active ingredient in Roundup, is so safe it can be used around trout and quail with no ill effects. Atrazine, while it bonds weakly to the soil and seasonally turns up in drinking water, is so safe that a person would have to drink 154,000 gallons of water per day containing the maximum allowable level—for 70 years—to get above the no-effect level. The sulfanylurea pesticides are no more toxic than table salt. One tablet, the size of an aspirin, treats a whole acre and they degrade into harmless compounds within weeks.

These types of herbicides are the only category of farm pesticides in which First World usage has been rising in recent decades.

Petroleum

Modern farming is criticised for using petroleum as a fuel. But agriculture accounts for only 2 per cent of US petroleum use. Another 1 per cent is used to transport foods from the farms to the table, but transportation allows us to grow food where yields are often two or three times higher. If farming had to produce its own fuel—as ethanol, or biodiesel or even pasture for horses—it would take more land from nature. The gasoline tractor reportedly released about 30 million acres of US farmland, which had been used for pasture for horses, to grow food for people. When the rest of the economy shifts away from fossil fuels to some new (and perhaps more expensive) energy source, so will farmers.

Chemical Fertilisers

Chemical fertilisers replace exactly the nutrients that are taken out of the soil by growing plants. Soil testing allows the farmer to tell exactly what nutrients need to be re-supplied.

Will we run out of fertilisers? Our nitrogen is taken from the air, which is mostly nitrogen; that will never run out. The world has very large deposits of potash. Reasonable estimates of our phosphate ore reserves suggest about 250 years' supply—after which we will have to start recovering phosphate from lower-grade deposits. There is no reason to believe that humanity will run out of plant nutrients.

Too Much 'Fixed' Nitrogen?

Is the world 'fixing' too much nitrogen? Will nitrogen oxides from farming disrupt ecosystems? It is true that our world today is fixing twice as much nitrogen as nature used to and that nitrous oxide is being redeposited on the earth's surface. However, even the worriers have been unable to come up with a credible threat. Nitrogen from chemical fertiliser, animal manure and legume crops is emanating from only about 15 per cent of the earth's surface—and being deposited across the entire surface. It would take truly heroic amounts of fixed nitrogen to alter the ecology of the forests and oceans. To date, the additional nitrogen being deposited is only about 4-6 kg per acre per year—about enough to stimulate forest and fish growth and mildly disadvantage wild legumes.

The Soil and Water Conservation Society of the US, which has often been critical of 'modern' farming, published a report in 1995 titled *Farming for a Better Environment.* The Society concluded that modern farmers were conducting the most sustainable agriculture in history, using high-yield seeds, chemical fertilisers, integrated pest management and conservation tillage.

What Are the Pesticide Impacts on Wildlife?

The claims that agricultural pesticides wreak havoc on natural ecosystems are unrealistic given today's highly specific, low-volume, rapidly-degrading pesticides and their precision application. There is relatively little wildlife in the fields themselves and the farmers make dedicated efforts not to waste their expensive pesticides outside the fields.

Some pesticides are, indeed, carried from the fields by heavy rains. However, the traces of pesticide found in ground and surface waters are very low, typically a few parts per billion and well below the safety limits. Less than 1 per cent of the herbicides applied in the US leave the root zone of the crops. The percentage for insecticides is probably even lower, since the insecticides are typically more expensive and targeted more directly at crop plants.

The State of Virginia, in the 1990s, proposed a ban on one granular soil insecticide because a study had found 6 per cent of the eagles in the James River estuary were dying of secondary pesticide poisoning. Doves ate the granules, eagles ate the doves and both died. The manufacturer solved the problem by withdrawing it from sale in areas where it impacted sensitive bird populations.

In Britain, reports indicate that the major impact of today's pesticides on birds is to locally reduce the number of insects on which they can feed.

The major bird problem in South Africa is that raptors, especially vultures, too often feed on poisoned baits put out by native farmers to protect their livestock from hyenas. There is now an aggressive education programme in place to teach the farmers safe ways to protect both the vultures and their livestock.

While efforts to reduce these losses are applauded and must be pursued, the wildlife impacts are trivial in comparison to the huge amounts of wildlife habitat saved from destruction by higher yields.

Can We Achieve Still-Higher Yields?

The prospects for raising yields still higher are excellent. The world could perhaps double its current average yields of major crops by extending known technologies to all of its farms and supporting all its farms with roads, input supply systems and competitive pricing.

As examples of potential, India averages 2.5 tons per hectare on its mostly-irrigated wheat and Pakistan 2 tons, while Chile averages 3.5 tons. Thanks to an excellent rice-breeding programme, China averages 6 tons per hectare of rice while India and Bangladesh average only half as much. America averages 7 tons per hectare of corn (mostly rain-fed) while the world corn yield average is 2.7 tons.

Dr Norman Borlaug, with the support of the Sasakawa Global 2000 Foundation, is proving that African farmers can double their yields using improved seeds, along with very modest levels of fertiliser and pesticide. (Borlaug won the Nobel Peace Prize in 1970 for his key plant-breeding role in the Green Revolution.)

Traditional approaches to raising crop yields are still gaining steadily: plant breeding continues to raise world grain yields by 1 to 2 per cent annually. Artificial insemination in dairy cattle is raising milk yields by 2 per cent annually. Integrated pest management is cost-effectively raising yields for some farmers.

However, there is no question that the rate of yield gains on the world's farms has slowed in the 1990s compared to the halcyon days of the Green Revolution. For one thing, the expansion of irrigation has virtually stopped. If the world is to save all its current wildlands, it will need to develop additional yield breakthroughs. . . .

Can We Save the Small Family Farm?

Saving the family farm has been the mantra of government farm policy in most of the world's affluent countries for at least 200 years. (Stalin's state farms and Mao's communal farms were important exceptions.)

This is one of the driving ethics behind the urbanites in the organic farming movement. Today's affluent urbanised democracies fanaticise that they can return to the traditional small hand-powered family farm of the last century, which is imagined as a more stable and comfortable alternative to today's large commercial farms. However, agricultural technology has not driven the decline of the small family farm.

The decline in the numbers of small family farms is a direct result of the rising value of off-farm jobs. When high urban wages attract farmers to town, they leave behind land and market demand which must be satisfied with less human labour. The result is the modern, high-tech farm, which substitutes technology for hand hoes and stoop labour.

We cannot 'save' the small family farm unless we are willing to subsidise small farmers through direct income payments to be rural residents; in effect, costumed guides in 'living museums.'

The current trends in affluent societies indicate that we are headed for still-larger and increasingly specialised commercial farms in most countries, with a concurrent increase in the number of 'sundowners'—people with off-farm income, who enjoy working small farms as hobbies. Their numbers are likely to grow rapidly as the electronic age permits more and more people to do their jobs from their homes and to live wherever they choose.

Such hobbyists are likely to fill more of our rural residences and to manage a modest percentage of the farmland in affluent countries. However, they will supply only a small proportion of the farm products.

Carping About Wonder Wheat

... In the 21st century, I believe that the debate should be framed by 1) the huge increase in farm output which will be demanded; and 2) the urgent need to save room for wildlife.

If we can triple the yields, again, on the land we are already farming, we can supply the three-fold increase in farm demand without ploughing additional wildlands. If we can use 5 per cent of the current wild forest area for high-yield trees, to supply the projected ten-fold increase in timber and paper demand, we can protect the other 95 per cent of the wild forests from ever being logged, let alone cleared. High-yield conservation thus promises to let us save more than 90 per cent of the current wildlands and more than 95 per cent of the existing wild species.

Organic farming offers no such lofty promise. Rather it pledges to keep more people working on more low-yield farms at a terrifying cost: huge tracts of wildlands ploughed, far more soil erosion and degradation, perhaps a million wildlife species driven to extinction and higher health risks for consumers.

With high costs, low returns and higher levels of pest damage, it is little wonder that organic food has captured less than 1 per cent of the food market in affluent countries, except where it has been heavily subsidised. American organic purchases in 1996 were $3.5 billion, out of a total grocery market of $430 billion. And, since organic foods tend to carry a price premium, it may be that organics supplied only about 0.5 per cent of the market volume.

In West European countries, where organic food production is subsidised by the government, the organic sector has expanded to as much as 3 per cent of the market. Ironically, however, Western Europe is subsidising organic food precisely because of its low yields. The governments hope that organic subsidies will be less expensive than the export subsidies currently used to dump the surpluses generated by farm price supports that are too high. Both the organic subsidies and the high price supports work against the freer farm trade that is needed to save tropical forests in densely populated Asia.

The critical factors in meeting the 21st century food challenge are:

- More public funding for sustainable higher-yield farming research in both the First and the Third Worlds.
- A regulatory welcome for safe and sustainable new farming systems and farming inputs, instead of applying a 'precautionary principle' which pretends the world already has plenty of food and no pressure to triple yields in the 21st Century.
- Free trade in farm products, so that the world can use its best land and highest-yielding farming systems to save as much wildlife habitat around the globe as possible.

POSTSCRIPT

Is Organically Grown Food Better Than Conventionally Grown Food?

It is worth examining the economic and policy implications of this debate. Huge agricultural and chemical companies hold stakes in the current farming system. A switch to organic farming methods would reduce sales of chemical fertilizers, pesticides, and herbicides, and affect the income of these industries as well as those that support the application of such products. Furthermore, if consumers perceive organic foods as beneficial, sales of organic foods will continue to increase at the expense of conventionally produced foods (as they are now doing in the United States). Further evidence for the economic and environmental superiority of organic farming methods might cause demands for a shift in farm supports to organic producers. Clearly, large amounts of money are at issue in this debate.

So are matters of social values. Some people might think a small reduction in yield or profit a worthwhile price to pay for reducing harm to the environment, maintaining the quality of soil, and retaining small organic farms in rural areas. Others, like Avery, value efficiency and productivity more highly.

Scientific matters also are at issue. The public, for example, views organic foods as more nutritious. Avery contends that they are not. Perhaps because nutritional differences between apple varieties are minimal, the Washington State study did not compare the nutrient content of fruit grown under the three conditions. On the other hand, few well-designed studies have addressed the question of nutritional differences, as noted in January 2002 reviews by Christine Williams (*Proceedings of the Nutrition Society*) and Deane Bourn and John Prescott (*Critical Reviews in Food Science and Nutrition*). Two studies in the *Journal of Agricultural and Food Chemistry* provide preliminary evidence for the nutritional superiority of organic peaches and pears (Marina Carbonaro et al., September 11, 2002) and organic berries (Danny Asami et al., February 26, 2003). Questions of yields, soil fertility, and pesticide use also are currently under investigation. As might be expected, B. P. Baker et al. have shown that organically grown fruits and vegetables have lower levels of pesticides than conventionally grown crops (*Food Additives and Contaminants*, May 2002). In May 2002 Paul Mäder et al. reported in *Science* that a 21-year review of organic systems research demonstrates a reduction of fertilizer and energy use by 34 to 53 percent, a reduction in pesticide use by 9 percent, and an overall improvement in soil fertility and biodiversity, with a reduction of 20 percent in crop yields. On this basis, these researchers conclude that organic methods are a "realistic alternative" to conventional agricultural methods.

ISSUE 16

Will Irradiation Improve the Safety of the Food Supply?

YES: Olivia Bennett Wood and Christine M. Bruhn, from "Position of the American Dietetic Association: Food Irradiation," *Journal of the American Dietetic Association* (February 2000)

NO: George L. Tritsch, from "Food Irradiation," *Nutrition* (July–August 2000)

ISSUE SUMMARY

YES: Nutritionists Olivia Bennett Wood and Christine M. Bruhn, speaking for the American Dietetic Association (ADA), say that irradiation enhances the safety and quality of the food supply and helps protect consumers from foodborne illness. They maintain that officials should educate the public that irradiated foods are safe and offer a wider variety of such foods in the marketplace.

NO: Cancer researcher George L. Tritsch argues that the principal beneficiary of food irradiation is the food industry; the public derives no tangible benefit from this technology but bears all of its safety risks. He concludes that the long-term consequences of food irradiation will be far worse than any disease against which it may have been directed.

Foods contaminated with viruses, bacteria, and protozoa are responsible for an estimated 76 million illnesses, 325,000 hospitalizations, and 5,200 deaths annually in the United States alone, according to the Centers for Disease Control and Prevention (CDC). Large as they may seem, these numbers surely *underestimate* the extent of the problem, as people tend to report only a small proportion of food "poisoning" episodes. Microbial contamination of food occurs as a result of poor sanitary practices. Animals or people that harbor harmful microorganisms excrete them in feces into the environment where they come in contact with food or with people who handle food. Because fecal contamination can occur at any stage of production, distribution, or preparation, everyone in the chain of food production and consumption shares the responsibility for producing safe food: commercial food producers, distributors, and food service establishments as well as home cooks. Because the precise source of an outbreak of foodborne illness is often difficult to identify, accountability for preventing contamination problems cannot always be determined. Furthermore, although most foodborne illnesses occur as a result of eating contaminated commercial food, most intervention efforts focus on education of home cooks about basic food safety procedures—cooking foods to appropriate temperatures, separating cooked from raw foods, keeping foods cold, and storing them properly.

Given the educational and accountability flaws in the current food safety system, irradiation has emerged as an alternative method for killing foodborne organisms. The process uses gamma rays, x-rays, or electron beams to bombard foods and disrupt the genetic material (DNA) of cells. Lower or shorter bouts of irradiation reduce the number of microbes on a food; higher and longer exposures can kill all of them. The process does not cause the foods themselves to become radioactive, although it does induce minor losses of nutrients as well as slight changes in food color, flavor, and odor.

Irradiation is a late-stage intervention that kills harmful organisms prior to sale. The sterility it induces is usually incomplete and, therefore, temporary. Foods must be irradiated in intact packages; once the packages are opened or damaged, the foods can be recontaminated. To remain safe, irradiated foods must be handled like fresh foods and may need to be refrigerated to retard microbial growth. Even so, irradiation is useful to food producers and processors because they do not need to worry about preventing contamination at earlier stages. The process destroys whatever pathogens are present at that moment, and it greatly extends the shelf life of packaged fresh foods.

Olivia Bennett Wood and Christine M. Bruhn argue that irradiated foods are indistinguishable in taste or nutritional content from fresh foods. They say that any changes in chemical structure that result from the process are similar to those caused by cooking and are benign.

Despite the ability of irradiation to kill microbes and extend food shelf life, the technology has been highly controversial and slow to gain acceptance. In addition to concerns about the incompleteness of irradiation-induced sterility, George L. Tritsch charges that irradiation alters chemicals in food and induces the formation of unusual compounds, some of them with the potential to cause genetic mutations or cancer. He argues that these compounds have not been tested adequately and that their effects on human health may not be known for years.

In reading the following selections, take particular note of the kinds of evidence chosen by the authors to bolster their positions. Which approach seems more compelling? Why, for example, does Tritsch introduce his selection with biographical comments? The points of view expressed here seem diametrically opposed, but on what facts do they agree? What additional information might help you decide whether or not irradiation will benefit consumers as well as it benefits the food industry?

**Olivia Bennett Wood and
Christine M. Bruhn**

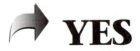

Position of the American Dietetic Association: Food Irradiation

Position Statement

It is the position of The American Dietetic Association (ADA) that food irradiation enhances the safety and quality of the food supply and helps protect consumers from foodborne illness. The ADA encourages the government, food manufacturers, food commodity groups, and qualified food and nutrition professionals to work together to educate consumers about this additional food safety tool and to make this choice available in the marketplace.

General Overview

Although the US food supply has achieved a high level of safety, microbiological risks exist. Because foods may contain harmful bacteria, mishandling—including improper cooking—can result in foodborne illness. The Centers for Disease Control and Prevention estimates that foodborne bacteria caused 76 million illnesses, 325,000 hospitalizations, and 5,000 deaths in the United States in 1998. Known foodborne pathogens accounted for an estimated 14 million illnesses, 60,000 hospitalizations, and 1,800 deaths. Outbreaks of *Escherichia coli 0157:H7* (*E coli*) from food sources are estimated to cause 62,458 illnesses, 1,843 hospitalizations, and 52 deaths yearly. Four pathogens—*Campylobacter spp, Listeria monocytogenes, Salmonella nontyphoidal,* and *Toxoplasma gondi*—are responsible for 3,420,000 illnesses and 1,526 deaths annually. Illnesses and death cost society monetarily and emotionally. . . . Pasteurization by irradiation has been identified as a solution that enhances food safety through the reduction of potential pathogens and has been recommended as part of a comprehensive program to enhance food safety.

The Food Irradiation Process

Irradiation exposes food to radiant energy (Box 1). . . . Food is passed through an irradiator—an enclosed chamber—where it is exposed to a source of ionizing energy. The sources of ionizing energy may be gamma rays from cobalt 60 (^{60}Co),

From Olivia Bennett Wood and Christine M. Bruhn, "Position of the American Dietetic Association: Food Irradiation," *Journal of the American Dietetic Association,* vol. 100, no. 2 (February 2000), pp. 246–251. Copyright © 2000 by The American Dietetic Association. Reprinted by permission of Elsevier. References omitted.

cesium 137 (^{137}Cs) x-rays, or electrons generated from machine sources. In 1999, food irradiation in the United States occurs exclusively from the use of ^{60}Co, which is contained in stainless steel rods placed in racks. The emitted gamma rays are very short wavelengths, similar to ultraviolet light and microwaves. Because gamma radiation does not elicit neutrons (ie, the subatomic particles that can make substances radioactive), irradiated foods and their packaging are not made radioactive. A self-contained, prefabricated cabinet loaded with ^{137}CS to provide an additional processing option is being developed. Electron beam facilities, widely used to irradiate medical equipment, have been built for food treatment. Energy penetration is about 1½ inches in food products, so the thickness of items to be treated is limited to about 3 inches with double-sided treatment. A combination electron beam and x-ray facility for food irradiation is being planned for construction in the northeastern United States. Regardless of source, the effect of ionizing energy on food is identical. Energy penetrates the food and its packaging but most of the energy simply passes through the food, similar to the way microwaves pass through food, leaving no residue. The small amount of energy that does not pass through the food is negligible and is retained as heat.

BOX 1. DEFINITIONS RELATED TO FOOD IRRADIATION

Cold pasteurization or electronic pasteurization   Irradiation at pasteurizing doses. Industry must demonstrate that all vegetative pathogens are destroyed.

Gray   The SI unit of measurement of absorbed radiation. One joule of energy is absorbed per kilogram of matter being irradiated. 1,000 Grays (Gy) = 1 kiloGray (1 kGy).

Ionizing radiation   Radiation capable of converting atoms and molecules to ions by removing electrons.

Irradiation   Treatment with radiation or treated by irradiation.

Irradiation dose   The amount of kiloGray used to irradiate a product.

Irradiator   The part of a radiation facility that houses the source of irradiation.

RAD   Term formerly used to measure radiation. 100 rad = 1 Gy.

Radiation   Ionizing radiation.

Radiolytic product   A substance produced from irradiation.

The duration of exposure to ionizing energy, density of food, and the amount of energy emitted by the irradiator determine the amount or dose of radiant energy to which the food is exposed. Regulated doses are set at the minimum levels necessary to achieve specified purposes or benefits. Radiation doses allowed by the US Food and Drug Administration (FDA) are the most restrictive of all countries in which irradiation is allowed. Low doses (up to 1 kiloGray [kGy]) control the *Trichina* parasite in fresh pork; inhibit maturation in fruits and vegetables; and control insects, mites, and other arthropod pests in food. Medium doses (up to 10 kGy) control bacteria in meat, poultry, and other foods, and high doses (above 10 kGy) control microorganisms in herbs, spices, teas, and other dried-vegetable substances.

Food irradiation does not replace proper food production or handling. Even with treatments that destroy 99.9% of a pathogen, some could still survive. Bacteria that cause spoilage are more resistant to irradiation than pathogens and requires a higher treatment. Therefore, the handling of foods processed by irradiation should be governed by the same food safety precautions as all other foods. Food irradiation cannot enhance the quality of a food that is not fresh or prevent contamination that occurs after irradiation.

Historical Summary of Food Irradiation

Food irradiation currently has a 50-year history of scientific research and testing, with more than 40 years preceding approval of the process for any foods in the United States. To date, no other food technology has had as long a history of scientific research and testing before gaining approval. Research has been comprehensive and has included toxicological and microbiological evaluation, as well as testing for wholesomeness. In 1955, the US Army Medical Department began to assess the safety of types of foods commonly irradiated in the US diet. Petitions to the FDA for approval of specific foods for irradiation soon followed; wheat and wheat powder received first approval in 1963. In the early 1970s, the National Aeronautics and Space Administration adopted the process to sterilize meats for astronauts to consume in space, and this practice has continued. The first products approved by the FDA were wheat and white potatoes in the 1960s. During the 1980s, the FDA approved petitions for irradiation of spices and seasonings, pork, fresh fruits, and dry or dehydrated substances. Poultry received FDA approval in 1990; red meats were approved in 1997. Worldwide, 40 countries permit irradiation of food, and more than half a million tons of food are irradiated annually. The United States has approximately 40 licensed irradiation facilities; most are used to sterilize medical and pharmaceutical supplies. Food irradiation has an impressive list of national and international endorsements: ADA, Centers for Disease Control and Prevention, American Council on Science and Health, American Medical Association (AMA), American Veterinary Medical Association, Council for Agricultural Science and Technology, International Atomic Energy Agency, Institute of Food Technologists, Scientific Committee of the European Union, United Nations Food and Agricultural Organization (FAO), and World Health Organization (WHO).

Benefits of Food Irradiation

Treating foods with ionizing energy offers many benefits to consumers, retailers, and food manufacturers. The benefits depend on the treatment used.

Certainly the most important benefit is improved microbiological quality of food. Additional benefits include the replacement of chemical treatments and extended shelf life. The following benefits are specified:

- Most spices and herbs are fumigated with ethylene oxide to improve microbiological quality. Irradiation replaces this chemical, which is being phased out for environmental and worker safety reasons.
- Because pathogens in raw poultry or meat can be reduced by 99.9% or more by a low "pasteurization" treatment, irradiation can help reduce the potential for cross-contamination in homes and foodservice kitchens (eg, schools, industry, groceries, hospitals, restaurants). Irradiation also provides an additional level of safety if food is not fully cooked.
- Transport of some fruits and vegetables is restricted or prohibited to prevent the spread of harmful insects such as the Mediterranean fruit fly. Current insect quarantine procedures require harvest and heat treatment of fruit that is not fully ripe. Irradiation is an approved quarantine treatment that results in a higher-quality fruit because it can be used on ripe fruit, does not cause hard spots, and does not increase susceptibility to mold. Additionally, irradiation can be used on fruits that do not tolerate heat treatments. Use of this quarantine method will increase availability of a wider variety and higher quality of tropical and semitropical fruits.
- Irradiation can replace chemical fumigants used to protect rice and grain from insect infestation.
- Irradiation retards the natural decay of fruit and vegetables, thus extending shelf life.
- Irradiation contributes to keeping down food costs as a result of less wastage and extended shelf life.

Because irradiated food is virtually indistinguishable from fresh items, food can be prepared in the traditional manner. The process can be considered a "win-win" situation for consumers, retailers, and food manufacturers.

Effect of Irradiation on Nutritive Value of Food

Irradiation has been compared to pasteurization because it destroys harmful bacteria. Since irradiation does not substantially raise the temperature of the food being processed, nutrient losses are small and often substantially less than other methods of preservation such as canning, drying, and heat pasteurization and sterilization. The relative sensitivity of the different vitamins to irradiation depends on the food source, and the combination of irradiation and cooking is not considered to produce losses of notable concern.

Proteins, fats, and carbohydrates are not notably altered by irradiation. In general, nutrients most sensitive to heat treatment, such as the B vitamins and ascorbic acid, are sensitive to irradiation. . . . Nutrient losses can be further minimized by irradiating food in an oxygen-free environment or a cold or frozen state. Fox and coworkers derived a formula to calculate predicted losses in cooked pork and chicken on the basis of data—derived from the second National Health and Nutrition Examination Survey—on quantities of these items in the US diet and irradiation doses allowed by the FDA. Predicted losses of riboflavin and niacin in pork, and of thiamin in both pork and chicken, ranged from 0.0 1% to 1.5%. . . .

Before approving irradiation of meat, the FDA evaluated an "extreme case" in which all meat, poultry, and fish were irradiated at the maximum permissible dose under conditions that led to maximum destruction of thiamin. Even in these extreme and unlikely circumstances, the average thiamin intake would still be above the Recommended Dietary Allowance (RDA) and now the Dietary Reference Intake (DRI). Thus, the FDA concluded there would be no deleterious effect on the total dietary intake of thiamin as a result of irradiating foods. Another study by Fox et al compared radiation reductions in B-vitamin levels in beef, lamb, pork, and turkey. The researchers reported losses of riboflavin that were virtually undetectable in all the tested meats at doses up to 3 kGy. Thiamin losses were detectable, and the losses varied among the meats tested, but the range was narrow, from a low of 8% loss to a high of 16% loss. . . . In a study of the ascorbic acid content of oranges, Nagai and Moy found no significant differences between irradiated and control fruit at dose levels up to 1 kGy throughout a 6-week storage period.

Sensory qualities such as appearance and flavor have been evaluated in the laboratory as well as in market studies with consumers. Consumers consistently rated irradiated fruit as equal to or better than nonirradiated fruits in appearance, freshness, and taste. However, irradiation may affect the color and odor of meat, depending on the irradiation dose, dose rate, temperature, packaging, and atmosphere during irradiation. Irradiated beef becomes a deeper red and pork and poultry become more pink. These changes are more pronounced at higher levels of ionizing energy. When meat is irradiated at low doses under specific conditions—such as low oxygen or no oxygen—with specific packaging such as vacuum sealed or in the frozen state, there is no notable development of off-odors or flavors. Studies have found that flavor in vacuum-packed raw or cured pork is not negatively affected by irradiation and that cooked pork ranks equally with nonirradiated samples for meatiness, freshness, tenderness, juiciness, and overall acceptance. Irradiation of chicken breast and thigh up to 10 kGy had little effect on sensory acceptability of appearance, odor, texture, and taste.

Food Safety

Food safety encompasses enhanced safety as a result of destruction of pathogenic microorganisms, as well as chemical and toxicological safety of foods that have been irradiated. The scientific literature clearly demonstrates that irradiation destroys common enteric pathogens including *Campylobacter jejuni, E coli, Listeria monocytogenes,* various *Salmonella spp,* and *Staphylococcus aureus* associated with meat, poultry, and fresh produce. An irradiation dose of 0.4 kGy destroys *Toxoplasma gondi* and *Cyclospora,* the latter of which has been associated with gastroenteritis linked to the ingestion of fresh raspberries, lettuce, and herbs. *Vibrio* infections associated with the consumption of raw molluscans shellfish can be prevented with irradiation pasteurization, but Norwalk-like viruses associated with raw shellfish and hepatitis A virus require higher doses than are approved for meat and poultry pasteurization. Irradiation does not protect against bovine spongiform encephalopathy.

Some people are concerned that irradiated food will not show signs of spoilage and people will inadvertently consume a harmful product. As with any food, proper handling and preparation—not taste or smell—ensures food safety. Some people have also inquired about the safety of irradiated food if postirradiation contamination were to occur. Meat or poultry contaminated after irradiation does not spoil more rapidly than a nonirradiated product. Irradiated and nonirradiated meats challenged with postirradiation application of pathogenic bacteria exhibited spoilage at virtually the same time when held at refrigerator temperatures or temperatures that would normally allow for bacterial growth. Some people have inquired about the viability of microorganisms that may survive low-dose or medium-dose treatment. The bacteria that survive irradiation are destroyed at a lower cooking temperature than the bacteria that have not been irradiated.

When evaluating the safety of irradiation, the FDA did not consider possible benefits to consumers or food processors. The agency must identify various effects that can result from irradiating food and assess whether these may pose a human health risk. The FDA review addresses potential toxicity, nutritional adequacy, and potential microbiological risks.

Irradiation does cause chemical changes in food, all of which have been found to be benign. More than 40 years of multispecies, multigenerational animal studies have shown no toxic effects from eating irradiated foods. Additionally, human volunteers consuming up to 100% of their diets as irradiated food have shown no ill effect. Irradiation produces such a minimal chemical change in food that it is difficult to design a test to determine whether a food has been irradiated.

A small number of new compounds are formed when food is irradiated, just as new compounds are formed when food is exposed to heat in other processing or cooking methods. Early research described these new compounds as "unique radiolytic products" because they were identified after food was irradiated. Subsequent investigations have determined that free radicals and other compounds produced during irradiation are identical to those formed during cooking, steaming, roasting, pasteurization, freezing, canning, and other forms of food preparation. Free radicals are even produced during the natural ripening of fruits and vegetables. All reliable scientific evidence based on animal feeding tests and consumption by human volunteers indicates these products pose no unique risk to human beings. In fact, people requiring the safest food—hospital patients receiving bone marrow transplants—are often served irradiated and/or pasteurized foods. Furthermore, because spices, being of tropical origin, are often microbe-laden, irradiated spices are preferred for routine use in hospital foodservice for patients. As with pasteurization, evidence suggests that food irradiation can make better a quality food supply.

AMA's Report of the Council on Scientific Affairs on Food Irradiation agreed with a FAO/WHO policy statement released in 1992. Irradiated food produced under established good manufacturing practices is to be considered safe and nutritionally adequate because:

> i) the process of irradiation will not introduce changes in the composition of the food which, from a toxicological point of view, would impose an adverse effect on human health; ii) the process of irradiation will not introduce changes in the microflora of the food which would increase the microbiological risk to the consumer; iii) the process of irradiation will not introduce nutrient losses in the composition of the food, which, from a nutritional point of view, would impose an adverse effect on the nutritional status of individuals or populations.

In a 1999 report, the WHO and allied organizations concluded on the basis of knowledge derived from over 50 years of research that irradiated foods are safe and wholesome at any radiation dose. The limitation at very high doses is palatability, not food safety.

Environmental Safety of Food Irradiation

Strict regulations govern the transportation and handling of radioactive material. Irradiation facilities using radioactive material are constructed to withstand earthquakes and other natural disasters without endangering the community or workers. Radioactive material is transported in canisters tested to withstand collisions, fires, and pressure. Worker safety is protected by a multifaceted protection system within the plant. USDA-proposed regulations mandate that workers be trained in the safe operation of irradiation equipment. Establishments choosing to irradiate meat or meat products will be required to comply not only with USDA Food Safety and Inspection Service (FSIS) and FDA requirements regarding the safety of irradiated products, but also with the Nuclear Regulatory Commission, Environmental Protection Agency, Occupational and Safety Health Administration, Department of Transportation, and state and local government requirements regulating the operation of irradiation facilities. These regulations include maintenance of appropriate environmental, worker safety, and public health protection.

The ^{60}Co used by US commercial facilities is specifically produced for use in irradiation of medical supplies and other materials. It is not a waste product of any other activity, and it cannot be used to make nuclear weapons. All the spent ^{60}Co to date—in such a small amount—could fit in an office desk. Disposal of ^{60}Co is carefully arranged by the producer. Electron beam radiators are operated by electricity and use no radioactive isotopes.

Regulation of Food Irradiation

Congress defined the sources of ionizing energy as food additives and included them in the Food Additives Amendment to the Federal Food, Drug, and Cosmetic

Act of 1958, thus delegating the main regulatory responsibility to the FDA. Additionally, 2 agencies within the USDA are involved in the process: the FSIS, which develops standards for the safe use of irradiation on meat and poultry products, and the Animal and Plant Health Inspection Service, which monitors programs that are designed to enhance animal and plant health (eg, using irradiation as an insect quarantine treatment in fresh produce) (48) . . . .

All irradiated foods sold at the retail level in the United States must be labeled with a Radura, an international symbol for irradiation (Figure 1), and the words "treated by irradiation" or "treated with radiation." Products that contain irradiated ingredients, including spices, are not required to be labeled as such. The ADA supports the present labeling rules, including use of the Radura and current wording on irradiated foods. The ADA also supports incentive labeling in which a specific pathogen is listed on the label as being reduced, such as "treated by irradiation to reduce *Salmonella* and other pathogens." However, the ADA is concerned about statements that imply the irradiated food is free of pathogens, such as "free of *Salmonella,*" because food irradiation does not prevent recontamination of the irradiated food. Incentive labeling as specified by USDA regulations stipulates that elimination of a pathogen must be scientifically documented. A continuing area of research is identification of scientific detection methods to verify that unlabeled foods have not been irradiated and that foods have received the intended dose. . . . In 1999, the operating US irradiation facilities process spices, citrus fruits, tropical fruits, strawberries, tomatoes, mushrooms, potatoes, onions, and poultry.

Any new application of irradiation must undergo food additive approval. . . . The ADA supports continued expansion of categories to include such products as fish, shellfish, eggs, produce, ready-to-eat products, and mixed foods.

Figure 1

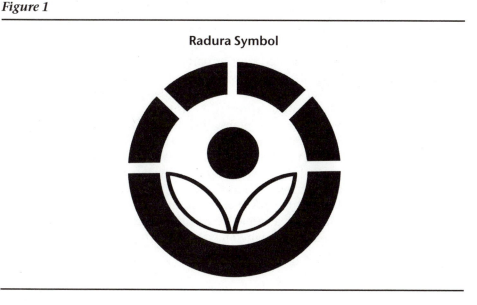

Radura Symbol

Consumer/Producer Issues

Despite repeated endorsements and regulatory approval, irradiated foods are not widely available in the United States. Although consumers are familiar with food irradiation, many have little knowledge of the process and its advantages. When consumers receive science-based information on food irradiation, however, most prefer irradiated to nonirradiated spices, poultry, pork, beef, and seafood. Concern about foodborne illness has increased consumer interest in irradiated food. A nationwide survey conducted in March 1998 found that almost 80% of the population sample said they would buy products labeled "irradiated to destroy harmful bacteria." Sixty-seven percent of consumers said it was "appropriate" to irradiate poultry; slightly fewer consumers deemed it "appropriate" to irradiate pork and ground beef. More than 60% thought irradiation was appropriate at a fast-food restaurant, and almost 50% considering it appropriate at the grocery store delicatessen or sit-down restaurant.

In another nationwide survey, consumers indicated they would pay a premium for irradiated ground beef. The increase in cost for irradiated foods is estimated at $0.02 to $0.03 cents per pound for fruits and vegetables and $0.03 to $0.08 cents per pound for meat products. Produce has been marketed without a price premium as a result of decreased losses and increased shelf life. Part of the cost for meat and poultry irradiation relates to packaging material. Currently only a limited number of materials are available and special, more expensive meat trays must be used. It has been estimated that the savings from the reduction of foodborne illness are substantially greater than the modest increase in food cost.

Consumer performance in the marketplace supports the results of attitudinal surveys. Mangoes labeled as irradiated sold successfully in Florida in 1986. In March 1987, irradiated Hawaiian papayas, available in a 1-day trial in Southern California, outsold the identically priced nonirradiated counterpart by greater than 10 to 1. Irradiated apples marketed in Missouri were also favorably received. Record amounts of irradiated strawberries were sold in Florida in 1992 and irradiated strawberries, grapefruit, juice oranges, and other products continue to outsell their nonirradiated counterparts in a specialty produce store in Chicago, Ill. Irradiated poultry, which is available in select markets, has experienced brisk sales. A University of Georgia shopping simulation test showed a significant increase in the proportion of consumers purchasing irradiated ground beef after they participated in an educational program on the benefits of food irradiation. After receiving information, 71% purchased irradiated beef, including 62% of the consumers who originally stated they would not purchase irradiated food. Consumers in Kansas have purchased labeled irradiated poultry in market tests in 1995 and 1996. The irradiated poultry captured 63% of the market share when priced 10% less than store brand, and 47% when priced equally. In 1997, after reading a brief description of irradiation, 80% of consumers selected irradiated poultry when it was priced the same as the nonirradiated house brand.

NO ↵

George L. Tritsch

Food Irradiation

In 1986, at a reunion of the Rockefeller University Hospital alumni, I was chatting with Lewis Thomas, then CEO of Sloan Kettering Cancer Institute. He invited me to join a group of scientists, the Media Resource Service of the Scientists' Institute for Medical Information, who were willing to provide the press with explanations and comments on scientific matters. This has resulted in my being invited to discuss possible relations between food irradiation and cancer before the Waxman Committee of the US Congress, and before legislative committees of the states of New York, New Jersey, and Hawaii. I have also participated in discussions with newspaper and television journalists and with food technology departments at Cornell University and the State University of New York at Buffalo. My comments are based on 45 y of experience since my doctorate at Cornell Medical College, Rockefeller University, and since 1959, at Roswell Park Cancer Institute, and are my own; they do not reflect official positions of the New York State Department of Health or the State University of New York at Buffalo.

At this point I should state that my comments and testimony have been that irradiation produces mutagenic and carcinogenic compounds in food, and that the testing design for irradiated food safety has been inadequate to detect carcinogenicity in humans. The most lethal food contaminants, the spores of *Clostridium botulinum* and the entity causing bovine spongiform encephalopathy (mad cow disease) are resistant to the permitted doses of radiation.

Because my arguments will not be accompanied by those of a proponent of food irradiation, I will attempt, with all the honesty and integrity at my command, to allude to both sides of this polemic, although, admittedly, probably with unequal intensity. Food irradiation is not just a scientific issue. The economic considerations are appreciable. It was stated in 1995, before US Food and Drug Administration (FDA) approval of food irradiation, that "Economic analysis shows that the public health benefits expected from the reduced number and severity of food-borne illness resulting from use of irradiation are greater than the costs associated with implementation of the irradiation process." I will not address economic issues in this [selection].

Irradiation has been proposed to control food contamination by microorganisms. *Escherichia coli* 0157:H7 among others, which have produced serious morbidity and even mortality during several outbreaks across the United States during the last two decades. With *E. coli* 0157:H7 it is evident that these bacteria, which normally inhabit the intestines of a small percentage of cattle, contaminate the meat as a result of puncture of the intestines during the slaughtering process.

Irradiation at the FDA-approved dose of 100 krad kills 90–99% of most organisms. The food is not sterilized by this dose. Higher doses would adversely alter the organoleptic acceptability of the food. Irradiation will extend the shelf life of the food appreciably, perhaps doubling it, but by no means indefinitely. The few percent of the remaining contaminating organisms will continue to divide during storage, and eventually the food will be "spoiled." Analyses of a *Salmonella* outbreak traced to contaminated cheese revealed that as little as one organism per 300 g of cheese sufficed to infect an individual. In a published study of irradiated fish fillets, the increase in the number of bacteria produced during cold storage of the irradiated and unirradiated fillets was tabulated. It is clear that bacteria can divide after irradiation, and can reach the same population levels after an extended time of storage as the unirradiated cells. In this instance, the storage time was increased by an additional 14 days until bacterial contamination equaled that of the unirradiated fillets. . . .

From these curve fittings, it is evident that bacteria in the irradiated fillets reproduced exponentially, whereas those in unirradiated fillets increased in a linear relation with time. Exponential growth results when cells divide and all progeny divide further. Linear growth results when only a fraction of the progeny divide. Thus, although irradiation lowers the bacterial contamination significantly, the surviving bacteria are able to divide to produce progeny. Hence, a new population of bacteria has been selected, which is of course, by definition, more radiation resistant than the population from which it was derived. It is not known whether this new population differs in other regards from the original population; the FDA has not investigated this aspect of the irradiation process. This is brought up because it has been stated that the survivors of irradiation have been so-called "weakened," but no further details were given. Recently, the most radiation-resistant organism known, *Deinococcus radiourans,* was isolated from irradiated canned meat. . . .

Exponentially dividing cells will amplify the cell population so that 20 cell divisions will produce one million progeny from each surviving cell. *E. coli* 0157:H7 divide rapidly, about every 20 min, so that about 7 h in a favorable environment such as the gastro-intestinal tract will provide a million-fold increase in cell number. Thus, irradiation will not eliminate morbidity related to bacterial contamination, but delay the onset of symptoms, provided of course that the pathologic properties of the radiation-resistant survivors remains unaltered and are not weakened. This delay would make it more difficult to trace the origin of the contamination, and thus provides a dubious benefit to consumers. The definitive test of this reasoning requires an experiment in a real-life setting, a proposal of questionable ethical implications. During testimony before a New York State legislative committee considering legalization of food irradiation, a representative interrupted my presentation with the following insightful observation. At the time when food in grocery stores is near its "expiration date," before it is considered spoiled, the price must be lowered drastically so that the food is sold quickly before overt spoilage. This would attract the poorer members of our society, making them the unwitting experimental subjects for field-testing the safety of irradiated food. In a democracy, this must be abhorrent to everyone. I must admit that this line of thought would not have occurred to me.

I bring up these arguments to indicate that the consuming public would derive no tangible benefit from food irradiation, but would bear all the potential risk related to the ultimate safety of this food. The food merchants and public health officers, the primary advocates of food irradiation, bear no risk other than as consumers themselves, and gain the benefits of extended storage time, and the public perception that government is doing something to protect the food supply. Should not the potential risk of an innovation be borne by the same groups that derive the benefits? Because of the understandable public aversion to things relating to radiation, some public health officials have proposed that the term *cold pasteurization* be used for food irradiation, an oxymoron when one considers that pasteurization implies heating.

Let us then examine the refereed scientific literature for clues about any potential risks to health from consumption of irradiated food. Unfortunately, proponents of food irradiation have published their studies primarily in consensus reports, internal memoranda, and the like, which are not readily available to the practicing scientist, and I am no doubt unaware of the existence of many of these studies.

Irradiation with high-energy beams splits chemical bonds in molecules to form free radicals and ions. When sufficient critical bonds are broken in organisms contaminating the food, the organisms are killed. Similar bonds are broken within the food. Free radicals contain an unpaired electron and will continue to react with stable molecules to form another free radical and another stable molecule after the radiation is turned off. This process will stop only when two free radicals react to form a stable molecule without unpaired electrons. The lower the dose of radiation, the fewer free radicals are formed and the longer it will take for two free radicals to find each other and collide to terminate these reactions. Different doses of radiation will therefore not only produce different amounts of new molecules, but different kinds as well. This has indeed been documented in actual practice with irradiated fish. As a model for these reactions, I have alluded to the mass spectrum of a pure compound. Here, a high-energy beam is focused on a pure compound and the resulting fragments are separated as a function of charge and mass. The pattern obtained is unique for any pure compound and will identify it unequivocally. In a complex mixture such as a food, this identification of all the constituents is technically not feasible because of their huge number and low concentration, but serves to illustrate that a very large number of new compounds is inevitable. The following example will illustrate the magnitude of new molecules formed during irradiation. It can be calculated that at a dose of 100 krad, 6 of 10 million chemical bonds are broken. This seems like a small number. If one considers the irradiation of water, which constitutes about 80% of many foods, it can be shown that for 100 mL, i.e., 5 g mole, there are a trillion trillion molecules. If 6 of 10 million bonds are broken, then in 100 mL water, one billion billion bonds will be broken. Thus, a very large number of new molecules may be expected to be introduced into food during irradiation with 100 krad. One of these, meta-hydroxyphenylalanine, has been proposed to monitor whether food had been irradiated. These theoretical considerations have been confirmed by looking at the products of irradiation of 280 g pure sucrose as a 2% aqueous solution. In addition to the recovery of 263 g unchanged sucrose, 476 mg of a white crystalline compound, identified as sodium formate, was found, and about 1 g crude yellow syrup, which was not resolved into pure compounds or identified. The formate suppressed the growth of cultured cells and produced chromosomal aberrations. I bring this up to emphasize and document that irradiation should not be considered to be a process, as advocated by proponents of food irradiation, but a means of adding a large number of new compounds to foods, as ruled by the FDA. The identification of all these compounds has not been attempted for technical reasons, but the formation from 1 mole sugar of almost 0.01 mole formate, no doubt derived from formaldehyde, a known mutagen, must give pause to anyone attempting to advocate irradiation as safe. The mutagenicity of formaldehyde has been documented with the Ames Test, which shows 0.05 mg as clearly mutagenic. Higher doses are toxic, as expected. From this experiment, it is evident that irradiation of 30 mg sucrose (1/250 of a teaspoon) will result in a mutagenic dose of formaldehyde. Although small amounts of formaldehyde are present in some foods, increasing its concentration by irradiation will increase the mutagenic burden and increase the incidence of neoplasia over and above what is now seen in population surveys. Thus, unique or ubiquitous, at least one harmful radiolytic product is produced during the irradiation of sugar.

A discussion of a study of irradiation of foods that contain unsaturated fats is timely because the American public is being advised to reduce fat intake, particularly saturated fats, in view of the high correlation between fat intake and cardiovascular disease and several forms of cancer. Irradiation of polyunsaturated fats produces peroxides, which oxidize benzopyrenes in the food to benzopyrene quinones in a dose-dependent manner. The carcinogenicity of these quinones has been documented, and is so potent that these compounds have been used to induce tumors in experimental animals. Unsaturated fats such as cod liver or mackerel oil showed greater quinone formation than saturated fats such as coconut oil or fats containing tocopherol (vitamin E), such as corn oil. The direct relation between quinone formation and peroxide content was documented with irradiation of herring flesh. Peroxidation of lipids results in their polymerization by cross-link formation. We are unable to digest these polymers, with the result that they will be deposited as insoluble plaques in blood vessels, akin to the deposition of insoluble cholesterol plaques, well-known to lead to high blood pressure and cardiovascular disease. In a consensus statement frequently quoted to document the safety of irradiated food by its proponents, the following is stated on page 17: "In this research, several anomalies appeared in the test animals (for example, hemorrhages, ruptured hearts, and vitamin deficiencies), but these were related to feeding the test animals food they did not customarily eat, and not to treating the foods with ionizing energy." Hemorrhages and ruptured hearts suggest acute elevation of blood pressure. Should a study be performed that involves feeding animals food they do not customarily eat, and then attribute adverse effects to this, rather than to the nature of the food that was eaten? This reasoning would not be acceptable in the refereed scientific literature. However, these observations illustrate acute effects of irradiated fat-containing foods; induction and detection of neoplasia would take much longer than the duration of this study. Another statement (page 18 of ref. 15) I find unacceptable in this publication is that ". . . when many experiments are conducted, an occasional statistically significant negative (and positive) outcome is to be expected, even in the absence of any real effect." I bring this up to illustrate the inherent danger of relying, as did the FDA, on studies not peer-reviewed by anonymous referees.

I would next mention the effects of irradiation on foods cured with nitrate (bacon, cold cuts, etc.). Irradiation converts nitrate to nitrite in a dose-dependent manner, and mutagenesis was found to be directly proportional to the nitrite concentration. Nitrite reacts with nucleic acids and various amino acids in proteins to form the recognized family of carcinogens known as nitrosamines. These are unequivocal and potent carcinogens in humans and have been used to induce tumors in experimental animals.

I would now like to turn to the most convincing and comprehensive group of studies to demonstrate the mutagenic effects of irradiated food. Some of these studies were performed in humans. In 1975 the results of feeding five malnourished Indian children wheat irradiated with 75 krad were reported. This wheat produced weight gain, and serum albumin and hemoglobin blood levels indistinguishable from what was found with unirradiated wheat. Food irradiation proponents might have used this part of the study to document the lack of adverse effects of irradiated wheat consumption. However, four of the five children showed gross chromosomal polyploidy 4 wk after initiation of the feeding program. Chromosome number returned to normal 26 weeks after feeding of irradiated wheat ended. This unequivocal evidence of mutagenesis in 80% of the test subjects can be contrasted with the highest cancer incidence in humans, lung cancer, of 80 per 100 000, or 0.08%. No statistical analysis is needed here! My one question would be what was different about the one child who showed no polyploidy. Based on lung cancer incidence, I would have predicted no observable polyploidy increase from a carcinogenic event unless at least 10 000 subjects were tested. Proponents of food irradiation have attempted to dismiss this study because only five subjects were involved; mercifully, no one has repeated this with greater numbers of children, considering that equivalent results were obtained when irradiated wheat was fed to monkeys and rats. In both of these studies, polyploidy was seen after several weeks of feeding and returned to normal about 2 mo after feeding irradiated wheat ended. During hearings before the US Congress, proponents of food irradiation referred to an abstract of a presentation of a Chinese study involving 382 medical students, which showed no statistically significant effects of irradiated food on chromosome number. Some irradiated foods, such as rice and potatoes, even reduced the number of polyploid cells! The most serious criticism of this study is that polyploidy was seen in 0–0.66% of the control subjects and in 0–1.03% of the experimental subjects. In several published studies of young children, not a single case of polyploidy was seen in 14,809 individuals. The Chinese findings of polyploidy suggest an inherent background of mutagenic stimulation in this population. This study has not been published in a refereed journal, certainly not in the American Journal of Clinical Nutrition, where the original findings were presented. This would be the accepted procedure for refuting a published study, and the editors of this prestigious journal would not have declined to publish reasonable data to set the record straight.

Let us now consider some of the studies that convinced the FDA to approve food irradiated with as much as 100 krad for human consumption. The criterion used by the FDA is safety of foods or drugs in terms of acute toxicity during short periods of exposure, i.e., months or a few years at most. I have already quoted from a publication that summarizes a series of studies. Weanling rats were fed irradiated food for 8 wk and showed decreased growth rates, which were not considered serious indications of toxicity. In another study, 41 young male volunteers were given irradiated food for 15 days without showing any unfavorable effects. Rats, mice, and dogs were fed irradiated food for 2 y or four generations and showed the previously cited hemorrhages and ruptured hearts, which were attributed to the fact that the animal ate food to which they were not accustomed and not to the fact that the food was irradiated. The details of these studies were not provided, and the manuscript was not reviewed by anonymous referees with competence in this field. However, all the studies were of much too short duration to demonstrate carcinogenicity of irradiated food; this takes several decades. . . .

Proponents of food irradiation have stated that no unique chemicals (radiolytic products) are introduced into food by irradiation. We do not know whether this is true because a biologic assay suitable to guide the purification of small amounts of materials introduced into the food by irradiation is not available. Nevertheless, unique or ubiquitous, an increase in concentration of a mutagen in food by irradiation will increase the incidence of cancer over and above what is presently observed during several decades of exposure. Formaldehyde and benzo(a)pyrene quinone are clearly increased in concentration by irradiation. If we knew nothing else, this suffices to advise against the consumption of irradiated food.

If consumption of irradiated food were to become widespread, it would take four to five decades to show statistically significant increases in cancer incidence. To recall . . . the parallel with smoking, the causation of lung cancer by smoking was first realized in the 1960s in the Surgeon General's report. . . . Even if all smoking ceased today, there are enough past smokers in the pipelines to keep lung cancer at the top of human cancer incidence. Likewise, with food irradiation. It will take four to six decades to demonstrate a statistically significant increase in cancer due to mutagens introduced into the food by irradiation. It will take years to convince the public and combat denials from a by then well-entrenched irradiation industry. When food irradiation is finally prohibited, several decades worth of people with increased cancer incidence will be in the pipelines. This will therefore be an experiment of a century's duration!

Is this worth the benefits irradiation will provide for the food industry? As shown previously, irradiation will not eliminate all the contaminating micro-organisms; it will only delay the onset of symptoms and will not affect severity and duration of illness.

The effective remedy is to cook food, especially ground beef, adequately (to 170°), not permit raw meat to come into contact with food that will be consumed uncooked, and to thoroughly wash all food that will be eaten raw. Keep in mind that excrement from infected cows could come into contact with produce in the field. However, the long-term consequences of irradiation will be far worse than any disease against which it may have been directed.

POSTSCRIPT

Will Irradiation Improve the Safety of the Food Supply?

Unsafe food causes millions of food poisoning episodes each year at enormous personal and economic cost to the public. The food industry also incurs enormous costs in recalls of contaminated products, legal liability, and reputation. It would seem to be in everyone's best interest to do everything possible to make sure that foods are safe at every stage of production, distribution, preparation, and consumption. As Marion Nestle discusses in *Safe Food: Bacteria, Biotechnology, and Bioterrorism* (University of California Press, 2003), the fact that foods are not always safe is a curious consequence of a food safety system of inadequate government oversight and shared responsibility—and, therefore, lack of accountability—among food producers, the food service industry, and consumers.

To fill the regulatory and accountability gap, the ADA and many other nutrition and health organizations suggest irradiating foods to kill contaminating pathogens. They view the safety and efficacy of the process as beyond dispute. They believe that nutrition professionals should be educating the public that the technology is safe and encouraging the production and purchase of irradiated foods. In contrast, Tritsch views the chemical changes induced in food by irradiation as a form of uncontrolled human experimentation.

Wood and Bruhn and Tritsch agree that irradiation kills microorganisms but that it does so incompletely. Both agree that irradiated foods require the same food safety precautions as other foods. Both also agree that irradiation induces the formation of new chemical compounds in foods. Beyond that, we enter the realm of science, values, and interpretation based on point of view.

Sorting out the differences in this case is particularly difficult without referring to the original studies on which the arguments are based. For example, Tritsch cites a February 1975 study in the *American Journal of Clinical Nutrition* as a crucial piece of evidence for the harm caused by irradiated foods. This study reported that malnourished children in India who ate freshly irradiated wheat exhibited "chromosomal polyploidy"—abnormal numbers of chromosomes—a feature related to an increased risk of cancer. Without actually reading the study, however, it is difficult to evaluate its significance. Only a small number of children participated in this study—five ate irradiated wheat, five ate stored irradiated wheat (and showed fewer abnormalities), and five ate wheat that was not irradiated (and showed no abnormalities). No information is available on the rate of chromosomal polyploidy in the general population of Indian children. Perhaps for ethical reasons, the study has not been repeated.

On the other hand, the statement by Wood and Bruhn that "irradiation contributes to keeping down food costs as a result of less wastage and extended shelf life" also can be questioned. Irradiation of foods is an expensive process because expensive equipment is needed and foods must be transported to and from central irradiation facilities. Higher costs are almost always passed along to consumers, and higher prices reduce consumption. For example, findings from a U.S. Department of Agriculture (USDA) analysis, reported in the Fall 1999 issue of *FoodReview*, show that a 10 percent premium for irradiated products would cause a 50 percent drop in the number of customers who would choose such products.

Because the food and irradiation industries have so much to gain from use of the process, they have pressured Congress to approve its widespread use. Because of fears that the public will reject irradiated foods, they also have pressured Congress to minimize labeling requirements. As a result, in the farm security bill of 2002, Congress authorized use of the word *pasteurized* for any process that reduces pathogens in meat and poultry and permitted substitution of this term for irradiation.

The irradiation experiment is now underway. As irradiated foods increasingly enter the marketplace, the degree of acceptance by industry and the public will soon become evident. Some food safety experts believe that even if the public does opt to buy irradiated foods, irradiation will not solve food safety problems. Unless contamination is prevented at earlier stages of production and distribution, irradiation will be a temporary and incomplete solution to the problem. Food safety advocates such as Carol Tucker Foreman are eloquent on this point. As she explained to *Consumer Reports* in March 1998, "After all, sterilized poop is still poop." Overall, the key to food safety is to prevent contamination with dangerous microbes at every stage of food production and consumption from farm to table.

ISSUE 17

Does the World Need Genetically Modified Foods?

YES: Robert B. Horsch, from "Does the World Need GM Foods? Yes," *Scientific American* (April 2001)

NO: Margaret Mellon, from "Does the World Need GM Foods? No," *Scientific American* (April 2001)

ISSUE SUMMARY

YES: Scientist-official Robert B. Horsch, of the Monsanto Corporation, says that use of biotechnology will allow more food to be produced on less land with less depletion or damage to water resources and biodiversity. He insists that agricultural biotechnology is imperative for meeting growing demands for food.

NO: Scientist-official Margaret Mellon, of the Union of Concerned Scientists, says that science has yet to demonstrate that the benefits of food biotechnology outweigh the risks. She concludes that biotechnology is no panacea for world hunger and that it diverts attention from more effective methods for solving world food problems.

$\mathbf{B}$iotechnology and its synonym, genetic engineering, are the processes by which scientists move genes (DNA) from one organism to another in order to transfer desirable traits from the donor to the recipient. Food or agricultural biotechnologists take genes from bacteria, viruses, or plants and insert them into the genetic structure of food plants. Foods containing the new genes are called by a variety of equivalent terms: transgenic, bioengineered, genetically engineered (GE), genetically modified (GM), genetically modified organisms (GMO), and, sometimes, the pejorative "Frankenfoods."

The rationale given by the food biotechnology industry and its scientists for use of this technology includes several basic elements. First, the world's population is increasing rapidly, and demands for food will greatly increase. Second, because the land available for growing food is limited, existing land must become more productive. Third, biotechnology is the best method for increasing food productivity; it is safe, good for the environment, and will lead to a less expensive food supply. Finally, the principal barrier to obtaining these benefits is public distrust of GM foods. As evidenced by the following selections, the first three points are debatable. The last point is not; in the United States, Europe, and throughout the world, people have been suspicious of bio-engineered foods. Some countries have banned them. Others have become involved in trade disputes over these foods.

From its inception, food biotechnology has raised issues about potential risks and benefits, how the risks and benefits are distributed to various sectors of society, and how decisions are made about who takes the potential risks and benefits. GE foods raise questions about how they might affect local, national, and international food systems and economies, how they should be regulated, whether or not they should be labeled, and whether or not their production is ethical. Questions about safety can be answered scientifically, but regulatory and ethical questions are matters of social values. Even if GM foods are safe for people and for the environment, they might not be acceptable on societal or ethical grounds. For this reason, debates about this technology involve both science and values and have been especially contentious.

Robert B. Horsch says that genetic engineering techniques are essential for meeting the food needs of the twenty-first century. The burgeoning world population requires farmers to produce more food on less land. Agricultural biotechnology is the only means to meet this goal, he believes, particularly because GM foods reduce use of fertilizer and pesticides, do little or no damage to the environment, and produce no measurable risks to human health. Margaret Mellon views genetically modified foods from a more critical perspective. She argues that the technology is not only unnecessary but is actually harmful. It diverts attention and resources away from seeking more effective solutions to world hunger problems. Agricultural biotechnology also is unlikely to be sustainable; insects will develop resistance to genetically engineered toxins in plants, and genes for herbicide resistance will get transferred into weeds. Furthermore, without adequate testing of these foods, there is no way to determine whether or not they are safe.

In the following selections, Horsch states that GM foods are necessary to solve world hunger problems. Mellon counters that although biotechnology may have uses, it is not the solution to current food problems.

Robert B. Horsch 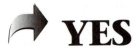 **YES**

Does the World Need GM Foods?

How did you become interested in the genetic modification of plants?

I started in this field with a strong interest in plants but with what you might call an academic interest in agriculture. I had this vague, naïve notion that if we could genetically improve plants with the new tools of molecular biology, we would find a way to make biotechnology relevant to agriculture.

That has now happened. Biotechnology is a great tool that will allow us to produce more food on less land and with less depletion or damage to water resources and biodiversity. I am convinced that biotechnology is not just relevant but imperative for helping us meet the rapidly growing demand for food and other agricultural products. The combination of more people and rising incomes will increase the demand for food by at least 50 percent in the next 25 years.

But critics of genetically modified foods point out that companies are not going to start giving products away. Can a corporation like Monsanto make biotechnology affordable for farmers in the developing world?

Cultivating commercial markets and applying technology to help the developing world are not mutually exclusive at all. One approach that works very well is to segment the market into three different areas. One is the pure commercial market. It makes economic sense, as a for-profit company, for us to invest in products and market developments in places where we can sell our products and where we think we can make a profit.

The other end of the spectrum is noncommercial technology transfer, which is largely focused on public-sector collaboration. Take, for example, our collaboration to put virus-resistance genes in the sweet potato. We will never have a commercial business in the sweet potato because it's just not a market economy crop. But by sharing our intellectual property and our technical knowledge with scientists from Kenya, we have helped them develop sweet potatoes that show resistance to the most serious sweet potato disease in Africa, which can cause the loss of 20 to 80 percent of the crop.

From Robert B. Horsch, "Does the World Need GM Foods? Yes," *Scientific American* (April 2001).

Then there's a third area, what I call a transitional market, where we have less experience related to biotechnology but that in the long run I think may be more powerful and beneficial for development efforts. We have used this approach with our older, nonbiotech products, such as high-yielding corn hybrids, and I think we can use it in the future with biotech products. Small farmers can see results in a demonstration plot and, if they want, try it themselves on a portion of their farm. If it works for them, they can expand or repeat it the next year. We have programs like this in Mexico, India and parts of Africa. By the third or fourth year, if it's working, the farmers will have made enough money from the experimentation phase to be able to run essentially on their own.

And what about profits for Monsanto?

We sell the seeds and the herbicide at market prices, and we subsidize the learning, the testing and the development of distribution channels so that we don't actually make a profit in the first several years. Only if the project is successful enough to become self-sustaining will we start making a profit. At this point, we haven't gotten that far with any of these programs.

Let's turn to the environmental effects of GM crops. What do you consider the most important benefits of the technology?

Lower use of pesticides is the environmental benefit that people relate to immediately, and it's huge for a product like Bt cotton. [*Editors' note: Bt crops have been genetically modified to produce a bacterial protein that kills certain insect pests.*] According to a recent report, 2.7 million pounds of pesticides have not been used in the past four years, and many, many more won't be used in the future as biotech expands in acreage and in traits.

Beyond that there are also yield benefits. The Bt corn we have today doesn't displace a whole lot of insecticides, but what it does do is boost the yields by a noticeable margin. It depends on the year and on the region, but the increase in yield can range from 5 to 15 percent. If you think about it, that leverages land use, water use, fertilizer use and all the pesticides that go into growing corn. You get a 10 percent greater corn harvest with the same resources that you were going to use anyway. You're getting more out of your resources.

Getting more from really good farmland, then setting aside land that is of marginal quality and returning it to habitat for wildlife is very beneficial to the environment. We can't continue to indefinitely expand our old practices—of chemical use, of water diversion, of plowing wild lands and converting them to farms, of nonagricultural sprawl and of the production of industrial waste.

One of the benefits of biotech that we first heard about was nutritionally enhanced foods. But despite promises of healthier broccoli, we have Bt corn. The famous "golden rice" is not available to consumers yet and is still in very early stages of testing. Will we ever have nutritionally enhanced foods?

We're seeing progress across industry, academia and the non-profit community. For example, we are collaborating with a non-profit group, TERI [Tata

Energy Research Institute] in India, on development of a product related to golden rice—golden mustard oil—that, like golden rice, is high in beta-carotene, a precursor of vitamin A. This may help alleviate vitamin A deficiencies in places where mustard oil is a staple in the local diet.

While making improvements to food for the industrial world is not a priority for Monsanto, other companies and university researchers are working hard in this area. For example, Du Pont has developed a modified oil with an increased amount of the fatty acid oleic acid. This product has reduced levels of polyunsaturated fatty acids and is more stable upon storage. Efforts are under way to modify other fatty acids to make oils more healthy for consumers. Also, there is research ongoing elsewhere to increase the amount of vitamin D in soybean oil.

Monsanto and other scientists have also been involved in research that may help reduce the likelihood of allergic responses to foods. We have been able to take a protein that is currently an allergen and modify specific amino acids in the protein to dramatically reduce the allergenic nature of the protein. Other scientists are using this and other methods to reduce the allergenic nature of some foods, such as peanuts and soybeans, which cause allergic reactions in a significant number of people.

Monsanto has been one of the most criticized, even despised, corporations because of its role in the development of genetically modified foods. Has it ever been hard to tell people you're an employee of Monsanto?

I've had a few people react negatively, but my experience is that when people meet you as a person, their reactions are very different than when they are commenting on the big nameless, faceless company.

I think the company is making an effort to address people's concerns about GM foods more openly. We've recognized that some genetic modifications are particularly bothersome. Among vegetarians, for instance, the idea of eating a vegetable that has an animal gene in it might raise questions. For certain cultures or religious groups, there could be similar concerns. So we decided it was better to avoid using animal genes in food crops.

I don't think it serves anybody's interest—including Monsanto's—to discount the potential risks of biotechnology. But for where we are today, and for what I see in the pipeline for the next few years, I really don't see a measurable risk from the GM products we are selling or developing. There have been numerous national and international scientific organizations that have reached this same conclusion, including the American Medical Association, the National Academy of Sciences, the World Health Organization and many others.

We at Monsanto have recently pledged to listen better to and engage in dialogue with concerned groups, to be more transparent in the methods we use and the data we have about safety, to respect the cultural and ethical concerns of others, to share our technology with developing countries, and to make sure we deliver real benefits to our customers and to the environment. I think this new attitude and new set of commitments will help improve both our company's image and the acceptance of this new technology.

NO ↵

Margaret Mellon

Does the World Need GM Foods?

How did you become interested in genetically modified foods?

I became aware of genetic engineering while running a program on toxic chemicals at the Environmental Law Institute in the 1980s. I was initially more positively disposed toward biotechnology than I came to be over the years. Like a lot of folks, I wasn't very critical. But the more I knew about the technology and the deeper the questions I asked about it, the less likely I was to accept at face value the extravagant promises made on its behalf.

I should also say, however, that my colleagues and I at the Union of Concerned Scientists are not opposed to biotechnology. We think its use in drug manufacture, for example, makes a lot of sense. The therapeutic benefits of the new drugs outweigh the risks, and often there aren't any alternatives. But in agriculture, it's different. So far, at least, there are only modest benefits associated with biotechnology products, and it has yet to be shown that the benefits outweigh the risks. And there are exciting alternatives to solving agricultural problems that we are simply ignoring.

Agriculture isn't like medicine. We in the U.S. produce far more food than we need. And we are so wealthy that whatever we can't produce we can buy from somebody else. As a result, there are about 300,000 food products on our grocery shelves and 10,000 new ones added every year. The notion that consumers in the U.S. fundamentally need new biotechnology foods isn't persuasive.

But, of course, many scientists and policy experts argue that we do need biotechnology to feed the world, especially the developing world.

That is an important question to ask because so many people—about 800 million—are undernourished or hungry. But is genetic engineering the best or only solution? We have sufficient food now, but it doesn't get to those who need it. Most hungry people simply can't afford to buy what's already out there even though commodity prices are at all-time lows. How does genetic engineering address the problems of income disparity?

The real tragedy is that the debate about biotechnology is diverting attention from solving the problem of world hunger. I'd like to see people seriously asking the question, "What can we do to help the world's hungry feed themselves?" and then make a list of answers. Better technology, including genetic engineering, would be somewhere on the list, but it would not be at the top. Trade policy, infrastructure and land reform are much more important, yet they are barely mentioned.

Genetic engineering has a place and should not be taken off the table, but I don't believe it is a panacea for world hunger. Treating it as if it is distorts this important debate. It is also amazing to me how quickly some have dismissed the virtues of traditional breeding—the technology that, after all, made us into an agricultural powerhouse.

Can we turn to another potential benefit that people claim for GM foods: agriculture that is more environmentally friendly?

Let's ask a question: What is a green agriculture? Is it one that doesn't depend on pesticides? I think it's a lot more than that, actually. But if we just consider avoiding pesticide use, we now have some data on the impacts of engineered crops. Surveys of American farmers by the Department of Agriculture show that the use of Bt [pest-resistant] corn aimed at the corn borer, for example, hasn't done much to reduce the application of pesticides to corn, because the vast majority of corn acreage isn't treated with pesticide to control that pest.

The introduction of Bt cotton, however, has resulted in a measurable drop in pesticide use. That's good for the environment and good for the farmers who cut their input costs. But this benefit will last only as long as the Bt trait keeps working. I think most scientists expect that the way Bt crops are being deployed will lead—sooner rather than later—to the evolution of resistance in the target pests, which means that the Bt cotton won't work anymore. We are likely to run through Bt cotton just like we ran through all the pesticides before it. So it isn't a durable path to a greener agriculture.

And there are environmental risks out there. Most scientists agree now that gene flow will occur—genes *will* go from engineered crops to nearby relatives. That means pollen will carry novel genes from the agricultural settings into neighbors' fields or into the wild. Gene flow from herbicide-resistant GM crops into the wild is already leading to the creation of herbicide-resistant weeds in Canada.

What about the health risks of GM foods? Do you see any looming problems?

I know of no reason to say the foods currently on the market are not safe to consume. But I don't have as much confidence as I should in that statement. There was a letter published in the journal *Science* last June from someone who had searched the literature for peer-reviewed studies comparing GM food to non-GM food. The researcher found something like five studies. That's not enough of a basis on which to claim, from a scientific standpoint, that we know enough to assure ourselves that these foods are going to be safe.

With the little we know about the food safety issue, I would say the biggest concern is allergenicity. Introducing new toxins into food is also a risk. Of course, breeders are going to try to avoid doing that, but plants have lots of toxins in them; as scientists manipulate systems that they don't completely understand, one of the unexpected effects could be turning on genes for toxins. There are rules that govern how genes come together and come apart in traditional breeding. We're not obeying those rules.

So you don't see genetic engineering of crops to be an extension of traditional breeding?

No, not at all. You just can't get an elephant to mate with a corn plant. Scientists are making combinations of genes that are not found in nature.

From a scientific standpoint, there is no dispute that this is fundamentally different from what has been done before. And that it is unnatural. Now, because it's new and unnatural doesn't *necessarily* mean that it will prove to be more risky. But it is certainly a big enough break with what we have done before to demand an extra measure of caution.

And caution is particularly appropriate where the technology involves our food supply. Lots and lots of people—virtually the whole population—could be exposed to genetically engineered foods, and yet we have only a handful of studies in the peer-reviewed literature addressing their safety. The question is, do we *assume* the technology is safe based on an argument that it's just a minor extension of traditional breeding, or do we prove it? The scientist in me wants to prove it's safe. Why rest on assumptions when you can go into the lab?

Science can never prove that any technology is 100 percent safe. Will you ever be satisfied that we've tested GM foods enough? And how much risk is acceptable?

Sure, I could be satisfied that GM foods have been adequately tested. But it's premature to address that question now. Nobody is saying, "Look, we've got this large body of peer-reviewed experimental data comparing GM with non-GM foods on a number of criteria that demonstrate the food is safe."

When we have generated such a body of evidence, *then* there will be an issue of whether what we have is enough. And eventually, if things go well, we'll get to a point where we say, we've been cautious, but now we're going to move ahead—we need to fish or cut bait. But we're nowhere near that point now.

Obviously, we take risks all the time. But why are we taking these risks? If we didn't have an abundant food supply, if we didn't have something like 300,000 food products on our shelves already, then we would have an argument for taking this society-wide risk. But we've got plenty of food. In fact, we've got too much. And although we have many problems associated with our food system, they are not going to be solved by biotechnology.

POSTSCRIPT

Does the World Need Genetically Modified Foods?

Arguments about food biotechnology are worth taking seriously because of their implications for the science of biotechnology, the economic viability of the agricultural biotechnology industry, the sustainability of the agricultural environment, and the health of the world's populations. The technical challenges of moving genes from one organism to another are daunting and make plant biotechnology as much of an art as a science. These methods are explained in a report from the Institute of Food Technologists in the August 2000 issue of *Food Technology*. Scientists able to perform these feats take pride in their accomplishments and tend to minimize suggestions of risk. The agricultural biotechnology industry is heavily invested in having its products succeed in an overabundant and highly competitive food marketplace. The Monsanto Company, for example, worked hard to create crop plants resistant to Roundup, a chemical weed killer also made by the company. The company benefits from sales of Roundup-resistant seeds as well as from the sales of Roundup. Monsanto officials like Horsch argue that the products are good for people and the environment as well as for the company. Furthermore, he says, the use of biotechnology is *imperative* for feeding a hungry world since food demands will increase by half in the next 25 years. These views support the economic interests of a company that has lobbied vigorously to influence government policies on genetically modified foods. Such issues are discussed in Gerald Nelson, ed., *Genetically Modified Organisms in Agriculture: Economics and Politics* (Academic Press, 2001), Peter Pringle's *Food, Inc.: Mendel to Monsanto—The Promises and Perils of the Biotech Harvest* (Simon & Schuster, 2003), and Marion Nestle's *Safe Food: Bacteria, Biotechnology, and Bioterrorism* (University of California Press, 2003).

Mellon argues that claims for the benefits of food biotechnology are "extravagant," that whatever benefits have occurred are modest, that the benefits have not been shown to outweigh the risks, and that such debates distract people from paying attention to more potentially useful alternatives to solving world hunger problems. In particular, she maintains that this technology has been so little studied that its safety cannot be determined. The real problem is that we have far too much food available already but that it is not distributed fairly; the poor do not have enough resources to buy the available food. Biotechnology, says Mellon, will not solve problems of income and political inequity.

Debates about food biotechnology encompass three main issues: necessity, human safety, and environmental benefit. Proponents of food biotechnology see genetic engineering techniques as the only way to meet world food needs in the future; opponents see biotechnology as one of a number of possible solutions to problems of agricultural productivity—but not necessarily the best one. Concerns about human safety focus on allergenicity. Since genes code for proteins, could the introduction of new genes cause formerly harmless plants to make proteins to which some people are allergic? Today, about 60 percent of supermarket products contain ingredients from genetically modified corn or soybeans but for reasons of politics do not carry "GM" labels. Thus, as Kathleen Hart discusses in *Eating in the Dark* (Pantheon, 2002), people have no way to avoid eating these foods even if they do not want to—for reasons of health or simply because they do not approve of biotechnology. Even if GM foods are safe, they still might not be acceptable to society.

At present, the most compelling safety concerns are environmental. Despite evidence that the use of genetically modified crops reduces use of pesticides (other than Roundup), environmental advocates have argued for years that insects will develop resistance to bioengineered toxins and that the genes for herbicide resistance will spread to related weeds. A 2002 report from the National Research Council, *Environmental Effects of Transgenic Plants,* discusses such concerns. Because plant pollen—particularly that from corn—is spread by wind and bees, it can be transported over long distances and "contaminate" organically grown corn and native and other varieties. Examples of such transfers already have occurred. Thus, genetically modified foods represent an experiment in progress with unknown consequences. Whether or not the experiment is worth unknown risks is the question in this debate.

Contributors to This Volume

EDITORS

MARION NESTLE is professor and chair of the Department of Nutrition, Food Studies, and Public Health at New York University. She holds a doctorate in molecular biology and a master's degree in public health nutrition, both from the University of California, Berkeley. Her previous faculty positions were at Brandeis University and the University of California San Francisco (UCSF) School of Medicine, where she was associate dean. She was the managing editor of the 1988 Surgeon General's Report on Nutrition and Health, has been a member of advisory committees to the Food and Drug Administration, and was a member of the government committee that prepared the 1995 Dietary Guidelines for Americans. Her research examines scientific, social, cultural, and economic factors that influence dietary recommendations and practices. She is the author of *Food Politics: How the Food Industry Influences Nutrition and Health* (University of California Press, 2002) and *Safe Food: Bacteria, Biotechnology, and Bioterrorism* (University of California Press, 2003). In 2003, *Food Politics* won awards from the Association for American Publishers (outstanding professional and scholarly title in nursing and allied health), the James Beard Foundation (literary), and World Hunger Year (Harry Chapin media).

L. BETH DIXON is assistant professor in the Department of Nutrition, Food Studies, and Public Health at New York University. She has a doctorate in nutrition from the Pennsylvania State University and a master's in public health with a specialization in epidemiology from the University of California, Berkeley. Before taking her current position, she completed fellowships in behavioral aspects of cardiovascular disease at the University of Minnesota and cancer prevention at the National Cancer Institute, and she received training in social epidemiology at Stanford University. She has published several articles on dietary assessment and dietary patterns of diverse populations, and she has given invited talks at the National Cancer Institute, Stanford University, and the Harvard School of Public Health.

STAFF

Jeffrey L. Hahn   Vice President/Publisher
Theodore Knight   Managing Editor
David Brackley   Senior Developmental Editor
Juliana Gribbins   Developmental Editor
Rose Gleich   Permissions Assistant
Brenda S. Filley   Director of Production/Manufacturing
Julie Marsh   Project Editor
Juliana Arbo   Typesetting Supervisor
Richard Tietjen   Publishing Systems Manager
Charles Vitelli   Designer

AUTHORS

DEMETRIUS ALBANES earned his B.S. in biology from the State University of New York at Stony Brook and holds a medical degree from the Medical School of Wisconsin. He now works at the National Cancer Institute as the chief of the Office of Education and as a senior investigator in the Division of Cancer Epidemiology and Genetics.

MARGARET ANDREWS works in the Food and Rural Economics Division of the Economic Research Service at the U.S. Department of Agriculture. She is the assistant deputy director for food stamp research in the Food Assistance and Nutrition Research Program.

DENNIS AVERY is the director of the Hudson Institute's Center for Global Food Issues and editor of the newsletter *Global Food Quarterly*. He studied agricultural economics at Michigan State University and the University of Wisconsin. Avery served as an agricultural analyst at the U.S. Department of State from 1980–1988 and is also a staff member of the President's National Advisory Commission on Food and Fiber. He is the author of a nationally syndicated column in the financial publication *Bridge News*.

ABBY S. BLOCH is an adjunct associate professor at New York University and at the University of Medicine and Dentistry of New Jersey. She directs a program that provides advanced training for dietitians in oncology. She is a registered dietitian and a fellow of the American Dietetic Association.

STEVEN BOOTH-BUTTERFIELD received his M.A. from Central Missouri State University and his doctorate in education from West Virginia University. He works for the Health Communications Research Branch, National Institute for Occupational Safety and Health, in Morgantown, West Virginia.

CHRISTINE M. BRUHN received her B.S. and master's degrees in home economics and her Ph.D. in consumer behavior from the University of California, Davis. She is the director of the Center for Consumer Research at the University of California, Davis. Her research focuses on consumer attitudes toward food safety and quality.

REBECCA J. BRYANT received her B.S. and master's degrees from Ball State University and her Ph.D. from Purdue University School of Consumer and Family Sciences. She is a faculty member at Meredith College. Her research focuses on calcium metabolism in adolescents, vitamin E, and diabetes.

JO CADOGAN holds a degree in zoology, and she holds a master's degree and a Ph.D. in human nutrition from Sheffield University in Britain, where she is an instructor. Her previous work focused on the role of nutrition in bone growth and metabolism in teenage girls and the effects of isoflavones on calcium metabolism in postmenopausal women. She is studying the development of biomarkers for folic acid and its role in cancer prevention.

STEVEN CARLSON is the director of family programs staff in the Office of Analysis, Nutrition, and Evaluation at the Food and Nutrition Service of the U.S. Department of Agriculture.

KATHLEEN M. FAIRFIELD received her medical degree from the Boston University School of Medicine and earned a master's of public health from the Harvard School of Public Health. She is pursuing a doctorate in public health at Harvard. She is an associate in medicine at the Beth Israel Deaconess Medical Center and instructor in medicine at the Harvard Medical School.

ALISON E. FIELD is an assistant professor at Harvard Medical School and an associate epidemiologist in the Department of Medicine at Brigham and Women's Hospital in Boston. Her research focuses on the causes and consequences of overweight and disordered eating in children, adolescents, and adult women.

ROBERT H. FLETCHER is a professor in the Department of Ambulatory Care and Preventive Medicine at Harvard Medical School and Harvard Pilgrim Health Care. He is coauthor of the newsletter *UpToDate in Adult Primary Care and Internal Medicine.*

STEPHEN P. FORTMANN graduated from Stanford University and obtained his M.D. from the University of California, San Francisco. He is the C.F. Rehnborg Professor of Preventive Medicine in the Department of Medicine at Stanford. He is also a professor of medicine in the General Internal Medicine Division. His principal research interest is in the prevention and control of cardiovascular disease in populations and individuals.

JEANNE FREELAND-GRAVES is Bess Heflin Centennial Professor in the College of Natural Sciences at the University of Texas at Austin. Her research focuses on obesity, women's health, vegetarian diets, minerals, and nutrient regulation. She is a coauthor of *Foundations of Food Preparation*, 6th ed. (Prentice-Hall, 1995). She received her doctoral degree in nutrition from Rutgers and is a registered dietitian.

CLARE M. HASLER earned a B.S. from Michigan State University, an M.S. from Pennsylvania State University, and a Ph.D. from Michigan State University. She is the associate director for outreach and industry relations of the Functional Foods for Health Program and an assistant professor of nutrition at the University of Illinois at Urbana-Champaign. Her research focuses on the role of soy products in health.

SUZANNE HAVALA is an assistant professor at the University of North Carolina at Chapel Hill from which she earned a doctoral degree in 2002. She is the author of several books about vegetarianism and vegetarian cooking, among them *Being Vegetarian* (Chronimed, 1996); *Vegetarian Cooking for Dummies* (John Wiley, 2001); and *Being Vegetarian for Dummies* (John Wiley, 2001). She is a registered dietitian.

ROBERT B. HORSCH received his Ph.D. in genetics at the University of California at Riverside, and he conducted postdoctoral work in plant physiology at the University of Saskatchewan. He is the head of the North American Stakeholder Dialogue Program and president of sustainable development for the Monsanto Company.

BARBARA V. HOWARD is president of the Medlantic Research Institute in Washington, D.C.

JEAN HUMPHREY is an associate professor at the Center for Human Nutrition at the Johns Hopkins Bloomberg School for Public Health. Her research focuses on the health effects of vitamin A supplementation.

PETER ILIFF is with the Department of Pediatrics and Child Health at the University of Zimbabwe and the SVITAMBO Project in Harare, Zimbabwe.

ANNEMARIE JUTEL is a registered nurse and earned a doctorate in physical education from the School of Sports Institute of Otago, New Zealand. She is a freelance journalist who has written four books about running as a sport.

PIERRE L. LE BARS is executive research director at the New York Institute for Medical Research in Tarrytown, New York.

I-MIN LEE is an associate professor in the Department of Epidemiology at the Harvard School of Public Health, who studies the role of physical activity in promoting the health of women.

BONNIE LIEBMAN holds an M.S. in nutritional sciences from Cornell University. She is director of nutrition at the Center for Science in the Public Interest in Washington, D.C.

DAVID S. LUDWIG is a professor at the Harvard Medical School and a member of the Division of Endocrinology at the Children's Hospital in Boston, Massachusetts. His research focuses on obesity, endocrinology, and nutrition.

ANNE L. MARDIS is an epidemiologist at the Centers for Disease Control and Prevention in Atlanta. She previously worked with the Center for Nutrition Policy and Promotion at the U.S. Department of Agriculture.

DOROTHY MBORI-NGACHA is a pediatrician and senior lecturer at the University of Nairobi, who trained in epidemiology at the University of Washington. She is senior clinical advisor to the Kenyan AIDS Vaccine Initiative in Nairobi. Her research career is devoted to finding ways to block mother-to-child transmission of the Human Immunodeficiency Virus (HIV).

MARGARET MELLON is director of the Food and Environment Program at the Union of Concerned Scientists in Washington, D.C. Her work focuses on the health effects of widespread use of antibiotics in raising farm animals and on the environmental effects of genetically modified foods.

SUSAN NITZKE is professor of nutritional sciences at the University of Wisconsin-Madison where her research focuses on development and evaluation of techniques to improve the effectiveness of nutrition education. She received her doctorate from that university and is a registered dietitian.

MARK NORD is team leader for food stamp and food security research in the Food and Rural Economics Division of the Economic Research Service at the U.S. Department of Agriculture.

B. E. CHRISTOPHER NORDIN is visiting professor in the Department of Medicine and Pathology at the University of Adelaide in South Australia. He is also a professor in the Department of Clinical Biochemistry at the Institute of Medical and Veterinary Sciences. His research focuses on calcium metabolism and its effects on bone density.

F. XAVIER PI-SUNYER is chief of endocrinology, diabetes, and nutrition and director of the Obesity Research Center at St. Luke's/Roosevelt Hospital Center in New York. He is professor of medicine at Columbia University College of Physicians and Surgeons.

ROBERT E. RECTOR is a policy analyst for The Heritage Foundation in Washington, D.C. He holds a master's degree in political science.

JOHN P. REGANOLD received his B.A. and his M.S. from the University of California, Berkeley and his Ph.D. from the University of California, Davis. He is professor and scientist at Washington State University, whose research interests are in land use and soil management.

BILL REGER earned his doctorate in education from West Virginia University where he holds a position in the Department of Community Health Promotion. He is an exercise physiologist who specializes in worksite wellness and communication approaches to community intervention.

PAUL R. SOLOMON received his Ph.D. from the University of Massachusetts. He is professor of psychology at Williams College in Massachusetts and studies the neuropsychology of memory and memory disorders.

GARY TAUBES is an award-winning journalist who writes about science, medicine, and health for publications such as *Science, Discover, The Atlantic Monthly,* and the *New York Times.* He is a contributing correspondent to *Science* and a contributing editor to *Technology Review*.

CYNDI THOMSON is a clinical nutrition research specialist at the University of Arizona Prevention Center. She is a registered dietitian.

GEORGE L. TRITSCH is with the Roswell Park Cancer Institute in Buffalo, New York.

ANN N. VARADAY is a biostatistical analyst with the Center for Research in Disease Prevention, Department of Medicine, Stanford University School of Medicine.

CONNIE M. WEAVER received her M.S. from Oregon State University and her Ph.D. from Florida State University. She is professor and chair of the Department of Foods and Nutrition at Purdue University in Indiana. She studies the chemical form and bioavailability of minerals from foods.

WALTER C. WILLETT is the Fredrick John Stare Professor of Epidemiology and Nutrition at the Harvard School of Public Health and professor of medicine at Harvard Medical School. He earned his M.D. degree from the University of Michigan and his doctorate in public health from Harvard. His research program employs epidemiological approaches to the prevention of chronic disease risk through large prospective cohort studies such as the Nurses Health Study and the Health Professionals Follow-Up Study. He is the author of *Nutritional Epidemiology,* 2d ed. (Oxford University Press, 1998), and *Eat, Drink, and Be Healthy* (Simon & Schuster, 2001).

OLIVIA BENNETT WOOD is a registered dietitian and an associate professor of foods and nutrition at Purdue University in Indiana. Her expertise is in clinical nutrition, with an emphasis on weight control, medical nutrition therapy, nutrition in the life cycle, and vegetarian diets.

MARGO G. WOOTAN is senior staff scientist and director of nutrition policy for science at the Center for Science in the Public Interest in Washington, D.C.

JUDITH WYLIE-ROSETT is a registered dietitian and a professor of epidemiology and social medicine at the Albert Einstein College of Medicine in New York. She is a member of the American Heart Association's Nutrition Committee.

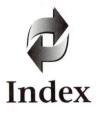

Index